PHARMACOTHERAPEUTICS

&

ADVANCED
NURSING PRACTICE

PHARMACOTHERAPEUTICS

&

ADVANCED NURSING PRACTICE

EDITORS

Laurel A. Eisenhauer, R.N., Ph.D., F.A.A.N.

Professor of Nursing
Boston College School of Nursing
Chestnut Hill, Massachusetts

Margaret A. Murphy, R.N.C.S., A.N.P., Ph.D.

Associate Professor of Nursing
Boston College School of Nursing
Chestnut Hill, Massachusetts

McGraw-Hill
Health Professions Division

New York St. Louis San Francisco Auckland Bogotá Caracas Lisbon
London Madrid Mexico City Milan Montreal New Delhi
San Juan Singapore Sydney Tokyo Toronto

McGraw-Hill
*A Division of The **McGraw-Hill** Companies*

PHARMACOTHERAPEUTICS
AND ADVANCED NURSING PRACTICE

1234567890 DOCDOC 9987

ISBN 0-07-105485-5

This book was set in Times Roman by V&M Graphics, Inc.
The editors were John J. Dolan and Lester A. Sheinis.
The production supervisor was Helene G. Landers.
The text and cover designer was Marsha Cohen / Parallelogram.
The indexer was Patricia Perrier.
R. R. Donnelley & Sons Company was the printer and binder.

This book is printed on acid-free paper.

Library of Congress Cataloging-in-Publication Data

Pharmacotherapeutics and advanced nursing practice / [edited by]
  Laurel A. Eisenhauer, Margaret A. Murphy.
        p. cm.
    Includes bibliographical references and index.
    ISBN 0-07-105485-5
    1. Pharmacology.   2. Therapeutics.   3. Nursing practitioners.
  I. Eisenhauer, Laurel A.   II. Murphy, Margaret A.
    [DNLM: 1. Drug Therapy—methods.   2. Primary Care—
  methods.   3. Drugs—administration & dosage—nurses' instruction.
  WB 330 P535   1997]
  RM300.P525   1997
  615.5′8—dc21
  DNLM/DLC
  for Library of Congress.   97-35644

CONTENTS

Part 2

DRUG THERAPY ISSUES AND APPLICATIONS 169

Part 3

CASE STUDY APPLICATIONS 407

CONTRIBUTORS

Susan Chase, R.N.C.S., Ed.D.
Associate Professor
Boston College School of Nursing
Chestnut Hill, Massachusetts
(Chapter 13)

Laurel A. Eisenhauer, R.N., Ph.D., F.A.A.N.
Professor of Nursing
Boston College School of Nursing
Chestnut Hill, Massachusetts.
(Chapters 1–7, 11, 14, 15)

Margaret A. Murphy, R.N.C.S., Ph.D.
Associate Professor
Boston College School of Nursing
Chestnut Hill, Massachusetts
(Chapters 9, 12)

Constance F. O'Connor, R.N.C.S., M.S.
Nurse Practitioner
Boston College Health Services
Boston College
Chestnut Hill, Massachusetts
(Chapter 10)

Anthony J. Rothschild, M.D.
Professor of Psychiatry
Director of Clinical Research
Department of Psychiatry
University of Massachusetts Medical Center
Worcester, Massachusetts
(Chapter 16)

Judith A. Shindul-Rothschild, Ph.D., R.N.C.S.
Assistant Professor
Boston College School of Nursing
Chestnut Hill, Massachusetts
(Chapter 16)

Patricia A. Stevenson, R.N.C.S., M.S.
Nurse Manager
Boston College Health Services
Boston College
Chestnut Hill, Massachusett
(Chapter 8)

Gail Wilkes, R.N.C., M.S.N.
Nurse Practitioner
Boston Medical Center
Boston, Massachusetts
(Chapter 17)

PREFACE

Nurses have had a critical role in the management of medications for many years. With the evolution of nurses into advanced practice roles, prescriptive authority has been legally permitted in most states. With this authority comes increased responsibility and accountability for the selection of appropriate drugs and the monitoring of drug therapy. This involves a greater knowledge of pharmacology and the development of clinical judgment skills in the choice of drug therapy for each individual patient.

This book provides advanced practice nurses (nurse practitioners) with the knowledge needed for understanding and integrating pharmacology into their clinical judgments. Emphasis is on adult patients and the prescribing *and* monitoring of drugs commonly used in adult patients being cared for in ambulatory or primary care settings. In this book the pharmacotherapeutic aspects of patient care and decision making are emphasized; the reader is encouraged to see his or her patients through the lens of drug therapy. There is a potential danger that this emphasis may overexaggerate the importance of drug therapy to the detriment of other considerations; however, this emphasis counterbalances what the authors believe to be the general insufficient attention in many clinical situations to the impact of drug effects on patients.

It is intended to provide content that is necessary but difficult to find in any one publication or that has not been published in an easily accessible form. This book is not intended to replace a basic medical or pharmacology book or drug reference book but rather to be used in conjunction with them. Its goal is to assist advanced practice nurses in developing "pharmacological thinking" within their clinical judgment process. It provides the materials that advanced practice nurses need in assessing and interpreting patient responses as well as a basis for prescribing.

Topical Coverage

Content focuses on those areas not fully covered in basic nursing pharmacology books or that are scattered in certain medical or pharmacology books or found primarily in other publications (books or journals). Integration of nursing, medical, and pharmacology is emphasized throughout. The organizing format of drug, patient, and contextual variables is used to provide a consistent approach to the discussions of drug therapy.

In Part 1, foundational aspects affecting the advanced practice nurse's role in pharmacotherapeutics and prescription writing are presented. Emphasis is on integrating the pharmacological and nursing aspects in assessment, monitoring/intervention, and evaluation of patients.

Part 2 covers selected categories of drug therapy with emphasis on those factors important and clinically relevant in individualizing and managing patients' medication regimens. Chapters are organized by pharmacological classification or medical diagnoses and/or symptoms, depending upon the most useful approach for discussing the particular drug therapy.

Part 3 has the case studies, an important feature of the book. The cases are of two types. One type is shorter and presents selected or focused patient data and asks specific questions related to the drug therapy discussed in the chapters and leading to decisions about the choice of drug, dose, route, etc. There are also complex cases with "full" patient assessment and other data provided. Complex data are presented so that students can recognize relevant data among all other assessment data; these types of cases are intended to facilitate the integration of nursing, medical, and pharmacologic knowledge.

ACKNOWLEDGMENTS

We would like to thank the many individuals who contributed to the development and publication of this book. First our thanks to our families for their patience and encouragement. Thanks also to the Boston College School of Nursing for its direct and indirect assistance during the writing and publication process. Our appreciation also goes to the editorial staff at McGraw-Hill, especially John J. Dolan and Lester A. Sheinis.

We especially thank the clinicians who were willing to share their expertise by contributing chapters: Susan Chase, Constance O'Connor, Patricia Stevenson, Anthony Rothschild, Judith Shindul-Rothschild, and Gail Wilkes. Thanks also to the advanced practice nurses who agreed to have their cases and case analyses included as learning tools for beginning advanced practice nurses: Joyce Barkin, Amy L. Borden, Elizabeth A. Casey, Susan Chase, Laura Delaney, Anne T. Ferguson, Lisa Kennedy-Sheldon, Kathleen B. O'Donnell, Kathleen McWha, Cecilia M. Mullen, Judith Shindul-Rothschild, Kathleen Salerno, Debra Swerda, and Cara Jean Yamamoto.

Our thanks also to our many students over the years who have helped us to refine the types of content needed by advanced practice nurses and nursing students as they enhance and transform their knowledge of pharmacology and nursing into the clinical judgments inherent in prescribing medications safely and appropriately.

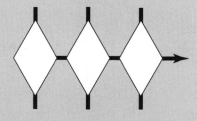

Part 1

GENERAL INFORMATION

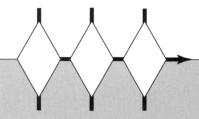

Chapter 1

MEDICATION MANAGEMENT AND PRESCRIBING IN ADVANCED NURSING PRACTICE

Laurel A. Eisenhauer

Prescribing drugs is the most recent evolution of the nurse's role in drug therapy. Although for many years nursing roles have involved clinical judgments related to drug therapy, only recently have APNs (advanced practice nurses) been given legal status to prescribe drugs in most states. APNs have some type of prescribing authority in 49 states.[1] Even before this legal expansion of the nurse's role, nurses and APNs have used their clinical judgment within standing orders or the administration of PRN medications.

With the responsibility for prescribing come additional responsibilities and accountability for the selection of the appropriate drug and dose for the particular patient and his or her problems. Ongoing responsibilities related to preventing and monitoring for drug interactions and side effects and patient/family teaching and counseling continue as inherent parts of the nursing role.

ESSENTIAL KNOWLEDGE

In assuming the role and responsibilities of prescribing, the APN must integrate in-depth knowledge of pharmacology and pharmacotherapeutics with his or her nursing expertise and expanded knowledge of medical diagnosis and therapeutics.

Knowledge of *pharmacology* has been an essential core of all levels of nursing practice. Even if a nurse is not involved directly in the administration or prescribing of drugs, the nurse is responsible for understanding drug effects on the patient. Drug therapy represents a variable in patients' responses; therefore, it is essential for the nurse to understand the bases for differences in patients' responses to drug therapy—differences in response either to the same drug in the same patient or the same drug in different patients.

Knowledge of the *patient* also is essential in order to prescribe drugs safely and appropriately. The physiological functioning of each individual based on his or her genetics, age, or pathophysiological conditions can alter the responses of the individual to a drug. Knowledge of the patient's psychosociocultural background provides insights valuable to planning a drug regimen with which the patient will comply and thereby to enhancing the likelihood of positive outcomes for the drug therapy.

Knowledge of the *contextual aspects* of drug therapy is needed by a prescribing clinician in order to understand factors that impact on the prescribing practices, on patient access to medication, and on delivery and administration of the prescribed drug.

These categories of knowledge needed by a prescribing clinician form the framework for this book.

SOURCES OF DRUG INFORMATION

APNs, especially those involved in prescription writing, need to be able to locate and use reliable, accurate, and up-to-date sources of information about drugs and drug therapy. Information sources include reference works, texts, databases, and the medical literature. Other resources are pharmacists and drug information centers. Clinicians also need to be aware of the latest research in order to provide up-to-date and safe care.

The location of information about drugs depends to a great extent on the type of information needed. A stepwise approach can be used:[2]

- Tertiary resources (e.g., texts and compendia, review articles, meta-analyses)
- Secondary literature (e.g., indexing and abstracting services)
- Primary (original research articles from biomedical journals)

The patient population served also may influence what types of drug information resources are available to the clinician in a particular setting. The 1990 Omnibus Budget Reconciliation Act (OBRA '90) indicates that *AHFS Drug Information, AMA Drug Evaluations, United States Pharmacopeia–Drug Information* (USPDI), and/or primary literature must be available for DUE (drug use evaluation) activities, including patient counseling.[2(p31)]

Clinicians also need to be cognizant of the information about drugs that is published in the lay media. Information about new drugs often appears first in the lay literature, often in the business section. Most newspapers and radio and television stations have regular coverage of medical research such as studies from the *New England Journal of Medicine* and the *Journal of the American Medical Association.* Since patients are consumers of this media coverage, they may ask their health care providers about their own treatment based on what they have heard from media reports.

Another trend that is increasing consumer awareness of drug information is the increasing use of prescription drug advertisements in the media to market prescription drugs directly to the public. Currently the Food and Drug Administration (FDA) has restrictions on how prescription drugs can be advertised to the public, but strategies to provide information about prescription drugs and specific brands directly to patients are being used by drug manufacturers. Therefore, clinicians need to be able to locate and critique original research reports in order to be able to interpret media reports and drug research reports for their patients.

With the advent of the Internet and computerized databases, patients have access to a great deal of information about health and drugs that previously was not readily accessible. CD-ROMs with drug databases are available for most home computers. Consumers can access most of the same World Wide Web drug information sources available to the health professional.

Pharmacists in hospitals, nursing homes or other health care agencies, or in the community are an invaluable source for information about drug therapy, both through their professional expertise and through their access to drug information sources. Pharmacists have assumed an increasingly important role in the counseling of patients about their drug therapy. Counseling about medications by the pharmacist was required by the 1990 OBRA regulations.

Drug information centers are available to answer questions. An example is the Drug Information Service at the University of Maryland which is accessible via the Internet (http://www.pharmacy.ab.umd.edu~umdi/umdi.html).

Other resources for obtaining current information include continuing education courses on drug therapy and/or clinical issues such as those sponsored by Nurse Practitioner Associates for Continuing Education (NPACE). Pharmaceutical company representatives also can provide information about their products that is helpful to the clinician. However, the clinician needs to evaluate this information in light of other data sources in order to have a balanced perspective on the particular company's drug product compared to other similar products or methods of treatment.

Tables 1-1, 1-2, and 1-3 list various resources for current drug information.

TABLE 1-1

Journals with Drug Therapy Information Useful to Clinicians

Annals of Internal Medicine
Archives of Internal Medicine
Clinical Pharmacology and Therapeutics
Clinician Reviews
Drugs
Drug Therapy
FDA Drug Bulletin
Journal of Clinical Pharmacology
Journal of the American Medical Association
Medical Letter on Drugs and Therapeutics
New England Journal of Medicine
Nurse Practitioner
Postgraduate Medicine
Yearbook of Drug Therapy

TABLE 1-2

Selected References Useful to Clinicians

Information Source	Comments
Facts and Comparisons	Extensive coverage of virtually every drug available in U.S. Available in bound version or looseleaf with monthly updates. Also available on CD-ROM. Has cost comparison index that is useful in determining relative cost of different brands.
USP Dispensing Information	Has 3 volumes published annually. Vol. I is written for health care professions; contains practical information about drugs, including signs and symptoms requiring immediate medical attention and what to do about missed doses. Vol. II contains drug information written for consumers. Also available in Spanish. Vol. III contains information on therapeutic equivalence and selected state and federal regulations related to prescriptions and regulation of prescription drugs and controlled substances.
Physicians' Desk Reference (PDR)	Fairly comprehensive listing of available drugs. However, information about specific drugs consists only of package inserts and these are included only if the drug's manufacturer has paid for the inserts to be published in the PDR; therefore, information about many older drugs or drugs marketed by several manufacturers may not be included. Also available in CD-ROM and handheld computer formats.

TABLE 1-2

Selected References Useful to Clinicians (continued)

Information Source	Comments
Goodman and Gilman's The Pharmacological Basis of Therapeutics	A classical reference on the pharmacology of drugs and updated research.
Remington's Pharmaceutical Sciences	Information on pharmacy practice, including aspects of compounding.
Drugs in Pregnancy and Lactation	Most complete resource on drug use in pregnancy and breastfeeding.
Martindale's: The Extra Pharmacopoeia	Monographs on domestic and foreign drugs as well as information on herbal and homeopathic medications.
American Drug Index	
AHFS Drug Information	Drug monographs with quarterly supplment. Also available in CD-ROM and on-line.
Drug Interactions (Hansten)	
Meyler's Side Effects of Drugs	Most comprehensive resource on drug adverse effects. Also available in CD-ROM format.
Physicians GenRX	Detailed monographs including informtion on drug pricing and therapeutic equivalency ratings, FDA approval dates, patent expiration dates.
Handbook of Nonprescription Drugs	Comprehensive information on over the counter drugs.

TABLE 1-3

Selected Computerized Databases Useful to Clinicians*

Database	Comments

MEDLARS (Medical Literature Analysis and Retrieval System)
    MEDLINE
    TOXLINE
    TOXLIT
	Available by subscription via Internet or in libraries using CD-ROMs such as Silver Platter.

Iowa Drug Information Service (IDIS)	Indexing service for retrieval of articles from more than 180 biomedical journals.
National Library of Medicine AIDS Databases: AIDSLINE, AIDSDRUGS, AIDSTRIALS, CANCERLIT	
MICRODEX Computerized Clinical Information Systems (CICS)	Combination of other publications, e.g., PDR, Martindale: The Extra Pharmacopeia, DRUGDEX.

*See also Table 1-6 on Internet drug information resources.

Drug Information Available via the Internet

A great amount of information is available to both consumers and professionals via the Internet. This makes information readily and easily available; however, not all information posted on the Internet is accurate or reliable. Users need to be careful in evaluating these sites. Even information from reputable sites may not have been subjected to the peer review process that helps to ensure the publication of valid information. Some sites may be sponsored by drug manufacturers or other persons or entities with a vested interest in the information; this information may be biased. Sometimes it is difficult to determine who is the author of the information and what are his or her credentials. Table 1-4 presents criteria to evaluate health information on the Internet, and Tables 1-5 and 1-6 give addresses and commentary on general medical-nursing sites and on drug-related information sites, respectively.

TABLE 1-4

Is This Site Reliable? Evaluating Health Information on the Internet

FDA staff and others familiar with Internet medical offerings suggest asking the following questions to help determine the reliability of a Web site:

Who maintains the site?

Government or university-run sites are among the best sources for scientifically sound health and medical information. Private practitioners or lay organizations may have marketing, social, or political agendas that can influence the type of material they offer on-site and which sites they link to.

Is there an editorial board or another listing of the names and credentials of those responsible for preparing and reviewing the site's contents?

Can these people be contacted by phone or through E-mail if visitors to the site have questions or want additional information?

Does the site link to other sources of medical information?

No reputable organization will position itself as the sole source of information on a particular health topic. However, links alone are not a guarantee of reliability, since anyone with a Web page can create links to any other site on the Internet. The owner of the site that is "linked to" has no say over who links to it. A person offering suspect medical advice could conceivably try to make his or her advice appear legitimate by, say, creating a link to FDA's Web site. What's more, health information produced by FDA or other government agencies is not copyrighted; therefore, someone can quote FDA information at a site and be perfectly within his or her rights. By citing a source such as FDA, experienced marketers using careful wording can make it appear as though FDA endorses their products.

When was the site last updated?

Generally, the more current the site, the more likely it is to provide timely material. Ideally, health and medical sites should be updated weekly or monthly.

Are informative graphics and multimedia files such as video or audio clips available?

Such features can assist in clarifying medical conditions and procedures. Bear in mind, however, that multimedia should be used to help explain medical information, not substitute for it. Some sites provide dazzling "bells and whistles" but little scientifically sound information.

Does the site charge an access fee?

Many reputable sites with health and medical information, including FDA and other government sites, offer access and materials for free. If a site does charge a fee, be sure that it offers value for the money. Use a searcher to see whether you can get the same information without paying additional fees.

SOURCE: Adapted from Larkin.[3]

TABLE 1-5

General Medical-Nursing Information Sites on the Internet

Site	Address	Comments
CliniWeb	www.ohsu.edu/ cliniweb/	Arranges medical subject categories by heading.
Internet Sleuth	www.isleuth.com/ heal.htm	Links to variety of health related resources.
MEDWEB	www.gen.emory.edu/ MEDWEB	
Mayo Health Oasis	www.mayo.ivi.com	Health information available from recent publications, expert opinions, multifaceted search library, medical centers, and the Mayo clinic purpose statement.
University of Washington Health Sciences Center	www.hslib.washington. edu	Links to personal, public, educational, and research areas. Access to university programs and services.
Achoo On-line Healthcare	www.achoo.com	Search agent for multiple health care information topics.
BU Alumni Medical Library	www.med- libwww.bu.edu	Access to on-line library, Medline, personal librarian contact, and links to medical information and other sites.
Briscoe Library University of Texas Health Sciences Center	www.briscoe. uthscsa. edu/library/	Offers a collection of books, journals, media, and microcomputer and software programs. Reference and staff available for information searches.
Laboratory Values	www.ghsl.nwu.edu/ Norm.html	Uses table format to present normal lab values for all body fluids.
National Library of Medicine	www.nlm.nih.gov	Information collected from federal and private agencies, organizations, institutions, and individuals on medical and related sciences. Links to electronic information services.
Department of Health and Human Services	www.os.dhhs.gov	Public affairs, consumer, policy research, and information. Link to all HHS agencies.

Site	Address	Comments
Online Clinical Calculator	www.intmed. mcw.edu/ clincalc.html	Converts and/or calculates patient information into other determinants, e.g., BMI, pounds to kilograms, etc.
National Institutes of Health	www.nih.gov	Selection of health indexes, specifically research at NIH.
Virtual Library (History/Science/ Technology/ Medicine)	www.asap.unimelb.edu. au/hstm	Comprehensive collection of abundant resources on the history of science, medicine, and technology. Link to Library of Congress.
Indiana University Ruth Lily Medical Library	www.medlib.iupui.edu	
Johns Hopkins University Welch Medical Library	www.welch.jhu.edu	
Physical Exam	www.medinfo.ufl.edu/ year1/bcs/clist/index. html	Textbook instructions and diagrams on how to take a complete health history.
Jonathan Tward's Multimedia Medical Reference Library	www.med-library.com	Collection of information for professionals, students, and patients.
Mt. Sinai Medical Library	www.mtsinai.org	
National Network of Libraries of Medicine	www.nnlm.nlm.nih.gov	
Virtual Hospital	vh.radiology.uiowa.edu	Access to textbooks, patient simulation, guidelines, and teaching files on many medical specialties.
Stanford University	www-med.stanford. edu/lane	
Texas A&M Med. Sciences Library		
Learn Well RNonline	www.learnwell.org/~edu/ rnonline.shtml	

TABLE 1-5

General Medical-Nursing Information Sites on the Internet (cont.)

Site	Address	Comments
HandiLinks	http://www.ahandyguide.com	Links to wide variety of health resources.
Centers for Disease Control and Prevention	www.cdc.gov	
Hospital Web	neuro-www.mgh.harvard.edu/ hospitalweb.nclk	
HELIX	http://helix.com	Information for consumers and professionals.
NP Web	http://unh:edu/npract/index.html	Links to resources for nurse practitioners.

TABLE 1-6

Drug-Related Information Sites on the Internet

Site	Address	Comments
Pharmacology Glossary—Boston University School of Medicine	http://med-www.bu.edu/ pharmacology/programmed/ glossary.html	Information on symbols and terms used in pharmacology.
Glaxo Wellcome Pharmacology Guide	http://www.glaxowellcome. co.uk/science/index.html	Quick reference guide to most of the important terms and concepts of pharmacology.
PharmWeb	http://www.pharmweb.net/	Provides links by subjects to other pharmacology related information sites for health professionals and patients.

TABLE 1-6

Drug-Related Information Sites on the Internet (continued)

Site	Address	Comments
PharmInfoNet	http://www.pharminfo.com/	Drug information and links to publications and disease centers.
"Virtual" Pharmacy Center—Martindale's Health Science	http://www-sci.lib.uci.edu:80/~martindale/Pharmacy.html#CPT	Variety of types of information about pharmacology and pharmacy around the world.
NP Web	http://www.unh.edu/npract/index.html	
NIH Clinical Alerts	gopher://gopher.nlm.nih.gov:70/11/alerts	Clinical alerts from clinical trials.
Drug FAQ Frequently Asked Questions about Drugs—PharmInfo	http://pharminfo.com/drugfaq/	Gives information about drugs, links to related articles and resources about the drug, and questions from patients and health professionals and the answers.
U.S. National Library of Medicine	http://text.nlm.nih.gov/ftrs/gateway	Links to AHCPR guidelines; AHCPR Technology Assessments and Reviews; NIH Concensus Development Program; NIH Clinical studies
Doctor's Guide to New Drugs or Indications	http://www.pslgroup.com/NEWDRUGS.HTM	Information about new drugs or new indications in US and worldwide.
Drug InfoNet	http://www.druginfonet.com/	Information about drugs, diseases, questions to experts, and links to other sites; names, addresses, and phone numbers for many pharmaceutical manufacturers.

TABLE 1-6

Drug-Related Information Sites on the Internet (continued)

Site	Address	Comments
Farmaweb	http://www.farmaweb.com/	Information about drugs in Spanish and English.
CenterWatch	http://www.centerwatch.com/	Information about clinical trials in US and internationally; also has information about newly approved drugs.
HealthA to Z-Pharmaceuticals and Drugs	http://www.healthatoz.com/categories/PC.htm	Information and links related to drug therapy.
Antibiotic Use Guidelines (University of Wisconsin)	http://www.biostat.wisc.edu/clinsci/amcg/amcg.html	Data on antibiotics by drug name, drug class, organism, empiric therapy by site, and antimicrobial treatment if HIV-infected patient.
Searle Health Net the Pipeline Game	http://www.searlehealthnet.com/pipeline.html	Interactive game that teaches about the process and pitfalls of drug development.
Agency for Health Care Policy and Research (AHCPR)	http://www.ahcpr.gov/	Information about research, policy, including clinical guidelines (e.g., acute pain and cancer pain).
Food and Drug Administration (FDA)	http://www.fda.gov/	Access to information about about drugs, foods, and devices regulated by FDA.
FDA Medical Bulletin	http://www.fda.gov/medbull/contents.html	Publication with information about drugs, devices, foods, and the MedWatch program.
	http://www.fda.gov/medwatch/index.html	Information about reporting adverse events from drugs and devices to FDA's MedWatch Program.

TABLE 1-6

Drug-Related Information Sites on the Internet (continued)

Site	Address	Comments
Pharmacokinetics Simulator	http://www.came.med. harvard.edu/pharm/	Computer-assisted learning modules on pharmacokinetics.
Internet Mental Health	http://mentalhealth.com	Drug monographs on psychotropics (Canadian).
University of Maryland Internet Drug Information Service	http://www.pharmacy.ab. umd.edu/~umdi/ umdi.html	Provides answers to questions submitted.
United States Pharmacopeia (USP)	http://www.usp.org	Information for physicians, nurses, pharmacists, patients/consumers, and others; medication counseling behaviors, medication error reporting (MER) program; drug products problem reporting (DPPR) program.
Merck Manual: Section 22: Clinical Pharmacology	http://www.merck.com	Section on clinical pharmacology available online: Click on publication and then Merck Manual Section 22 Clinical Pharmacology.
Internet Self-Assessment in Pharmacology (ISAP)	http://www.cs.umn.edu/ Research/GIMME/ isap.html	Various types of information and self-assessment guides in pharmacology.
Nursing the Internet-Pharmacy	http://home1.inet.tele.dk/	Links to a variety of information and tutorial sources related to pharmacology from around the world.

EVALUATING SOURCES OF DRUG INFORMATION

Whether it is in print or computer database or Internet form, the health professional can use the following criteria to judge the accuracy and reliability of the information source.

Is It Clear Who Has Written or Compiled the Information and from Where?

The source is important not only in terms of evaluating expertise but in identifying a possible source of bias. Some drug information is written and published by the drug manufacturer, which should alert the reader to potential biases in the information.

Package inserts are another important source of information about a particular drug; however, they may not include more recent data that have appeared in the research literature. Information in package inserts is written by the manufacturer but approved by the FDA in light of the data presented to the FDA as part of the drug approval process.

Internet resources are somewhat more difficult to judge since it is not always clear who has compiled the information. However, one usually can have confidence in information provided through major universities. Also, in a reliable site there usually is a contact person listed who can be contacted about the information (see also Table 1-4).

Is the Information Up-to-Date?

The copyright date of a book provides one clue to the probable age of information; however, books typically take a year to publish so information may be a year or more old. Journals usually have a time lag from the time of the submission of a manuscript to the time of publication due to the time necessary for the peer review process; even after approval and editing of manuscripts there can still be a time lag of two months or more before publication and distribution. On-line journals can decrease the time lag related to printing and distribution.

References used within journal articles or books should be checked for date as another clue to the currency of the information.

Computerized databases such as those on CD-ROMs need to be updated periodically.

Is There a Source of Potential Bias in the Information?

Drug information written by an author or investigator employed by a drug company, an Internet site sponsored by a drug manufacturer, or a study sponsored by a drug company should be scrutinized carefully for possible bias. Some journals now require that funding sources of the research be published along with the article. Journals may also require the authors or investigators to disclose any financial interests related to the drug or if they are employees or consultants with the manufacturer of a drug being studied.

Research journals tend to be biased in their publication of results of studies with positive findings as opposed to those with negative findings or findings of "no differences."

Some drug manufacturers provide free reprints of journal articles describing research favoring their product. While the study may have been conducted totally independently of the manufacturers, the clinician should be able to put the positive report in the context of other research on that drug; i.e., what do other research studies say about this drug? Was the study in the reprint the only one with positive results?

Is the Information Relevant?

The clinician needs to consider if the information is relevant to his or her patient population and/or to the individual patient. This requires careful analysis of the research design to determine which patients were included and which were excluded and why. This provides a basis for deciding if the findings are relevant to a particular patient or patient population. The clinician also needs to be familiar with the body of research in order to determine if research findings should be applied to practice; generally it is not appropriate or responsible to use the results of only one study as a basis for changes in practice.

Another consideration in evaluating relevance is whether or not the research showed a *clinically* significant difference. Clinical significance is different than the statistical significance that takes up a major part of many research reports. Statistical significance indicates whether or not the changes or differences observed were due to chance. Clinical significance refers to the difference the research makes in patient care. A drug study could have statistical significance but little clinical significance. For example, a drug could cause a decrease in blood glucose that was statistically significant, i.e., most likely caused by the drug and not by chance, but the decrease may not have clinical significance in that it would not require any need for additional drug therapy in diabetics. As a general rule of thumb, the larger the sample, the more likely the likelihood that there could be a statistical difference; therefore, it is important for the clinician to look even more carefully at the clinical significance—the amount of change and its implications for treatment or care.

EVALUATING DRUG RESEARCH

Research related to a drug has various purposes and takes various forms during the process of drug development and later after a drug has been approved for use. A key point related to research leading to the approval of a new drug is that the drug may have been studied in only 3000 to 5000 people before its approval by the FDA and its release for approved use. Therefore, many side effects are not known initially but will appear as the drug is used in greater numbers of patients and in patients with varied ethnic or genetic backgrounds and with a wider variety of concomitant conditions and other therapies.

Evaluating Research on Drug Therapy

The clinician should be familiar with basic research methods and approaches to the critique of basic research. These standards and criteria also apply to drug research. Some useful references to review involving drug therapy research are those by Ascione, Manifold, and Parenti[4] and Malone, Mosdell, Kier, and Stanovich.[2]

In drug research some aspects of research design have special importance or require special attention. Obtaining *informed consent of the research subjects* is important and required for virtually any type of drug research. An important element of informed consent that needs to be considered is the potential sense of coercion that a patient might feel when approached to be in a drug study. Research subjects need to be assured that they can refuse without endangering their ongoing regular health care. They need to be informed not only of the potential benefits but also the possible risks. The elements of informed consent are as follows: The research subject must:

1. Be competent to give consent, i.e., be able to understand information provided and make decisions and not be under influence of drugs that may cloud judgment.
2. Be informed of both risks and benefits.
3. Understand that he or she may receive a placebo and not the drug (if this is the research design).
4. Understand that he or she has the right to refuse to participate initially and to withdraw from the research at any point without risking the right to medical care.
5. Not feel coerced by other factors such as perceived obligation to the physician/clinician or researcher or the magnitude of rewards for participating (e.g., early release time for prisoners).

Information about the research must be provided in writing and signed by the patient.

It is particularly important to consider how the research design has *controlled* for the possibility that other factors than the drug are producing the effects being studied. One method for accounting for unknown influences is to use randomization of patients into control or experimental groups. Randomization presumably "randomizes" or equally distributes unknown factors into both groups. Even with randomization, however, the groups may not be identical in their characteristics. Researchers should compare (and report) the demographic or other characteristics of both the experimental and the control groups. This allows the reader to interpret the study findings in light of any significant difference in the two groups. Researchers also can control some differences statistically (e.g., by analysis of covariance—ANOVA) when they are analyzing the data.

The power of *psychological influences* on drug effects can cause actual physiological effects. This is the reason for the use of the placebo in most drug research, especially when the outcomes are subjective rather than objective in nature, in order to establish that effects are the result of the drug and not from expectations or other influences. Additionally, the patient or researcher consciously or unconsciously may overreport beneficial effects or minimize adverse effects. Control for this is usually accomplished through the use of double-blind studies in which neither the patient nor the researchers know whether the particular patient is receiving the experimental drug or a placebo. Table 1-7 illustrates the types of blinding used in experimental studies.

TABLE 1-7

Types of Blinding

Single-blind	Either the investigators or the subjects are unaware of assignment of subjects to the active or control group.
Double-blind	Both subjects and investigators are unaware of assignment of subjects to the active or control group.
Triple-blind	Both subjects and investigators as well as the group involved in interpretation of the data are unaware of assignments of subjects to the active or control group.

SOURCE: Malone et al.[2]

Types of Research Designs Used in Drug Research

Various types of research designs are used in the development and ongoing evaluation of drugs and drug therapy. Table 1-8 summarizes different research designs and their purpose.

Two common research designs are parallel and crossover. In a parallel study subjects receive only one treatment. In a crossover study each subject receives more than one treatment; a washout period (usually of at least five half-lives of the study drug) is necessary between the treatments. Table 1-9 compares parallel and crossover designs.

TABLE 1-8

Study Designs Used in Drug Research

Study Design	Study Purpose
True experiment	Determine cause and effect relationships
Follow-up (cohort) study	Determine association between various factors and disease state development
Case-control (trohoc) study	Determine association between disease states and exposure to various risk factors
Cross-sectional study	Identify prevalence of characteristics of diseases in populations
Meta-analysis	Combine, statistically evaluate, and summarize data from multiple studies
Case study or series	Report observations in a single patient or several patients

TABLE 1-8

Study Designs Used in Drug Research (continued)

Study Design	Study Purpose
N-of-1 study	Compare effects of drug to control during multiple observation periods in a single patient
Stability study	Evaluate stability of drugs in various preparations (e.g., ophthalmologic, intravenous, topical, oral)
Survey research	Study the incidence, distribution, and relationships of sociological and psychological variables through use of questionnaires applied to various populations
Postmarketing surveillance study	Evaluate use of and adverse effects associated with newly approved drug therapies
Pharmacoeconomic analysis	Compare outcomes and costs of drug therapies or services
Programmatic research	Determine impact and/or economic value of pharmaceutical services

SOURCE: Malone et al., p. 72.[2]

Sample

The sample is important not only in judging adequacy of the sampling the research population but also in evaluating whether research findings can or should be applied to a particular patient population. Historically, women and minorities have been underrepresented in drug research. Now, research funded by the National Institutes of Health must specifically include these underrepresented groups or explain why this is not necessary. Amazingly, drugs have rarely been tested on elderly persons before approval; it is all the more amazing since the elderly consume a much greater proportion of medications than any other age groups. The alterations in drug pharmacodynamics and kinetics resulting from normal aging processes make the elderly especially vulnerable to both known and unknown drug effects.

Inclusion and exclusion criteria are important to note. Often patients with conditions other than the one being treated are excluded. Therefore, the use of the drug in patients with multiple conditions and/or on multiple drug therapy will not have been tested, and this can be a factor in evaluating whether the drug research findings should be applied to a different or even a similar patient population.

How the patients were recruited into the study may influence the results. If they were recruited from specialists or academic health centers, the patients may represent sicker patients than those recruited from a rural family practice. If subjects responded to an advertisement in a newspaper or on a bulletin board, they may have certain character-

TABLE 1-9

Parallel versus Crossover Designs

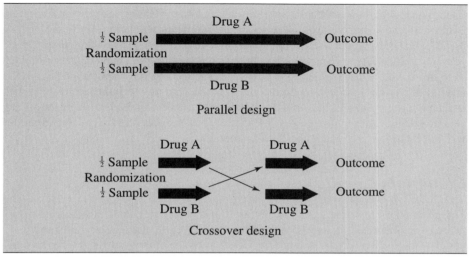

SOURCE: Malone et al., p. 96.[2]

istics that make them different from other patients who might eventually use the drug. Geographical location may play a role. One study of the use of herbal medicines reported a relatively high incidence of use; however, the study was conducted in a city in which there was a school of alternative medicine.[5]

The time of year that the study was conducted could be an important variable with certain drugs such as antihistamines and other antiallergy or antiasthma drugs. A study involving photosensitivity of a drug probably would have poor results if done during the winter in the snowbelt states (or Alaska!).

How were patients entered into the study? Were they randomized into the control and the experimental groups? If so, how? *Randomization* must ensure that each patient has an equal chance of being in either or any of the research groups. Usually the demographic and other relevant characteristics of the control and experimental groups are compared statistically and hopefully will show no statistically significant difference. Even with randomization, however, assigned groups can end up with different characteristics that could influence results.

Did any patients drop out, and if so, is this reported and explained? Patients' dropping out of a study because of inability to tolerate side effects would skew results. The level of compliance of the subjects with the drug regimen should be evaluated and reported by the researchers in order to determine the possible influence on the study results.

RULE OF THUMB: A basic key question the reader or consumer of drug research (or actually any research) should ask is: What else besides the drug (or intervention) could have produced the effect or outcome?

PRESCRIBING

Each state regulates the practice of the various health professions, including prescribing. Because of the variations from state to state in the legal regulation of the prescribing role of advanced practice nurses, it is impossible to cover each state's regulations. Each year the journal *Nurse Practitioner* publishes the results of its annual survey of each state in relation to the regulation of scope of practice and prescription writing. APNs need to be aware of the laws and regulations in the state in which they practice as well as the policies, protocols, etc., in their specific practice setting. Federal regulations may also impact prescribing practices of APNs. Some of the general patterns and variations will be discussed later under contextual variables.

Clinical Judgment

The decision to prescribe a drug is the result of therapeutic judgment based upon adequate assessment and diagnosis of the patient, therapeutic alternatives, and knowledge of pharmacology of drugs. Knowledge of the pathophysiology of the patient's condition, especially in terms of its usual trajectory (usual length, waxing and waning) is important in deciding if and what to prescribe. In weighing drug versus nondrug interventions, the clinician needs to weigh the cost of *not* prescribing to treat the condition as well as the cost of the drug and the cost of any monitoring for adverse effects. Table 1-10 lists questions to be asked in determining the appropriateness of a medication.

The decision to prescribe a drug also assumes that nondrug interventions have been considered, have been ruled out, or have been used or will be used concurrently. APNs should integrate their expertise in the assessment, nursing, and medical treatment of the whole person into the therapeutic plan.

TABLE 1-10

Medication Appropriateness Index

Is there an indication for the drug?
Is the medication effective for the condition?
Is the dosage correct?
Are the directions correct?
Are the directions practical?
Are there clinically significant drug–drug interactions?
Are there clinically significant drug–disease condition interactions?
Is there unnecessary duplication with other drug(s)?
Is the duration of therapy acceptable?
Is this drug the least expensive alternative compared with others of equal utility?

SOURCE: Schmader et al.[6]

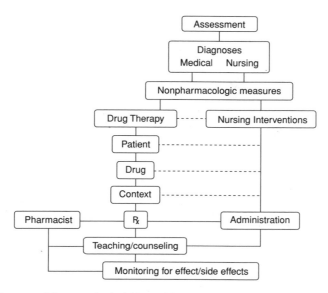

Figure 1-1 Process of therapeutic decision making by the advanced practice nurse.

Figure 1-1 outlines the process of decision making leading to prescribing a drug and how prescribing by the APN relates to nursing assessment and nursing interventions. It also shows the role of the pharmacist.

Once a decision has been made to treat the patient with a medication, the clinician and the patient need to be clear about the therapeutic goal and how it will be evaluated and monitored. For some drugs the goal is to control symptoms and/or improve lifestyle versus the more definitive "cure" or treatment of the underlying condition. The degree or type of side effects that can be tolerated is also important.

Choosing a Drug

When considering which drug to prescribe, the clinician needs to take into account a variety of factors. These may be clustered around the *D*rug variables, *P*atient variables, and *C*ontextual variables (DPC).

Drug variables are the pharmacodynamic and pharmacokinetic information about a drug as well as its available formulations.

Patient variables are the individual physiological and pathophysiological characteristics unique to each patient which may affect response and/or the choice of route, dose, or formulation.

Contextual variables are other factors that may influence the choice of a medication such as cost, insurance coverage, availability through an agency formulary, and the patient's lifestyle or occupation. An APN's choice of a medication may also be limited by state regulations or law or by protocols (e.g., if she or he is not allowed to prescribe opioid analgesics).

This approach to thinking about selecting drug therapy will be used within the chapters in Part 2 that discuss specific drug groups.

Prescription, Controlled, and Over-the-Counter Drugs

Drugs requiring a prescription are sometimes referred to as "legend" drugs. This term arises from the legal requirement of the FDA that the manufacturer's label have the ℞ legend: "CAUTION: Federal Law Prohibits Dispensing Without Prescription."

Certain prescription drugs, sometimes referred to as "controlled substances" or "controlled drugs" are regulated by the Controlled Substances Act of 1970. The Controlled Substances Act classifies drugs based on their potential for abuse; the resulting "schedules" have specifications for prescribing drugs as summarized in Table 1-11. States also may impose additional regulations on these or other drugs; practitioners need to be aware of the regulations in each state and setting that affect prescribing. Depending upon the laws in a state, the APN may or may not be able to prescribe controlled substances.

In order to prescribe these controlled drugs, the prescriber must have a Drug Enforcement Administration (DEA) number. Whether or not a DEA number will be

TABLE 1-11

Controlled Substance Schedule

Schedule	Examples	Prescribing Implications
Schedule I (no approved medical use, high potential for abuse)	Heroin, marijuana, LSD, peyote	
Schedule II* (high potential for abuse but have currently accepted medical use)	*Amphetamine-like products*: amphetamine, dextroamphetamine, methamphetamine, methylphenidate, phenmetrazine *Barbiturate-like products*: amobarbital, glutethimide, pentobarbital, secobarbital *Narcotic-like products*: alphaprodine, anileridine, cocaine, codeine, fentanyl, hydromorphone, levomorphone, meperidine, methadone, opium alkaloids (e.g., morphine), oxymorphone	Cannot be refilled. Prescriptions must be in writing. In an emergency a telephone prescription for an amount needed to treat the patient during the emergency period may be permitted. A written signed prescription for the prescribed substance must be provided within 72 h.

TABLE 1-11

Controlled Substance Schedule (continued)

Schedule	Examples	Prescribing Implications
Schedule III* (have accepted medical use and potential for abuse less than those in Schedule II)	Acetaminophen or aspirin with codeine, Fiorinal, hydrocodone bitartrate combinations, paregoric, Synalgos-DC, Tussionex *Sedatives:* aprobarbital, butabarbital sodium, pentobarbital suppositories *Anorectics:* benzphetamine hydrochloride, phendimetrazine tartrate *Anabolic steroids:* fluoxymesterone, methyltestosterone, testosterone	Cannot be refilled more than 5 times or more than 6 months after the original date.
Schedule IV* (drugs with accepted medical use and low potential for abuse relative to those in Schedules II and III)	*Examples:* alprazolam, chloral hydrate, chlordiazepoxide, diazepam, estazolam, fenfluramine hydrochloride, flurazepam hydrochloride, lorazepam, meprobamate, oxazepam, paraldehyde, pentazocine, propoxyphene, triazolam	Cannot be refilled more than 5 times or more than 6 months after the original date.
Schedule V* (formerly called Class X or exempt narcotic). If product contains codeine, it must have at least one other non-narcotic active medicinal ingredient and must not have more than 200 mg of codeine per 100 mL or per 100 g.	Ambenyl Cough Syrup, Actifed with Codeine Cough Syrup, Calcidrine Syrup, Dimetane D C Cough Syrup, diphenoxylate hydrochloride with atropine sulfate, Donnagel PG, Novahistine DH, Parepectolin, Pediacol Cough Syrup, Phenergan with Codeine Syrup, Robitussin A C Syrup, Tussar-2 Cough Syrup	Can be dispensed without a prescription after consultation with the pharmacist, limit on quantity of product that can be purchased in a given period of time; patient must sign for the purchase.

*For Schedules II to V: Prescriber's DEA number, printed name, signature in ink, and address are required. State laws may further regulate drugs and prescription provisions.

issued by DEA depends on the regulations of the state of the practitioner as to the scope of prescribing practices allowed to APNs, the scope of practice of the individual practitioner, and the "agreement" with the supervising physician (if this is required in the state). The required form for obtaining a DEA number (FORM DEA-224) can be obtained from the Drug Enforcement Administration, Registration Unit, PO Box 28083 Central Station, Washington, D.C. 20005, or from any DEA field office.

Resource

The Drug Enforcement Administration (DEA) of the U.S. Department of Justice publishes a manual with essential information for APNs or other clinicians involved in prescribing controlled drugs: *Midlevel Practitioner's Manual. An Informational Outline of the Controlled Substances Act of 1970.*

Nonprescription drugs are also called over-the-counter (OTC) drugs. They are approved by the FDA for specific uses and in specific dosages for use by the layperson. There must be adequate directions for use and warnings about misuse by the layperson. Recently an increased number of prescription drugs have been approved as OTC. Drugs are usually approved for OTC use in doses less than those for the same drug as a prescription drug. An additional issue here is that most third-party payers do not pay or reimburse for OTC drugs; therefore, in not prescribing the prescription form of a drug, the clinician may increase the cost to the patient. The clinician also needs to be aware of which drugs are available without prescription, since the patient may be taking these independently and may not have informed the clinician because the patient may not consider them to be "real" drugs. The use of OTC drugs obviously could lead to drug interactions if the clinician is not aware of their use. Similarly, the clinician should know about the use of herbs, home remedies, and other "health food store" preparations because of the active ingredients in many of these preparations. For example, high levels of vitamin C (ascorbic acid) may acidify the urine, which can affect the renal excretion of drugs. See further discussion in Chap. 2.

Writing the Prescription

The writing of a prescription involves some fairly standard components (see Table 1-12). Some details may vary according to state law or agency policy.

Sublingual nitroglycerin and certain aspirin-containing products are automatically exempted from the Poison Prevention Packaging Act of 1970, which mandated special packaging for prescription drugs, all controlled drugs, aspirin, acetaminophen, and many household products. Practitioners as well as patients may request a waiver from the childproof packaging; however, the decision is that of the pharmacist.

Substitution of another entity other than that indicated by the prescriber has become an increasing area for concern. *Generic substitution* (of a generic brand for a trade name brand) has become common practice and is often mandated or allowed by federal or state laws unless the prescriber specifically indicates "no substitutions" or writes "dispense as written." Usually, a generic brand is less expensive; however, certain brands of drugs may not achieve the same outcomes. See Chap. 3 for a discussion of drugs in which interchange of brands may produce clinically significant differences in bioavailability.

TABLE 1-12

Guidelines for Writing Prescriptions

Components of Prescription	Comments
Patient's name, address, date of birth	Age is of particular importance for pharmacist to determine appropriateness of medication or dose, especially in children and elderly.
Patient's weight	Might be needed in children and elderly.
Date of prescription	Some states place limit on time in which a prescription can be filled (e.g., within 30 days).
Name of drug	May be written as generic or brand name; however, will need to indicate "no substitution" if want a specific brand. Do not use abbreviations for drugs.
Dosage form and strength of drug (if applicable)	
Dose	Use metric systems; do not use apothecary names or symbols; spell out "unit" (rather than U which could be misread as a 0 and result in tenfold increase); write out micrograms.
	If a whole number, do not use decimal and zero with it (could be misinterpreted as ten times intended dose; e.g., use 3 mg rather than 3.0 mg).
	If number is less than 1, always place a zero and decimal, e.g., 0.1 ml.
Route and frequency	Write out "once daily." Avoid use of QOD (could look like QID).
Quantity to be dispensed	May restrict if concerned about potential danger to patient, e.g., use in suicide.
Directions for use	Any special directions; avoid use of "take as directed."
Number of refills (if any)	May need to restrict if danger to patient. PRN not usually acceptable to indicate number of refills. Spell out words for the numbers (or circle a printed number) to make it more difficult for patient to alter the number.
Prescriber's name, title,* address, phone number; name of supervising physician*	
Prescriber's signature	Must be in ink. Should never be signed in advance.
DEA registration number of prescriber*	
Substitution allowed or not allowed	Indicate whether you want patient to receive a particular brand of the medication or if a generic substitution is allowed.

*Will vary according to each state's laws and regulations for APN prescribing.

Certain references can be used to determine equivalence. *USP Dispensing Information–Volume 3: Approved Drug Products and Legal Requirements* provides information about therapeutic equivalence ratings. This information is also included in the *Physicians GenRx* monographs.

Pharmaceutical substitution may be done by a pharmacist. This may consist of dispensing a drug that is a different salt, ester, or dosage form (e.g., a suspension rather than capsules).[7]

More recently *therapeutic substitution* has come into prominence because of the increase in cost containment measures. In therapeutic substitution, a therapeutic alternate, not the same drug, may be dispensed instead of the drug ordered. In some situations this is the result of the use of formulary systems (see discussion below) in institutions and managed care plans. The prescribing clinician needs to be aware of this possibility and of the policies and situations in which this may occur. Often a particular drug is prescribed for a patient because of the specific characteristics and needs of the individual patient. Therapeutic substitution done without consulting the prescribing clinician could result not only in the possibility of adverse effects but also lack of effect in that patient. There have been some reported instances where physicians acting on behalf of drug manufacturers have been asked to allow therapeutic substitutions by pharmacists.

Practical Aspects

Prescription Pads

Prescription pads should be stored in a secure place; only one prescription pad at a time should be used. States may require certain statements or configurations of the prescription pad information, e.g., need for the name of the supervising physician, substitution of a generic brand allowed or not allowed, signature required—no stamps. Only one prescription can be written on each prescription page. Some states allow the actual writing of the prescription to be done by another person, but the prescriber must sign with his or her signature and is responsible for the accuracy of the whole prescription. Prescriptions must be written and signed in ink.

Prescriptions by Phone

The legal legitimacy of telephone prescriptions varies from state to state. Oral prescriptions must be written down by the pharmacist and filed. Telephone prescriptions may be conveyed to the pharmacist by the prescribing practitioner or by his or her legally authorized representative, who may be a nurse or secretary. The agent is communicating the prescription and is not making the prescription decision. Telephone orders or use of an agent to communicate the prescription may not be allowed in certain states. Certain controlled substances (e.g., Schedule II) may be dispensed only with a written order (see Table 1-11).

Record Keeping

The prescription essentials need to be recorded in some way in the patient's record. In some settings a duplicate of the original is placed in the record. In addition, any clinician prescribing controlled substances needs to keep written records of these transactions.

Practitioners involved in the purchase, storage, disposal, and actual administration of controlled substances will have additional recording and reporting requirements according to DEA and/or state regulations.

Refills

The quantity dispensed and the number of refills can be an issue of concern when there is a danger that the patient is suicidal and may amass a large quantity of a drug. The quantity allowed to be dispensed or allowed through refills should be restricted—usually to less than the total amount that could produce a lethal dose. Limiting the amount prescribed and/or number of refills is also a way to ensure that the patient will contact the clinician for follow-up. On the other hand, managed care drug plans usually restrict the amount dispensed at any one time to a 30-day supply; the pharmacist can adjust the number of refills for a longer prescription to 30-day refills in order to meet this requirement. Drug prescriptions refilled through the mail sometimes provide a larger supply at one time, depending on the third-party payer.

Drug Samples

The 1987 Prescription Drug Marketing Act regulates the distribution of drug samples. Written requests must be made by the prescribing practitioner to the manufacturer providing the following information: name, address, professional designation, signature of practitioner making request, identity of drug sample requested, quantity requested, name of manufacturer of drug sample, and date of request. The practitioner must provide written receipt to the manufacturer or distributor.

Teaching and Patient Instruction

Teaching the patient about the medication prescribed is very important from both a clinical and a legal perspective. Patients need to be fully informed about possible side effects and which of those should be reported. If a drug causes drowsiness, the clinician needs to warn patients not to drive or operate dangerous machinery or engage in other potentially dangerous situations. Warnings about taking a medication with alcohol are also important. Many prescribers and pharmacists have written information about a drug that they give to patients when they prescribe or dispense the medication. Counseling patients about their medication regimen is discussed further in Chap. 2.

Contextual Aspects

Scope of Practice

As mentioned previously, each state determines who may prescribe, dispense, and administer drugs. The traditional professions that have prescribed in the past have been medicine, dentistry, and veterinary medicine. More recently, APNs and physicians' assistants have been given prescribing privileges in some states. All but one state has had some form of prescribing authority for APNs.[1] States in which there is a nurse practitioner (NP) committee of the board of nursing and/or medicine were found in one study to be more likely to have NP prescriptive authority.[8] APNs usually included in legislation allowing prescribing are nurse practitioners (pediatric, adult, family, ob/gyn, women's health, geriatric), mental health clinical nurse specialists, nurse midwives, and nurse anesthetists. Nurse anesthetists have been prescribing within their scope of practice for many years. Clinical nurse specialists other than psychiatric–mental health clinical nurse specialists have had less success in obtaining prescribing authority.

The way in which legislation gives APNs prescribing privileges varies from state to state; the political processes involved have not always resulted in the ideal form of legislation, i.e., where APNs are awarded prescribing privileges based on the nursing practice act or board of nursing with no requirements for physician collaboration or supervision. Other mechanisms for establishing the legal basis of APN prescribing may involve requirements for physician collaboration or supervision, requirements for joint agreement and authorization between boards of nursing and medicine, limitations on prescription of some or all controlled substances, the use of written protocols, and prescribing authority based on delegation of prescription writing from physicians. Some states require a certain number of hours of postbasic pharmacology education. Prescribing by clinical nurse specialists (CNSs) is excluded in some states. APNs need to be aware of the legal requirements and regulations in the state and setting in which they practice and prescribe. APNs also need to be alert to the other barriers—some old and some new—to APN roles.

Numerous barriers have prevented APNs from obtaining or exercising their prescriptive role even in states where this role is legal. The Drug Enforcement Administration initially refused to provide DEA prescribing numbers to APNs; this policy was eventually changed. APNs who are authorized by their state to prescribe controlled substances now may obtain a DEA number.

Some physicians continue to attempt to control nurses and APNs by proposing limitations on the number of APNs a physician can supervise. The need to limit the number has been further aggravated by the increased costs of malpractice insurance for MDs supervising prescribing by APNs. The American Medical Association House of Delegates has adopted guidelines that include statement that, "The physician is responsible for the supervision of nurse practitioners in all settings."

More recently, the barriers to APN prescribing have shifted from the legal basis to the employment arena. APNs have found that some employers have not encouraged or allowed APNs to obtain or use prescribing privileges. APNs also have found that the processes involved in obtaining these privileges may be cumbersome—from the intricacies of paperwork for authorization to the need to rewrite policies, procedures, and protocols to incorporate the APN role in prescribing in their practice setting.[9]

Research on Advanced Practice Nurses as Prescribers

Research has been done on the various aspects of the APN role in prescribing. As described by Mahoney,[10] the research evolved from small-scale studies focusing on similarities to MDs, protocol adherence, and client and physician acceptance to large-scale national studies focusing on practice issues, regulatory policy, decision-making styles, client outcomes, and cost-effectiveness. Several studies have shown that APNs prescribe fewer drugs than MDs. However, many studies did not control for differences in case mix. In an attempt to address this issue, Brown and Grimes[11] conducted a meta-analysis of studies of nurse practitioners and nurse midwives in primary care. They conducted separate analyses of studies with varying degrees of control for severity of illness. In randomized studies, the only statistically significant effect size for NPs versus MDs was in patient compliance. In the analyses that included both randomized and controlled studies no statistically significance effect size between NPs and MDs was found.

IMPLICATIONS OF COST AND QUALITY MEASURES

In this era of increased concern for control of costs and quality, there are various mechanisms in place to monitor the prescription and/or use of medications. Prescribers from all disciplines are subject to a variety of factors affecting their prescribing. Formularies are being used by managed care providers, insurers, and some Medicaid programs as a mechanism for cost containment.

Formularies specify the drugs which may be prescribed in the particular setting. In some cases these are considered open formularies with a list of drugs that are recommended; in other situations the cost of a drug not in the formulary will not be reimbursed unless the prescriber has obtained prior authorization.[12] Managed care programs and drug use review (DUR) also may monitor the prescribing patterns of prescribers, providing periodic reports to prescribers on how their prescribing patterns compare with other prescribers or the percentage of prescriptions that were for drugs from the formulary.

Drug Use Review

The Omnibus Budget Reconciliation Act of 1990 (OBRA 90) resulted in various measures to control the cost of health care and of drug therapy for Medicaid patients. One measure involved rebates from pharmaceutical companies, i.e., that Medicaid would pay only the lowest price paid by any customer for a given medication. OBRA also required DUR as a quality improvement system for drug usage. This federal legislation covered only Medicaid patients, but it directed the states to develop the programs; many states then developed DUR programs that affect other types of patients.

DUR is retrospective or prospective. In retrospective DUR large numbers of drug orders are analyzed to identify potential problems. The review may look at prescriptions that fall outside of DUR criteria or it may look at prescriber practice patterns. The goal is to look at current data to prevent future problems; the prevention occurs through prescriber-focused educational interventions. Each state is to establish a DUR board with membership consisting of 33 to 51 percent pharmacists and 33 to 51 percent physicians.[13]

A prospective DUR under OBRA places responsibility on the pharmacist to screen prescriptions before dispensing in order to prevent and resolve problems due to prescription duplication, drug or disease contraindication, drug-drug interactions (including serious interaction with OTC drugs), incorrect dosage or duration, drug-allergy interactions, and clinical abuse or misuse.

Patient counseling by the pharmacist is also mandated by OBRA and has been adopted by most states for all patients. The pharmacist is obliged to initiate the discussion with the patient (not just wait until a patient asks for drug information).

Economic Variables: Pharmacoeconomics

Pharmacoeconomics uses the principles and methods of economic analysis in evaluating drug therapy. It incorporates both costs and clinical outcomes in a variety of methods to determine the therapeutic approach that produces the best outcomes for the resources invested.

The particular analysis used may incorporate the various perspectives of the patient, provider, hospital or health system, third-party or managed care system, government, or society.

Table 1-13 delineates the types of the costs usually used in pharmacoeconomic analyses, and Table 1-14 identifies different types of methods used in pharmacoeconomics.

Outcomes may be measured as improvements in indices of a patient's medical diagnoses and/or more general measures that reflect improvements in life span or improvement in the quality of life. Quality-of-life (QOL) measures may be general, such as the Medical Outcomes Study 36-item (SF-36) Health Survey,[15] or they may be specifically developed for a particular patient population, such as cancer patients.

Patient Contextual Variables

A patient's living or financial situation, especially his or her health insurance coverage, can impact on the choice of a drug and on patient compliance. The ability to pay for medi-

TABLE 1-13

Categories of Health Care Costs or Economic Outcomes

Direct medical: costs of products and services to prevent, detect, and/or treat disease, e.g., drugs, laboratories, hospitalization
Direct nonmedical: e.g., costs of transportation, hotel room near treatment
Indirect nonmedical: costs of reduced productivity (morbidity, mortality)
Intangible other financial outcomes: pain, suffering, grief
Opportunity costs: the economic benefit forgone when using one therapy instead of the next best alternative

SOURCE: Sanchez.[14]

TABLE 1-14

Pharmacoeconomic Methods

Economic Evaluations	Humanistic Evaluations
Cost of illness (estimates the cost of a disease in defined population)	Quality of life (physical, social, and emotional aspects of patient's well-being that are relevant and important to the patient)
Cost minimization (finds the least expensive alternative)	Patient preferences
Cost benefit (measures benefit in monetary units and computes a net gain)	Patient satisfaction
Cost-effectiveness (compares alternatives with therapeutic effects measured in physical units and computes a C/E ratio)	
Cost utility (measures therapeutic consequences in utility units rather than physical units; computes a C/U ratio)	

SOURCE: Sanchez.[14]

cations is a major concern, especially if the patient does not have prescription coverage or has a large number of prescription medications with copayments. As a rule of thumb, a month's supply of a prescription drug will cost a patient about $50 to $60 for each drug. Even when prescriptions are covered by a third party, the copayments can be as high as $10 to $15 per prescription; some plans require a copayment at time of dispensing. Some third-party plans reimburse after the patient pays out of pocket for the drug, which can impose a need for a cash outlay and the submission of paperwork for compensation.

Patients' physical limitations such as visual impairments or loss of hand function from arthritis or stroke, may impact on their ability to handle medications in general or by certain routes. This may also result in the need to consider the ability of the patient's caregiver to manage the medication regimen. Patients' living arrangement as well as occupational activities could impact on storage of medications and on their ability to take medications on a certain schedule.

SUMMARY

As the chapter has illustrated, the decision to prescribe a medication requires clinical judgment as well as consideration of a variety of legal, social, and economic factors. Schwinghammer[16] has identified a series of steps that are useful in focusing on the aspects of prescribing.

Steps in Solving Drug-Related Problems

1. Identification of real or potential drug-related problems
2. Determination of the desired therapeutic outcome
    Primary outcomes:
       Cure of disease (e.g., bacterial infection)
       Reduction or elimination of symptoms (e.g., pain from cancer)
       Arresting or slowing of the progression of disease (e.g., rheumatoid arthritis)
       Preventing a disease or symptom (e.g., cardiovascular disease)
    Other outcomes of pharmacotherapy:
       Not complicating or aggravating other existing disease states
       Avoiding or minimizing adverse effects of treatment
       Providing cost-effective therapy
       Maintaining the patient's quality of life
3. Determination of therapeutic alternatives
4. Design of optimal individualized pharmacotherapy plan—best drug, dosage, dosage form, schedule, and duration of therapy for a given patient
5. Identification of assessment parameters
6. Provision of patient counseling
    Name and description of the medication (including the indication)
    Dosage, dosage form, route of administration
    Special directions or procedures for preparation, administration, and use
    Techniques for self-monitoring
    Proper storage
    Prescription refill information
    Action to be taken in the event of missed doses

REFERENCES

1. Pearson LJ: Annual update of how each state stands on legislative issues affecting advanced nursing practice. *Nurse Pract* 22(1): 18, 1997.
2. Malone PM, Mosdell KW, Kier KL, Stanovich JE: *Drug Information: A Guide for Pharmacists.* Stamford, CT: Appleton & Lange, 1996, p 31.
3. Larkin M: Health information on-line. *FDA Consumer Magazine,* June 1996.
4. Ascione FJ, Manifold CC, Parenti MA: *Principles of drug information and scientific literature evaluation.* Hamilton, IL: Drug Intelligence Publications, 1994.
5. Brown JS, Marcy SA: The use of botanicals for health purposes by members of a prepaid health plan. *Res Nurs Health* (14(5): 339–359, 1991.

6. Schmader K, Hanlon JT, Weinberger M, et al: Appropriateness of medication prescribing in ambulatory elderly patients. *JA Geriatr Soc* 42:1241–1247, 1994.

7. Eckel FM: Prescription writing, in Munson PL (ed): *Principles of Pharmacology: Basic Concepts and Clinical Applications*. New York: Chapman and Hall, 1995.

8. Wilken M: State regulatory board structure, regulations, and nurse practitioner availability. *Nurse Pract* 20(10):68, 1995.

9. Mahoney, DF: Employer resistance to state authorized prescriptive authority for NPs. Results from a pilot study. *Nurse Pract* 20(1):58, 1995.

10. Mahoney DF: Nurse practitioners as prescribers: Past research trends and future study needs. *Nurse Pract* 17(1):44, 1992.

11. Brown SA, Grimes DE: A meta-analysis of nurse practitioners and nurse midwives in primary care. *Nurs Res* 44(6): 332–329, 1995.

12. Brydolf C: Prescriptions under scrutiny. Is a formulary coming to your setting? *Advance Nurse Pract*: April 17, 1994.

13. Bushwood DB: OBRA 90 and managed care pharmacy. Internet: Medscape, 1995.

14. Sanchez LA: Pharmacoeconomics: Principles, methods, and application to pharmacotherapy in DiPiro JT, Talbert RL, Yee GC, et al (eds): *Pharmacotherapy: A Pathophysiological Approach*. Stamford, CT: Appleton & Lange, 1997.

15. Ware JE Jr, Sherbourne CD: The MOS 36-item short-form Health Survey (SF-36). *Med Care* 30:473–482, 1992.

16. Schwinghammer TL: *Pharmacotherapy: A Patient-Focused Approach*. Stamford, CT: Appleton & Lange, 1997.

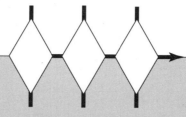

Chapter 2

PSYCHOSOCIOCULTURAL ASPECTS OF DRUG THERAPY

Laurel A. Eisenhauer

INTRODUCTION

This chapter focuses on the various factors which may influence the success of drug therapy. Beliefs about health, disease, and therapy, including cultural or ethnic beliefs, the use of self-care practices, and alternative medicine, are discussed. Strategies for promoting compliance/adherence and patient teaching are also included.

BELIEFS ABOUT DRUG THERAPY

The beliefs of individuals about the role of drug therapy in curing or controlling their disease or in promoting their health are intimately linked to their beliefs about disease causation. Often these beliefs are based on religious or cultural beliefs.

Beliefs may influence the degree of trust in the efficacy of a drug and therefore can strongly influence either positively or negatively the operation of a "placebo" effect. These beliefs may also translate into health care practices outside of mainstream conventional medicine, such as the use of home and other ethnic health remedies, herbs, and alternative medicine therapies. Beliefs also can influence compliance with prescribed drugs and influence the success of patient education.

The current trend toward self-care also contributes to individuals seeking out and using a wide variety of remedies for promoting and maintaining health as well as treatment of disease.

Resources:

Print

Bergan FW: Cultural aspects of drug therapy, in Eisenhauer LA, Spencer RT, Nichols W, Bergan FW: *Clinical Pharmacology and Nursing Management.* Philadelphia: Lippincott, 1998.

Dossey BM, Keegan L, Guzzetta CE, Kolkmeier LG: *Holistic Nursing: A Handbook for Practice,* 2d ed. Frederick, MD: Aspen, 1995.

Youngkin EQ, Israel DS: A review and critique of common herbal alternative therapies. *Nurse Pract* 21(10): 39, 43–44, 48, 49–52, 54–56, 59–60, 62, 1996.

Internet

Alternative Medicine Homepage: http://www.pitt.edu/~cbw/altm.html (Information source from Falk Library of Health Sciences at University of Pittsburgh.)

Dr. Bower's Complementary and Alternative Medicine Homepage: http://galen.med.virginia.edu/~pjb3s/ComplementaryHomepage.html (Information and links to other sites.)

Homeopathy Homepage: http://www.dungeon.com/home/cam/homeo.html (Resources and links on homeopathy and complementary medicine.)

NIH Office of Alternative Medicine: http://altmed.od.nih.gov/

Ethnic Beliefs

Beliefs about health, disease, and treatment are often closely tied to an individual's ethnic background. With the increase in the number of immigrants from an increasing variety of countries and cultures, there is a potential increase in the variety of ethnic practices and beliefs that may influence drug therapy. However, caution is needed in making generalization or assumptions about these without assessing each individual patient. It is also important to realize that individuals from "majority" American ethnic backgrounds also practice home remedies and have beliefs that influence their health behaviors. Therefore, individual assessment is key to understanding an individual and eliciting data of potential relevance for drug therapy—either for choice of drug or for estimating impact on compliance or patient learning.

By using two of the Functional Health Patterns (see Chap. 4), the Health Perception-Health Belief Pattern and the Value-Belief Pattern, clinicians can elicit important data related to individual beliefs and health practices. The following questions may be useful in eliciting information about self-medication based on ethnic or cultural beliefs or the use of alternative therapies:

- When you have a cold (or fever, rash, constipation, diarrhea, cough, headache, menstrual cramps, bleeding, etc.), what do you usually do to treat it?
- Do you use herbs or herbal teas?
- Do you use any homeopathic medicines?
- What nonprescription drugs do you use?
- What vitamin and minerals do you use?
- Are there any particular types of drugs or brands of drugs that you will not use? If so, why?

- What kinds of health practitioners (e.g., homeopath, naturopath, chiropractor, herbalist, nutritionist, medicine man, etc.) have you consulted?
- What do you believe about the cause of illness (or this illness)?
- What kinds of things do you believe can help to cure it or make it better?
- Do you use any healing practices?

HEALTH CARE FRAUD AND USE OF UNPROVEN THERAPIES

With the increase in self-care and interest in prevention has come a proliferation of therapies being advocated, usually for commercial purposes.

The APN can have an important role in helping patients to evaluate claims of therapies, including those not within mainstream conventional medicine. A major point should be made that the FDA considers anything that makes a health claim to be a drug and anything claiming to alter body function to be a drug. Despite this, many products not approved by the FDA as drugs are being marketed with cleverly worded claims that may have avoided FDA detection or control.

EXHIBIT 2-1

Avoiding Fraud

According to the FDA, these red flags should make you think twice about remedies not prescribed by your doctor:

- Celebrity endorsements
- Inadequate labeling (a legitimate nonprescription medication is labeled with indications for use, as well as how to use it and when to seek medical help)
- Claims that the product works by a secret formula
- Promotion of the treatment only in the back pages of magazines, over the phone, by direct mail, in newspaper ads in the format of new stories, or 30-minute commercials in talk show format

The Arthritis Foundation says the following claims are also warning signs that a "cure" has but questionable therapeutic value:

- It's effective for a wide range of disorders, such as cancer, arthritis, and sexual dysfunction.
- It's all natural.
- It's inexpensive and has no side effects.
- It works immediately and permanently, making a visit to the doctor unnecessary.

SOURCE: Adapted from Napier K: FDA Consumer Publication No. (FDA) 94–1218, 1994.

ALTERNATIVE OR
COMPLEMENTARY MEDICINE

Alternative medicine is a term that refers to the use of a variety of nontraditional approaches to the treatment of illness that are alternatives to the practice of traditional allopathic Western medicine. Alternative medicine has been described as any medical practice or intervention that lacks sufficient documentation of its safety and effectiveness against specific diseases and conditions, is not generally taught in U.S. medical schools, and is not generally reimbursable by health insurance providers.[1]

Some prefer to call this complementary medicine rather than alternative medicine to reflect the idea that these practices should be seen as supplemental to traditional medical treatment.

Recently, interest in alternative medicine has increased dramatically along with increased interest in the self-care movement. The National Institutes of Health (NIH) has established the Office of Alternative Medicine, which is providing funding to study the outcomes of some of the approaches of alternative medicine. The nurse needs to be able to promote sound decision making by clients and families by teaching them how to evaluate the benefits and limitations of various alternative medicine practices and the importance of early detection and appropriate treatment that may be delayed by the injudicious or sole use of alternative medicine (see Table 2-1).

The nurse especially needs to be aware of a client's use of alternative medicine that may interact with prescribed medications. The types of alternative medicine approaches that are most likely to interact with pharmaceutical medications are herbal medicines, use of vitamin, minerals, and nutrients, and homeopathy.

TABLE 2-1

Considerations Related to Use of Alternative Medicine

The National Institutes of Health (NIH) Office of Alternative Medicine recommends the following before getting involved in any alternative therapy:

- Obtain objective information about the therapy. Besides talking with the person promoting the approach, speak with people who have gone through the treatment—preferably both those who were treated recently and those treated in the past. Ask about the advantages and disadvantages, risks, side effects, costs, results, and over what time span results can be expected.
- Inquire about the training and expertise of the person administering the treatment (e.g., certification).
- Consider the costs. Alternative treatments may not be reimbursable by health insurance.
- Discuss all treatments with your primary care provider, who needs this information in order to have a complete picture of your treatment plan.

SOURCE: Stehlin.[1]

Herbal Medicine

Herbs are plants, and plants have been and continue to be a source of conventional medicines. Until 1962 herbs were considered to be drugs; however, it then became required that all drugs be evaluated for both efficacy and safety. Herbs then were sold as "food" products through health food stores. Only a few herbs (out of 1400) have been approved (see Table 2-2) as being both safe and having therapeutic actions by the FDA.[2] The 1994 Dietary Supplement Health and Education Act allows labels on herbs to have information about their effects on body structure and function; however, the labels also have to state that the herb is not intended to be used as a drug and that it has not been reviewed by the FDA.

Purity and standardization of ingredients are problems since there are no government standards. Some herbal products have been found to contain a wide variation in the amount of the "active ingredient," and contaminants have been found to have had deleterious effects (e.g., eosinophilia from a contaminant in tryptophan). Herbs and plants may vary in their potency according to conditions where they are grown; imported products may contain prescription drugs or toxic agents not identified as such when they were sent to the United States.[2]

It is important to emphasize to patients that just because an herb is "natural," this does not mean that it is not harmful; many of our pharmaceutical drugs (e.g., digitalis glycosides) have been purified from herbs, plants, and other substances found in nature. Table 2-3 contains some guidelines for using herbs. In 1995 the FDA issued a warning about a product containing ma huang (which contains ephedrine) and kola nut (which contains caffeine) that caused serious adverse effects and deaths. Herbal teas are a potential source of adverse effects, especially if an individual is using them repeatedly or in excess amounts.

Vitamins and Minerals and Dietary Supplements

The public is increasingly using vitamins and minerals as well as food supplements as part of health regimens. Some of the increase in their use is due to the increased advertising of "foods" containing them as having health benefits. Although the FDA controls both foods and drugs, the requirements for approval of a drug are much more rigorous, lengthy, and expensive. Food products cannot make health claims without FDA approval. Therefore, the advertisements for health benefits for food supplements and other nondrug products are usually very carefully worded and can be confusing to the public. Food supplements also are not as closely regulated for purity and standardization of dosage as are drugs. Tryptophan's connection to a fatal blood dyscrasia was found to be caused by a contaminant in the production process. A further basis for potential confusion is that many drugstores also sell these food supplements as well as homeopathic remedies.

Clinicians need to teach patients about the limitations of nondrug products. They also need to make patients aware of the potential dangers of excess use of vitamins,

TABLE 2-2

Herbs Approved by FDA

Herb	Use
Aloe	Laxative
Capsicum	Topical analgesic
Cascara	Laxative
Psyllium	Laxative
Senna	Laxative
Slippery Elm	Oral demulcent
Witch Hazel	Astringent

SOURCE: Adapted from Youngkin and Israel.[2]

especially those that are fat-soluble. Vitamins and minerals can affect the pharmaco-kinetics of drug therapy; for example, excess use of vitamin C (ascorbic acid) can acidify the urine and therefore impact on the excretion of drugs.

Use of Nonprescription Drugs

The use of nonprescription (OTC) drugs has increased; many prescription drugs are becoming available as nonprescription drugs. This increases the availability of medicines for the consumer but also can result in inappropriate use, delay in obtaining accurate diagnosis and treatment, and possible interference with prescribed medications. Careful assessment and specific questioning about nonprescription medications are important; patients may not think of nonprescription drugs as "real" drugs when they are asked about medication use. Oral contraceptives, vitamins, and minerals are commonly not mentioned by patients.

Table 2-4 provides a guide for patient decision making about the use of nonprescription medications.

TABLE 2-3

Guidelines for Patients Concerning Use of Herbs

- Do not take herbs if pregnant
- Do not take herbs if nursing
- Do not give herbs to your baby or young children
- Do not take a large quantity of any one herbal preparation
- Do not take any herb on a daily basis
- Buy only preparations with the plants and their quantities listed on the packet (no guarantee of safety)
- Do not take anything containing comfrey

SOURCE: Huxtable.[3]

TABLE 2-4

Guide to Client Decision Making about Nonprescription Drugs

Do I need to treat my symptoms with a medication?

1. Are my symptoms minor, self-limiting, and not interfering significantly with my functioning? — Yes —> Stop—consider not using any medication to treat symptoms

2. Do my symptoms indicate a possibly serious health problem (e.g., fever > 101°F; sudden onset of acute abdominal pain, chest pain, or pain radiating down arm)? — Yes —> Consult physician

3. Have my symptoms continued or increased despite my use of OTC and/or prescription medications? — Yes —> Consult physician

4. Am I pregnant or nursing an infant? — Yes —> Consult physician

5. Will use of OTC drug relieve my symptoms, increase my comfort, and/or increase my ability to perform my daily activities? — Yes —> Consider using OTC drug

Evaluate the OTC Drug

Evaluate OTC drug under consideration in relation to:
   My current symptoms and other health problems
   Allergies I have
   Interactions with other drugs I am taking
   Concerns about alcohol, sugar, or sodium contents
   My functioning (e.g., producing sedation)
Evaluate specific OTC product for:
   Tamper-resistant feature
   Name of product
   Active and inactive ingredients
   Indications for use
   Warnings, contraindications, and interactions
   Expiration date
Compare several similar products for:
   Active and inactive ingredients
   Costs (especially differences between brand name and generic products)

SOURCE: Eisenhauer et al.[4]

Homeopathy

Homeopathy is a system of medicine practiced more widely in Europe and India than in the United States. It was established by a German physician, Samuel Hahnemann, in the early 1800s. Its underlying belief is that the treatment of illness consists of administering remedies that reproduce the client's symptoms. The name "homeopathy" derives from *homoios*, the Greek word for "similar," and *pathos*, the Greek word for "suffering." "Allopathic medicine" refers to conventional medicine where the search is for a medicine to oppose the symptoms.[5]

A homeopathic remedy is considered to be a substance that causes the same symptom that a sick person has. The remedies are diluted; the more diluted a homeopathic remedy is, the more effective it is ("potentization by dilution"). When administered, these remedies may produce side effects or an increase in the client's symptoms that homeopaths believe indicates that the remedy is producing its intended effect.

The process by which homeopathic remedies are prepared is described in *Homeopathic Pharmacopeia of the United States* (HPUS). Prescribed homeopathic products are prepared by repeatedly diluting active ingredients by a factor of 10. The degree of dilution is noted on the label by the Roman numeral X. A preparation labeled 6X means that a 1-to-10 dilution of the original hydroalcoholic solution was done 6 times. After each dilution, the product undergoes succussion, which is the act of shaking violently.[6] Homeopathic remedies are available in many health food stores and in some pharmacies in the United States.

Since homeopathic drugs are very diluted, there is usually no interference with the effectiveness of conventional drugs. However, homeopathic liquid drugs commonly do contain alcohol as a preservative. On the other hand, most conventional medicines are considered detrimental to the effectiveness of homeopathic medicines because conventional medicines are believed to suppress the patient's symptoms without strengthening the person as a whole. In particular, the use of caffeine, camphor, hormones or birth control pills, large doses of vitamins, or therapeutically prescribed herbs is considered to be detrimental to the effects of homeopathic medicine.[7]

Interpretations of an increase in a patient's symptoms may differ from the conventional (allopathic) and homeopathic perspectives. Homeopathic medicine considers the worsening of symptoms after treatment with a homeopathic therapy as a beneficial "healing crisis." This could result in differing interpretations of the significance of symptoms and could lead to a possible delay in obtaining medical diagnosis and treatment of serious conditions.

Table 2-5 presents a summary of alternative medicine practices and their implications for drug therapy.

TABLE 2-5

Alternative Medicine Practices and Drug Therapy

Alternative Medicine Practice	Comments/Implications for Drug Therapy
Acupuncture	Has been effective in relief of pain, reducing amount of drug needed for analgesia, assisting in detoxification/withdrawal from substance abuse, relief of some types of nausea and vomiting.
Relaxation and biofeedback	Can reduce blood pressure in hypertension and reduce or eliminate need for antihypertensive medications.
Vitamins and minerals	High doses may affect drug pharmacokinetics by causing liver toxicity (e.g., niacin) or affecting renal excretion [e.g., ascorbic acid (vitamin C) can acidify urine and thereby affect the excretion of drugs]. They may also interfere with diagnostic tests (e.g., high doses of folic acid can interfere with diagnostic tests for pernicious anemia).
Herbal medicines	Herbs may contain pharmacologically active ingredients; about one fourth of pharmaceutical drugs are derived from herbs. Ingredients may interact with pharmaceutical drugs (e.g., natural licorice contains glycyrrhiza, which interferes with cortisol metabolism; this can interfere with effectiveness of antihypertensive medications by causing sodium retention. Ma huang contains ephedrine and produces sympathomimetic effects that can increase blood pressure. Preparations may not be pure and have varying amounts of ingredients since preparations are not standardized or approved by FDA as drugs.
Homeopathy	Homeopathic medicines are well diluted and are unlikely to interact with conventional medications. Some liquid preparations, however, may contain alcohol as a preservative. Conventional medicines in general and in particular caffeine, camphor, hormones/birth control pills, large doses of vitamins, or therapeutically prescribed herbs are considered to be detrimental to the effects of homeopathic medicine.

COMPLIANCE/ADHERENCE
TO DRUG THERAPY

The willingness and ability of the patient to take medications as prescribed is a major variable in the success of drug therapy. Therefore, compliance is an area of concern to all clinicians and particularly to those prescribing medications; the prescriber can influence the degree of compliance by consideration of drug variables such as route, frequency, formulation, and side effects of a drug. Equally of concern are patient variables that can influence the successful administration of drugs. These patient variables include physical factors as well as motivation and health beliefs. The National Pharmaceutical Council (1992) has stated that "noncompliance with treatment for chronic disease is itself a chronic disease, and needs sustained or periodic attention at periodic intervals."[8(p7)]

Costs of noncompliance have been estimated to be $100 billion or more annually. Costs include initial prescriptions, additional prescriptions, additional office/clinic visits, additional care for uncontrolled chronic diseases, emergency room visits, hospitalizations, additional diagnostic tests, nursing home admissions, and home health care services. Indirect costs include lost productivity, absenteeism, lost earnings (of patients during illness, to pharmaceutical industry from unsold medications, to physicians when patients drop out of system), and employee turnover due to premature death and disability.[8(pp 13, 14)]

Health consequences of noncompliance include the worsening and spread of disease (e.g., spread of tuberculosis and other contagious diseases, increased morbidity and mortality from insufficient treatment). In a study of a beta blocker, women who took less than 75 percent of the medication were 2.5 times more likely to die following a heart attack. In a study of asthma deaths, 61 percent had unsatisfactory compliance.[8]

Noncompliance makes evaluation of the effectiveness of therapy difficult to judge; continued prescribing of medications which are not taken at therapeutic levels is not only costly because of unnecessary further diagnostic tests and medications but also may expose the patient taking subtherapeutic dosing to adverse side effects or the development of sensitization without beneficial effects.

Terminology

The term "compliance" is widely used; however, it is controversial since it is believed to connote that the patient must accede to the wishes of the clinician. Others prefer the use of the term "adherence," while still others prefer to use the phrase "enhancement of therapeutic alliance." The concept of "intelligent noncompliance" has been used to describe the behavior of patients who make conscious decisions to cease or adapt their therapeutic regimens, usually because of side effects. The National Council on Patient Information and Education (NCPIE) defines compliance as "following a medicine treatment plan developed and agreed on by the patient and his/her health professional(s)."[8(p7)]

This controversy on terminology exists also within nursing with disagreement about the use of the nursing diagnosis "noncompliance."[9,10] "Ineffective management of therapeutic regimen" has been offered as a more satisfactory nursing diagnosis. The therapeutic regimen is seen as that of patient, including the patient's values and goals and not just the therapeutic recommendations of a health care professional. The health care professional's recommendations are viewed as advice that can be followed or disregarded by the patient. In this view, therefore, noncompliant patients can be viewed as effectively managing their therapeutic regimen.[11]

Research on Noncompliance

While much research has been done on compliance in a variety of disciplines, there have been no definitive or consistent findings. Some of this is due to differences in the definition of (and method of measuring) compliance.

A review of the literature on noncompliance by the NCPIE indicated that more than 200 factors have been studied. This review also concluded that there is no stronger theoretical model to explain compliance (see Table 2-6).

TABLE 2-6

Factors Related to Noncompliance

1. Inadequate patient/health professional communication about medicines and medicine compliance
2. Unresolved patient concerns
3. Health care professional issues

Patients

Patient's perception about the seriousness of illness and their susceptibility

Disagreement about the diagnosis or treatment or lack of belief in the effectiveness of the treatment

Dissatisfaction with the health professional's attitude, communication, or perceived skill

Negative patient attitudes about medicine use in general

Dislike of the sick role and worries about the social stigma of taking medicines

Fear of side effects or becoming dependent on a drug

Desire to exert control over one's health and health care

Media influence on creating fears and confusion

Health care professionals

Overestimating their patient's compliance by as much as 50 percent.

Not recognizing their role in promoting compliance

Blaming patient

Inadequate training in communication, interpersonal skills, and behavior change strategies

Practical issues such as lack of time and lack of reimbursement for counseling

Need for collaboration among many health care professionals in treating patients with chronic diseases

TABLE 2-6

Factors Related to Noncompliance (continued)

4. Special population issues
   Older patients, children, parents, teenagers, culturally diverse patients, and
      the hearing- and sight-impaired
5. Regimen-related barriers
   Even one daily dose involves over 65 separate tasks over a 2-month
      period—taking the drug each day and having it refilled on time takes four
      or five separate actions
6. Environmental barriers
   Safety closures
   Social isolation
   Lack of transportation to pharmacy, doctor, or health care facility
   Homelessness problems such as storage, privacy, and lack of a regular
      schedule
   Use of multiple pharmacies
   Language difference and/or illiteracy

SOURCE: Adapted from National Council on Patient Information and Education.[8]

Strategies for Promoting Compliance/Adherence

In a study on strategies used by nurse practitioners, Kolton and Piccolo[12] studied the extent to which NPs used 24 behaviors identified in the literature as important for compliance. Fifteen of these behaviors were identified by more than 70 percent as important or very important; 11 of these were used by the NPs more than 60 percent of the time. Strategies not used by NPs were patient support groups for medication compliance, offering group classes for patients on medications, and employing contingency contracts.

Nurses generally have been successful in promoting compliance. In a meta-analysis of randomized studies comparing nurse practitioners and physicians, Brown and Grimes[13] found that promoting compliance had the only statistically significant effect size for NPs versus MDs.

Strategies of particular usefulness to the APN as a prescriber include simplification of the drug regimen to the fewest number of doses of medications a day, timing administration to mealtimes (unless contraindicated) or other daily events, and clustering the times for taking multiple medications (if feasible) to a minimum. Listening carefully to the patient and paying attention to side effects can help with establishing and maintaining a therapeutic alliance with the patient. Asking questions in a nonthreatening way is important: How do you usually take your medications? How have you been feeling since you have been taking this medication? These are broad questions that encourage the patient to share his or her concerns and set the stage for requesting more specific

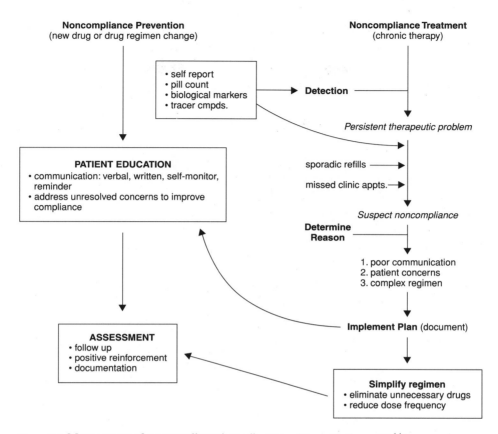

Noncompliance Prevention
(new drug or drug regimen change)

Noncompliance Treatment
(chronic therapy)

- self report
- pill count
- biological markers
- tracer cmpds.

Detection

Persistent therapeutic problem

PATIENT EDUCATION
- communication: verbal, written, self-monitor, reminder
- address unresolved concerns to improve compliance

sporadic refills

missed clinic appts.

Suspect noncompliance

Determine Reason

1. poor communication
2. patient concerns
3. complex regimen

ASSESSMENT
- follow up
- positive reinforcement
- documentation

Implement Plan (document)

Simplify regimen
- eliminate unnecessary drugs
- reduce dose frequency

Figure 2-1 Management of noncompliance/nonadherence. (*From Fuchs, p. 33.*[14])

information. Consideration should be given to economic or other contextual barriers that may be affecting compliance but that the patient may be reluctant to discuss. Including spouses or other family caretakers in medication teaching is also important.

Figure 2-1 illustrates processes for prevention and management of noncompliance/nonadherence.

PATIENT EDUCATION AND MEDICATION COUNSELING

Patient education about medications is an essential component of the role of the prescribing clinician. However, providing information is not always sufficient to ensure appropriate and safe use of medications.

Medication counseling is a broader approach that incorporates the health beliefs and values of the patient as well as the physical, psychological, sociocultural, emotional, and intellectual aspects. Emphasis is on promoting effective medication management by the patient in order to improve or maintain quality of health and quality of life.*

Key information about medications (see Table 2-7) needs to be provided in writing in the language of the patient and at the appropriate reading level. Many pharmacies and prescribing clinicians use drug monographs to provide essential information. For some drugs the FDA has required that patients be given a patient package insert.

Resources

Facts and Comparisons. *Patient drug information. A companion to Nurses Drug Facts.* St. Louis: Facts and Comparisons, 1997. (One-page monographs that can be copied and distributed without charge to patients.)

United States Pharmacopeia Dispensing Information (USP DI). Volume II: For Patients. Rockville, MD: United States Pharmacopeial Convention, Inc. (Available also in Spanish.) (Published annually.) United States Pharmacopeia Medication Counseling Behavior Guidelines (www.usp.com).

Patient education needs to be ongoing throughout the drug therapy. A variety of teaching-learning approaches should be used, depending on the patient's learning style and preferences. Written materials may need to be supplemented with graphics, audiotapes, videotapes, or special individual or group teaching programs about medications and/or disease management.

Pharmaceutical manufacturers often have useful materials for patient teaching; of course, the materials promote the manufacturer's brand of medication. Brochures, booklets, posters, slides, audiotapes, and videotapes are examples of materials commonly available from many pharmaceutical manufacturers.

Some companies have developed compliance programs in which the company communicates directly with the patient (e.g., newsletters, reminders for refills). Examples are listed in Table 2-8. Pharmaceutical companies will become more actively involved with the monitoring of actual drug therapy as they become more involved in managed pharmaceutical care and in the concept of disease management.

TABLE 2-7

Essential Medication Information for Patients

Drug name and intended therapeutic effect
How it is to be taken
Common side effects and side effects to be reported immediately
What to do if a dose is missed
Storage and refill information

*United States Pharmacopeia Medication Counseling Behavior Guidelines, 1997. (Internet: www.usp.com).

TABLE 2-8

Examples of Pharmaceutical Companies with Compliance Programs

Pharmaceutical Company	Medication
1. Zeneca	Tenormin, Tenoretic
2. Stuart	Zestril, Zestoretic
3. Marion Merrell Dow	Cardizem CD and SR
4. Lederle Labs	ProStep
5. Wyeth-Ayerst	Premarin
6. Merck & Co.	Proscar
7. Sandoz	Miacalcin
8. Becton-Dickinson	Insulin syringes
9. Schering-Plough	Nitro-Dur
10. Glaxo	Ventolin, Beclovent, Beconase

SOURCE: Fuchs, p. 34.[14]

SUMMARY

A variety of factors influence what an individual will use to treat his or her illness or to maintain health. These factors influence both the use of practices not prescribed and whether or not an individual will adhere to a prescribed medication and therapeutic regimen. Careful and skillful assessment by the APN can lead to an understanding of the unique beliefs of an individual that can impact on successful drug therapy and the safe integration of alternative health practices with the prescribed therapeutic regimen.

REFERENCES

1. Stehlin IB: *An FDA Guide to Choosing Medical Treatments.* Internet, http://www. the body.com/fda/medical.html (1996).
2. Youngkin EO, Israel DS: A review and critique of common herbal alternative therapies. *Nurse Pract* 21 (10): 39, 43–44, 48, 49–52, 54–56, 59–60, 62, 1996.
3. Huxtable R: The myth of beneficent nature: The risks of herbal preparations. *Ann Int Med* 117: 165–166, 1992.
4. Eisenhauer LA, Spencer RT, Nichols LW, Bergan FW: *Clinical Pharmacology and Nursing Management,* (5th ed.) Philadelphia: Lippincott, 1998.
5. Fugh-Berman AF: *Alternative Medicine: What Works.* Tucson, AZ: Odonian Press, 1996.
6. Ingraham SL: Homeopathic remedies may cause problems. Internet document, Health Science Center Office of Information Technology, (904) 392–7430, webmaster@vpha. health.ufl.edu, May 8, 1996.

7. Ulman D: *The consumer's guide to homeopathy.* New York: Putnam, 1995.

8. National Council on Patient Information and Education: *Prescription medicine compliance: A review of the baseline of knowledge. A report of the National Council on Patient Information and Education.* Washington, DC: The Association; August 1995.

9. Keeling A, Williams S, Shuster G, Boyle A: Noncompliance revisited: A disciplinary perspective of a nursing diagnosis. *Nurs Diag* 4:91–98, 1993.

10. Lunney M: Ineffective management of therapeutic regimen, in McFarland G, McFarlane E (eds): *Nursing Diagnosis and Intervention.* St. Louis: Mosby, 1993, pp 79–86.

11. Bakker RH, Kastermans MC, Dassen TWN: An analysis of the nursing diagnosis ineffective management of therapeutic regimen compared to noncompliance and Orem's self-care deficit theory of nursing. *Nurs Diag* 6(4): 161–166, 1995.

12. Kolton KA, Piccolo P: Patient compliance: A challenge in practice. *Nurse Pract.* 13 (12): 37–50, 1988.

13. Brown SA, Grimes DE: A meta-analysis of nurse practitioners and nurse midwives in primary care. *Nurs Res* 44(6): 332–339, 1995.

14. Fuchs J Jr: Managing medication nonadherence, in Muma RD, Lyons BA, Newman TA, Carnes BA (eds): *Patient Education: A Practical Approach.* Stamford, CT: Appleton & Lange, 1996, pp 31–35.

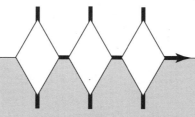

Chapter 3

VARIATIONS IN PATIENT RESPONSES TO DRUG THERAPY: ROLE OF PHARMACODYNAMICS AND PHARMACOKINETICS

Laurel A. Eisenhauer

INTRODUCTION

An understanding of pharmacodynamics and pharmacokinetics provides a basis for understanding how drugs produce their effects and how there can be different responses in different patients and/or different effects in the same patient at different times. For a prescribing clinician this information is critical for selecting the appropriate drug, dose, formulation, route, and frequency for a specific patient, as well as for monitoring of the patient for both drug effect and adverse effects. Understanding pharmacokinetics and pharmacodynamics also allows the clinician to understand the basis for many types of drug interactions.

A drug produces its effects when it reaches its sites of action; how the drug gets there and how much of the administered drug reaches the area depend on a variety of factors. There are many variables that influence the extent to which a drug reaches the site or sites of activity in the body and produces effects.

Pharmacokinetics describes what the body does to the drug; it involves the processes of drug absorption, biotransformation/metabolism, distribution, and elimination. *Pharmacodynamics* describes what the drug does to the body, i.e., how and where a drug acts to produce its effects.

The purpose of this chapter is to provide the APN with an understanding of the clinical application of this knowledge. The APN may need to read, study, and review a standard pharmacology text or computer tutorials for the more theoretical (and pharmacological) details. The reader may find it useful to consult these resources before and/or after reading this chapter.

Resources

Books

DiPiro J, Talbert RL, Yee GC, et al (eds): *Pharmacotherapy: A Pathophysiological Approach.* New York: Elsevier, 1997.

Hardman JG, Limbird LE (eds): *Goodman & Gilman's The Pharmacological Basis of Therapeutics*, 9th ed. New York: McGraw-Hill, 1996.

Herfindal ET, Gourley DR (eds): *Clinical Pharmacy and Therapeutics,* 6th ed. Baltimore: Williams & Wilkins, 1996.

Katzung BG: *Basic and Clinical Pharmacology,* 6th ed. Norwalk, CT: Appleton & Lange, 1995.

Melmon KL, Morrelli HF, Hoffman BB, Nierenberg DW (eds): *Melmon and Morrelli's Clinical Pharmacology. Basic Principles in Therapeutics*, 3d ed. New York: McGraw-Hill, 1992.

Munson PL (ed.): *Principles of Pharmacology. Basic Concepts and Clinical Applications.* New York: Chapman & Hall, 1995.

Mycek MA, Harvey RA, Champe PC (eds): *Lippincott's Illustrated Reviews: Pharmacology.* Philadelphia: Lippincott, 1997.

Smith CH, Reynard AM: *Essentials of Pharmacology.* Philadelphia: WB Saunders, 1995.

Smith CH, Reynard AM: *Textbook of Pharmacology.* Philadelphia: WB Saunders, 1992.

Young LY, Koda-Kimble MA (eds): *Applied Therapeutics: The Clinical Use of Drugs.* 6th ed. Vancouver, WA: Applied Therapeutics, Inc., 1995.

Audiovisuals

Pharmakinetics (videotape). Spokane, WA: Intercollegiate Nursing Education, 1986.

Internet/World Wide Web

Courses on pharmacokinetics:

University of Oklahoma: http://www.cpb.uokhsc.edu/gaps/pkbiol

Thomas Jefferson University: http://aisv.lib.tju.edu/cwis/oac/pharmacology/index.html

Virtual Pharmacy: http://www-sci.lib.uci.edu.80/n martindale/pharmacy.html#pp2

OVERVIEW

Pharmacodynamics and pharmacokinetics will be discussed under the framework of drug variables, patient variables, and contextual variables.

Drug variables include dose, route of administration, molecular weight, lipid versus water solubility, whether the drug is an acid or alkaline drug, the degree of protein binding, the mechanisms and pathways for biotransformation/metabolism, elimination, and therapeutic index and margin of safety.

Patient variables include normal versus abnormal physiological functioning, age, sex, organ functioning (especially liver and renal function), genetic makeup, pathophysiological conditions, such as state of hydration and serum albumin levels, allergy, pregnancy status, and other drug therapy. These all can play a major role in individualized responses to a drug and thus are a major consideration in choosing a specific drug for a given patient.

Contextual variables are those factors that are external to the drug-patient interface but which play a role in the patient's response. They include differences in manufacturing, storage, cost considerations, and correct use of the drug.

DRUG VARIABLES AFFECTING PHARMACOKINETICS AND PHARMACODYNAMICS

Bioavailability is a term used to describe the amount of the drug that reaches the systemic circulation in a chemically unchanged form. It thus reflects the amount of the drug available to produce effects and/or to go to other tissues to produce effects. Bioavailability is determined by comparing the amount of the drug in the plasma when given by a specific route compared to the amount when the drug is given directly into the blood, i.e., intravenously. When the plasma concentrations of a drug are plotted on a graph, the area under the curve (AUC) reflects the degree of absorption of the drug (Fig. 3-1). Concentrations of the drug in the plasma or serum are used rather than the amount in whole blood since the "concentration of the drug in the plasma ultimately determines and is in equilibrium with the concentration of the drug at its sites of action."[1(p7)]

Bioavailability is the result of a number of dynamic processes often occurring simultaneously. These processes include absorption, biotransformation/metabolism, protein and tissue binding, distribution, and elimination. These processes are subject to variation according to the characteristics of the drug as well as the characteristics of the patient.

The ability of a drug to cross membranes determines much of its fate—whether it is absorbed, where it is distributed, and how it is excreted. Drugs may cross membranes

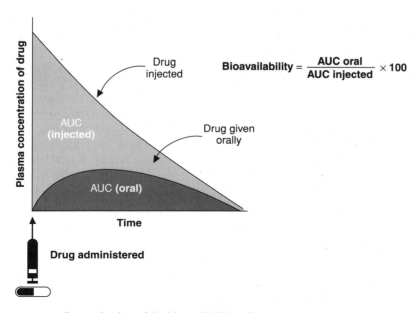

$$\text{Bioavailability} = \frac{\text{AUC oral}}{\text{AUC injected}} \times 100$$

Figure 3-1 Determination of the bioavailability of a drug. AUC equals area under curve. (*From Mycek MJ, Harvey RA, Champe PC, Fisher BD, Cooper M: Lippincott's Illustrated Reviews: Pharmacology, 2d ed. Philadelphia: Lippincott-Raven. Used with permission.*[5])

by passive diffusion, which is greatly affected by the drug's lipid solubility; size-limited diffusion through pores (drugs with smaller molecular size diffuse more readily than those of larger molecular size); or by carrier-mediated transport.

Acidity or Alkalinity

The ionization state of a drug is a major determinant of its pharmacokinetics. Drugs pass through membranes more readily if they are not ionized, i.e., if they have not separated into a negatively or positively charged component. Whether ionization occurs depends on the pH of the drug in relation to the pH of its environment. Most drugs are either weak acids or weak bases. Each drug has a pKa that reflects the strength of its interaction with a proton. The pKa is "that pH at which equal amounts of ionized and nonionized forms are present."[2(p42)] With a weakly acidic drug, if the pH is greater than its pKa, the drug will tend to ionize and therefore passes membranes with greater difficulty. Similarly, a weakly basic drug in an environment where the pH is less than its pKa will ionize and not pass through membranes as readily as if the pH were higher than its pKa. Acidity or alkalinity also affects the protein binding of the drug (see below).

RULE OF THUMB: A weakly acid drug in an acid environment will pass through membranes more readily than if it is in an alkaline environment. A weakly basic (alkaline) drug in an alkaline environment will pass through membranes more readily in an alkaline environment than if it is in an acidic environment.

Water versus Lipid Solubility

Because most cell membranes contain lipids, drugs that are lipid-soluble will pass through these membranes more readily than drugs that are water-soluble. Drugs that are uncharged (nonionized) are more lipid-soluble.[3] Lipid-soluble drugs generally can pass through the blood-brain barrier. The blood-brain barrier protects the brain from exposure to substances in the blood. This barrier prevents many drugs or other substances from crossing into the brain. When the meninges are inflamed, the blood-brain barrier may allow some drugs to pass into the brain that normally do not. Some antibiotics, for example, cross the blood-brain barrier only when the meninges are inflamed. Some drugs cannot pass in one form but may pass through the barrier in another form. Dopamine does not pass that blood-brain barrier; however, L-dopa, its levorotatory or mirror-image form, does pass through the blood-brain barrier and is then converted by the brain into dopamine.

Lipid solubility versus water solubility of a drug also influences where a drug will distribute in the body. Lipid-soluble drugs distribute to and may be stored in body fat. Therefore, individuals with more fat than normal may require higher doses and a longer time to reach therapeutic serum levels may be needed; drugs may also retain the drug longer in the body, and drugs may have a longer duration of action as the drug is released from fat storage sites. Likewise, in patients with less fat than normal, a lipid-soluble drug might require a reduction in dose because there would be less fat tissue for the drug to distribute to or to be stored in; the resulting higher amount of circulating drug could lead to toxicity. The proportionately greater amount of fat in women than in men may account for some differences in drug response. The aging process alters the fat and water distribution in the body and therefore can affect response to drugs (see aging effects below and in Chap. 7).

Distribution

In addition to factors related to alkalinity or acidity and lipid and water solubility, other areas of distribution of a given drug need to be taken into account. Some drugs enter the bone marrow and this can produce effects on blood components, potentially producing leukopenia, anemia, and thrombocytopenia. Some drugs may deposit in the bone affecting the growth of bones in children and adolescents.

Distribution of a drug to the placenta and thus to the fetus is a major concern in terms of its potential for producing teratogenic effects. Fluid shifts that occur in women during pregnancy affect pharmacokinetics. Chapter 6 discusses the issues related to teratogenicity and pregnancy.

Volume of Distribution

An important concept in understanding drug pharmacokinetics is the apparent volume of distribution (Vd) of a drug. This term refers to the hypothetical amount of a drug in the body. It includes the amount of the drug within the vascular tree, the interstitial space, and the cells and tissues. The Vd is the "hypothetical volume in which a dose (D) of a drug would have to be placed to yield the observed initial plasma concentration."[2 (p40)]

The total body water in a 70-kg adult is estimated at 42 L. The amount in plasma is about 4 percent of body weight; in interstitial space this amount is 20 percent. The total body water in an adult is about 60 percent of body weight. The plasma volume is 3 L; blood volume, 5.5 L; extracellular volume, 12 L; and total body water, 12 L. Some drugs have a Vd that is higher than the actual volume of the fluid in the body; a high Vd reflects a high degree of sequestration of the drug in the tissues. For example, a drug with a Vd of 3 L would be distributed only in the plasma; a drug with a high Vd (more than 42 L) would be likely to be sequestered in a depot such as fat or bone.

Knowledge of a drug's Vd is important in

1. Determining how much of a loading dose should be given
2. Estimating the amount of an additional dose needed to achieve a certain therapeutic level (desired concentration = dose/volume of distribution)
3. Estimating any changes in the half-life of a drug

A drug with a high Vd will have a more prolonged half-life since proportionately more of it is in other body compartments (e.g., interstitial and cellular) and therefore is not as concentrated in the blood to be taken to kidney or other organs for excretion. Patient variables that may alter a drug's volume of distribution include age, gender, disease, and body composition.

Table 3-1 provides examples of drugs with varying volumes of distribution.

TABLE 3-1

Distributional Characteristics of Some Pharmacological Agents

Agent	Vd (L)*	Comments
heparin	4.1	Extensively bound to albumin, distributed predominantly in plasma compartment
warfarin	7.7	Extensively bound to albumin, distribution consistent with its extravascular sites of action
acetylsalicylic acid	10.5	Binding to plasma protein relatively low (50%), exists largely in ionized form at physiologic pH, distribution volume approximates that of extracellular water
ethanol	38	Negligible binding to plasma albumin, accessible to most aqueous compartments within the body
metoprolol	294	Minimal binding to plasma proteins (13%), extensive accumulation in tissues is reflected in high Vd value
propranolol	273	Despite a high degree of binding to plasma protein (93%), high affinity for tissues gives rise to a high Vd value

*Values for apparent volume of distribution (Vd) are with reference to a standard 70-kg individual.
SOURCE: Godin D: Pharmacokinetics, in Munson PL (ed): *Principles of Pharmacology*. New York: Chapman & Hall, 1995. Used with permission.[6]

RULES OF THUMB: Drugs with a low Vd are more likely to be involved in drug interactions affecting plasma proteins.

Drugs with a high Vd may need to have a reduction in dosage under conditions of severe circulatory impairment, e.g., congestive heart failure (CHF).[2]

Half-life

The half-life ($t_{1/2}$) of a drug refers to the time it takes a dose of the drug to be reduced by half in the plasma. It reflects the rate of elimination of the drug from the plasma, primarily through distribution through tissues, biotransformation by the liver, or renal excretion. The half-life of a drug can provide guidance as to the frequency of multiple doses of a drug. The time required to attain such a steady state with multiple dosing is about five times the $t_{1/2}$ value. The volume of distribution and the half-life of a drug are quantitative indicators of the distribution and elimination phases of drug disposition. They provide answers to the questions of how much and how often.[2]

Loading Dose

Use of a loading dose is desirable when it is necessary to achieve therapeutic plasma levels rapidly. In general, the following formula can be used to estimate the loading dose: Loading dose = (Vd) (desired steady-state plasma concentration).[2] A steady state occurs when there is a balance between drug elimination and drug intake; plasma concentrations of the drug remain constant when maintenance doses are provided to replace the amount of drug that is eliminated.

RULES OF THUMB: When drugs are administered at regular dosing intervals approximately equal to their elimination half-lives, a steady state is reached wherein the amount of drug eliminated becomes equal to the amount administered; this is referred to as the maintenance dose.

After four half-lives, the peak plasma levels usually are greater than 90 percent. Dosing with a loading dose followed by maintenance doses results in the same steady state as dosing by regular maintenance doses; use of a loading dose should involve consideration of the urgency of the situation, margin of safety of the drug, and half-life (loading doses often are used for drugs with a very long half-life).[2]

Standard Vd and $t_{1/2}$ values for individual drugs can be found in many drug references (e.g., see the appendix of Hardman JG, Limbird LE, eds. *Goodman & Gilman's The Pharmacological Basis of Therapeutics*, 9th ed. New York: McGraw-Hill, 1996). However, the clinician also needs to consider the many patient variables that may affect a drug's half-life and volume of distribution.

The *route of administration* determines the extent and rapidity of absorption into the blood. The more membranes that need to be passed before a drug reaches the systemic circulation, the slower is the absorption. Topical drugs applied to the skin are less rapidly absorbed than when they are given IV; orally administered drugs are subject to a variety of variables that can alter the rate and extent of absorption.

Bioavailability is a term that reflects the fraction of the drug dose that reaches the system circulation in a chemically unchanged form. See Fig. 3-1 and Table 3-7.

RULE OF THUMB: The more membranes that need to be passed before a drug reaches the systemic circulation, the slower is the absorption.

Formulation of Drug

The formulation of the drug affects the speed of absorption. To pass through membranes, a drug needs to be in solution. For a solid drug such as a tablet to be able to be absorbed, it first must be dissolved. Bioavailability of oral dosage forms occurs in the following descending order: solutions, suspensions, oil-in-water emulsions, capsules, tablets, and controlled-released capsules/tablets. As mentioned above, other ingredients (e.g., binders or dispersing agents, coatings) in a particular product also may influence the speed and degree of dissolution of a drug. Drugs given by other routes may have added ingredients designed to slow down their absorption from that site and thus provide a longer period of action and allow for less frequent dosing, e.g., transdermal patches, insulin other than regular, procaine penicillin.

Protein Binding

Drugs may bind to proteins in the blood, and the degree to which they do affects much of their activity in the body. The most prevalent blood protein is albumin (4 to 5 g/100 mL. Others are lipoproteins, in particular α_1-acid glycoprotein. Some drugs bind to one or the other; acidic drugs bind to albumin and basic drugs bind to glycoproteins.[4] Protein binding has many implications for drug responses and for understanding many drug interactions. The portion of a drug that is bound to protein is stored temporarily on the protein and is pharmacologically inactive while stored. The unbound or "free" portion is free to cross membranes and exert pharmacological effects. The protein binding of a drug also influences the rate of drug removal during hemodialysis and peritoneal dialysis; there is an inverse relationship (e.g., the greater the protein binding, the slower is the rate of removal of the drug).[2]

The degree to which a drug binds with blood protein is indicated by the percentage of the drug in the blood that binds to the protein at any given time. Drugs in which a high percentage binds to blood proteins are referred to as highly protein bound. The *percentage* of the drug bound remains constant, but the *amount* bound and the *amount* in the plasma vary over time. For example, a drug that is 90 percent bound will always have 90 percent of whatever amount of the drug is in the blood bound to the blood proteins; as some of the "free" (unbound) drug passes out of the blood into the interstitial space or other tissues, more of the bound drug leaves the blood protein and becomes "free" drug. The amount of a given drug decreases but the percentage that is bound and the percentage that is "free" remains constant.

Highly protein bound drugs compete with other protein-bound drugs for binding sites on the blood proteins. Drugs vary in their affinity for blood proteins. They may displace other bound drugs, resulting in the sudden release of the other drug and possible toxic levels of that drug. A highly bound drug that normally has a large percentage bound to blood proteins may not be able to bind to the protein because of the saturation of binding sites from other bound drugs, resulting in possible toxic levels of the drug. Whether the displacement of drugs from the protein-binding sites results in toxic levels depends upon how rapidly the "free" amounts are distributed, metabolized, or excreted from the body. In the case of a drug with a large volume of distribution, this increased amount of "free" drug leaves the blood and goes to other tissues in greater amounts than usual. Its Vd is increased and its half-life is prolonged because a proportionately greater amount remains in the tissues rather than being excreted. The drug in the tissues takes longer to be excreted. Drugs that are highly protein bound (but not distributed extensively in tissues) usually have a volume of distribution similar to that of plasma.[4]

Whether protein binding causes clinically significant changes depends on the particular drug and the characteristics of the patient. Increased amounts of free or unbound drug in the plasma may be readily biotransformed or eliminated in a healthy individual

TABLE 3-2

Criteria Predictive of Clinically Relevant Drug Interactions at the Level of Plasma Albumin

1. The drug is extensively bound to albumin (usually in excess of 90 to 95 percent). Under these conditions, a small decrease in binding produced by a competing ligand causes a proportionally large increase in the pharmacologically active (unbound) component of the displaced drug.
2. The increase in the plasma level of the unbound drug cannot be readily dissipated. Such is the case when the displaced drug has a relatively long plasma half-life or when its elimination is decreased in the presence of the displacing ligand.
3. The displaced drug has a narrow margin of safety.

SOURCE: Godin D: Pharmacokinetics, in Munson PL (ed): *Principles of Pharmacology:* New York: Chapman & Hall, 1995. Used with permission.[2]

but could cause toxic effects in patients with pathological conditions, especially those affecting the liver and kidneys. Displacement of a drug with a narrow therapeutic index (see Table 3-7) from the plasma proteins would be more likely to cause toxic effects than a drug with a wider therapeutic index. Table 3-2 delineates some factors that may cause significant drug interactions based on protein binding.

Protein binding serves as a storage depot for many drugs, allowing for doses to be given that then become "unbound" over a period of time. Highly bound drugs generally have a longer duration of action than drugs that have little or no binding. For example, digitoxin is highly protein bound (90 to 100 percent) and has a longer half-life (118 to 216 hours) than digoxin (20 to 25 percent bound and a half-life of 30 hours).

RULE OF THUMB: Any drug that is highly protein bound has a greater potential for causing clinically relevant drug interactions:

When given with other drugs that are also highly protein bound because of increased risk of competition for binding sites

When elimination of the drug is decreased because excretion of unbound drug may be impeded

When the drug has a narrow margin of safety

Drug Biotransformation

Biotransformation refers to the process of converting a drug to another entity. Usually this means the metabolism of drugs, i.e., breaking them down into metabolites or other inactive forms that can then be eliminated. Usually drugs are converted to a more water-soluble form to facilitate excretion from the body.

Some references use the term drug *metabolism* rather than drug *transformation.* Biotransformation is a broader term that encompasses both drug metabolism as well as the conversion of some drugs (called pro-drugs) from an inactive to an active form. Most drugs are metabolized or broken down into other substances, which may or may not be pharmacologically active. Some drugs (pro-drugs) are initially inactive when administered and are then converted into active forms. The use of a pro-drug in a patient with impaired liver function would result in a nontherapeutic response (as well as possible toxicity). For example, prednisone in its oral form is inactive and needs to be metabolized to prednisolone by the liver to exert its pharmacological effects.

The biotransformation of many drugs occurs in the liver; however, the skin, kidneys, GI tract, and lungs, as well as other tissues, also may carry out metabolic processes with selected drugs. For example, in some diabetic patients, up to 50 percent of insulin administered subcutaneously may undergo extensive proteolysis before absorption into the bloodstream.[2]

Biotransformation takes place in two phases. In *Phase I reactions*, oxidation, dehydrogenation, and hydrolysis occur; drugs may become inactive, active, or unchanged. Also, in Phase I lipophilic molecules are converted into more polar molecules.[5] A group of enzymes regulate these Phase I processes. These enzymes are referred to as microsomal enzymes, or the cytochrome P-450 system or complex. This system is "named for the absorption peak at 450 nm that appears when hepatic microsomal metabolism is inhibited by carbon monoxide."[2(p54)] Families and subfamilies of P-450 have been identified for certain drugs. CYP3A4 metabolizes the greatest proportion of drugs in humans; it is found in the liver as well as in the GI tract.[6]

Some drugs may increase or induce the level of microsomal enzyme activity and thereby increase the rate of metabolism of other drugs metabolized by this system (Table 3-3). This results in lower than usual serum levels of the other drugs. An example is the decreased sedative effect of barbiturates seen in chronic alcohol abusers. This is due at least in part to the increased rate of metabolism of the barbiturate through the P-450 system whose activity has been increased by the chronic alcohol ingestion.[7]

Some other drugs inhibit the activity of these enzymes; this inhibition then can result in slowed metabolism of other drugs, leading to higher and possibly toxic serum levels. For example, cimetidine (Tagamet) is an inhibitor of microsomal enzymes; therefore, there is a possibility that its use could result in increased serum levels of other drugs taken concurrently by the patient.

Some drugs induce the speed of their own metabolism (autoinduction), which may result in the need for increasing doses to achieve the same effect. This may be one mechanism for the development of drug tolerance.

RULES OF THUMB: When a drug inhibits microsomal enzymes, or the P-450 system, the dosage of other drugs usually metabolized by that system may need to be decreased in order to prevent toxic effects.

When a drug induces microsomal enzymes, or the P-450 system, other drugs metabolized by that system will be metabolized more rapidly, resulting in lower serum levels and decreased effects; an increased dose may be required.

In Phase II reactions, drugs are conjugated with other substances, such as glucuronic acid or an amino acid, and become more water-soluble and usually become inactive.

TABLE 3-3

Examples of Enzyme Inducers and Inhibitors

Enzyme Inducers (increase the rate of drug metabolism)	Enzyme Inhibitors (decrease the rate of drug metabolism)	Autoinducers (affect the rate of their own metabolism)
Cigarette smoke	Cimetidine	Hexobarbital
Charcoal-broiled meats	Allopurinol	Meprobamate
Polycyclic hydrocarbons from industrial pollutants	Aspirin	Glutethimide
	Chloramphenicol	Phenobarbital
Glucocorticoids	Codeine	Nitroglycerin
Anticonvulsants	Cyclophosphamide	Probenecid
Alcohol (chronic use)	Desipramine	Tolbutamide
Acetone	Meperidine	Phenylbutazone
Isoniazid (INH)	MAO inhibitors	
Phenobarbital/barbiturates	Morphine	
Phenytoin	Nortriptyline	
Antihistamines		
Glutethimide		
Griseofulvin		
Meprobamate		
Tolbutamide		
PCBs		

Conjugation generally results in a substance that is more water-soluble and therefore more easily excreted from the body. Most drugs that have been conjugated become pharmacologically inert.[8]

Drugs do not necessarily follow these phases in sequence; they may enter Phase I or II and then be excreted, or they may enter Phase II and then Phase I.

First-Pass Effect

Some drugs are considered "first-pass effect" drugs, meaning that a large proportion of a dose is metabolized the first time it passes through the liver. For orally administered drugs this usually occurs right after absorption from the GI tract. In order to decrease this effect and allow for greater systemic effects before metabolism, these drugs are sometimes given IV, sublingually, or transdermally. When given by these routes, the drug usually will circulate to most of the body once before reaching the liver, where it is largely deactivated. When given orally, these first-pass effect drugs usually must be given in much higher doses compared to doses for other routes in order to compensate for the amount removed by the liver. The first-pass effect also may be avoided by giving a drug rectally rather than orally since blood returning from the lower part of the rectum largely bypasses the liver. An estimated 50 percent of the drug absorbed from the rectum bypasses the liver.[4] Examples of first-pass effect drugs are coumadin, dopamine, imipramine, lidocaine, morphine, nitroglycerin, propranolol, and reserpine.

Storage of Drugs in Tissues

After absorption into the bloodstream, drugs distribute first to organs and tissues that are well perfused. Subsequently, a drug may then distribute to the less well-perfused areas. Some drugs may accumulate in certain parts of the body. For instance, fat-soluble drugs will accumulate in fat in the body; this accounts for the prolonged effects of fat-soluble anesthetics.

Some drugs accumulate in bones (e.g., tetracyclines and heavy metals). The accumulation of lead in bones results in a slow release, which then prolongs the effects of lead poisoning.

Crossing the Placenta

The ability of a drug to cross the placenta to the fetus is of concern because of the danger of teratogenic effects on the fetus during pregnancy, as well as potential adverse effects of drugs administered just before delivery of the neonate. Transfer of a drug across the placenta occurs by diffusion, with lipid-soluble, nonionized drugs transferring readily from the maternal circulation to the fetal blood. (The use of drugs during pregnancy is discussed in further detail in Chap. 6.)

Elimination of Drugs from the Body

The kidney is the route of excretion for the majority of drugs. However, other routes of drug excretion need to be considered when assessing the appropriateness of a particular drug in a particular patient.

Some drugs may be partially eliminated through the lungs; the most common and obvious (because of the odor) are general inhalation anesthetics and alcohol. Paraldehyde also is eliminated by the lungs.

Drugs eliminated by the skin include alcohol and the anti-infective rifampin; with the latter drug this excretion can be seen visually by the yellow-orange discoloration of skin perspiration as well as other body fluids (saliva, tears). Excretion of drugs and/or their metabolites in breast milk is a concern for the nursing mother because of the possible inability of an infant with its underdeveloped liver and renal function to metabolize the drug or its metabolites. Chapter 6 discusses the issues related to drug therapy and breastfeeding.

Some drugs are excreted from the GI tract, including drugs that produce local effects in the GI tract (e.g., antacids, laxatives, certain antibiotics), and are not absorbed into the bloodstream. Other drugs or metabolites are excreted by the liver into the bile. Some drugs (e.g., digitoxin, morphine, tetracyclines) undergo enterohepatic cycling in which they are excreted by the liver into the bile, excreted with the bile into the duodenum, and partially reabsorbed and returned to the liver where they reenter the cycle. This recycling can result in a prolonged presence of the drug in the body; fat-soluble drugs are more likely to undergo enterohepatic recycling.

Renal Excretion

The kidneys are the major route of excretion for many drugs. Some drugs are excreted in their active form and others are converted into a metabolite (usually in the liver) capable of being excreted by the kidney. Therefore, the adequacy of a patient's kidney and liver function is a major consideration in the selection of a drug and the determination of dosage. (See Chaps. 4 and 5 for discussion of methods to assess renal function and adjustment of dosage.)

The adequacy of blood flow to the kidney affects the amount of the drug that can reach the kidney for renal excretion. Excretion of drugs from the kidney occurs through three mechanisms: glomerular filtration, tubular secretion, and tubular reabsorption (see Table 3-4). Approximately 20 percent of the plasma enters into the glomerulus. Unbound "free" drug and ionized drugs are in the ultrafiltrate. These drugs can be excreted into the urine via tubular secretion. Tubular secretion occurs in the proximal tubules and requires active transport systems. Drugs need to compete for tubular secretion; this can result in drug interactions—either desired or undesired. "Tying up the tubules" by one drug can result in another drug not being as readily excreted. Sometimes this interaction is used intentionally as when a patient on penicillin is also given probenecid (Benemid), an antigout or uricosuric agent, in order to prolong and maintain serum levels of penicillin. In other situations this type of interaction can result in toxic levels of the second drug (e.g., ASA and methotrexate).

Once in the tubules, the fate of a drug/metabolite in terms of the extent to which it is reabsorbed by passive tubular reabsorption or excreted in the urine depends upon certain characteristics of the drug and the urine. The pH of the drug or metabolite in relation to the pH of the urine will determine the extent of distal tubular reabsorption. The same principle of acid-base relationships as described earlier in this chapter with absorption applies here also. If the urine is acidic and the drug/metabolite is weakly acidic, the drug/metabolite remains nonionized and will return to the body by passing through the tubular membranes. If the pH of the urine is weakly basic, then the drug/metabolite would remain in the urine and be excreted from the body. In cases of overdosing with weakly acidic drugs, alkalinization of the urine (administration of sodium bicarbonate) can be used to enhance excretion of the acidic drug (e.g., phenobarbital, salicylates) from the body. Alkalinization of the urine from 6.4 to 8.0 can result in as much as a sixfold increase in excretion of a relatively strong acid such as salicylate.[4(p17)]

Although an acidifying agent such as ammonium chloride has been used to enhance the excretion of alkaline drugs (e.g., amphetamine, chloroquine, codeine, imipramine, meperidine), this practice is no longer recommended because it has caused tubular damage. The effect on drugs of altering the urine pH is greatest for those that are weakly

TABLE 3-4

Renal Processes that Influence Drug Excretion

Process	Transport Route	Drugs Transported	Notes
Glomerular filtration	Drugs pass from the blood into the nephron by perfusing across the fenestrated capillaries of Bowman's capsule.	Diffusion process. Small, nonionic drugs pass more readily. Drugs bound to plasma proteins cannot pass.	Rate of filtration depends in part on blood pressure.
Tubular secretion	Drugs secreted into the nephron tubule from the efferent arteriole.	Active transport (drug carriers and energy). Drugs which specifically bind to carriers (transporters) are transported. Size and charge are less important.	Drugs may compete with one another for the carrier. A drug with a low margin of safety might reach toxic levels. Therapeutically, drugs which compete for transporters can be coadministered to increase plasma half-life.
Tubular reabsorption	Drugs are reabsorbed into the blood stream from the nephron tubule.	Diffusion process. Small, nonionic drugs pass more readily.	Because ionic agents are poorly reabsorbed, drug metabolites which are more ionic than the parent drug will be passed into the urine more easily. Urinary pH can be purposely altered to increase the rate of drug excretion (e.g., administration of bicarbonate).

SOURCE: Olson J: *Clinical Pharmacology Made Ridiculously Simple*. Miami, FL: MedMaster, 1997. Used with permission.[4a]

acidic or basic; there is little or no effect on strong acids or bases. Large doses of vitamin C acidify the urine and may then affect renal excretion of other drugs.

Dose

The amount of a drug given has obvious influences on the effects produced; some drugs, however, may vary in their effect and clinical use by the dose used. Examples are the use of low doses of milk of magnesia for antacid effect and larger doses for cathartic effects, or the use of antidepressants in low doses for treatment of neurological pain and higher regular doses for treating depression.

Clearance

The concept of clearance is an important part of pharmacokinetics. Clearance refers to the amount of plasma from which all of a drug is removed in a given time. Knowing the clearance of a drug allows the clinician to achieve a steady-state therapeutic level in the plasma or blood. The clearance of most drugs in the concentration commonly used clinically is usually constant. In *first-order kinetics*, a constant *fraction* of drug is eliminated per unit of time. The rate of metabolism or excretion may vary in proportion to the concentration of the drug present, i.e., the more drug the greater the rate of excretion. However, if the drug becomes more concentrated (as may occur if a patient on long-term drug therapy becomes dehydrated or if drug dosage is increased), enzymes or carrier-mediated processes may become saturated. *Zero-order kinetics* occur when mechanisms of elimination become saturated and the body can handle only a specific *amount* of drug per unit of time to be eliminated; when this occurs a small increase in dose or serum concentration results in disproportionately greater (or more variable) levels of the drug and possible toxicity from "delayed" excretion.

The transition from first order to zero order kinetics can result in potential serious toxicity from relatively minor dosage increases. Examples are the high incidence of salicylism in patients with rheumatoid arthritis being treated on 4 to 6 g of aspirin daily. Phenytoin transitions from first order to zero order kinetics in elimination at plasma concentrations between 10 and 20 micrograms per mL (which also is its optimal therapeutic range).[2]

Therapeutic Index/ Margin of Safety

The therapeutic index (TI) reflects the safety of a drug—the wider the range of doses producing either toxicity or death (depending on which formula is used), the safer the drug is considered to be. A drug with a narrow therapeutic index is considered less safe and means that dosing must be very carefully considered and effects monitored more closely, possibly through serum levels.

The therapeutic index does not provide complete information because it does not reflect the distribution of responses at the levels measured; i.e., it does not reflect the variability of responses in patients (a level that may be therapeutic to one patient may be toxic to another) and any overlap in the curves of the two levels. It is also important to note that, since all drugs have more than one effect, a specific drug may have different therapeutic indexes, depending on the intended therapeutic effect (see also Table 3-7) at end of this chapter for definitions of other selected pharmacological terms.

Pharmacodynamics

Pharmacodynamics is what a drug does to the body. It is concerned with what occurs to bring about pharmacologic effects. Drugs produce their effects by a variety of mechanisms. Drugs have multiple effects on the various cells and tissues of the body; however, most drugs do not act everywhere—they produce effects on certain cells or tissues and not on others. This can be explained by the receptor theory. This theory explains the selectivity of effect by the presence of receptors with a high affinity for the drug. Receptors may be enzymes, nucleic acids, or specialized membrane-bound proteins.[3]

If the receptor has an affinity for the drug molecule, the receptor and molecule bind together. The analogy often used is that of a lock (receptor) and key (drug)—if the molecular structure of the drug fits the receptor, it will be attracted to that receptor. If the result of this binding produces a cellular response, the drug is called an *agonist*. Some receptors are on the cell surface and may produce effects there or by signaling messengers (usually proteins) into the cell; other receptors may be located within the cell. The magnitude of response is proportional to the number of receptors occupied by the agonist. Some drugs are *partial agonists* in that they can only achieve a partial response even at high doses.

Some drug-receptor combinations do not produce a change in cellular function but rather block another substance (or drug) from interacting with the receptor; these drugs are called antagonists. Examples are antihistamines, H_2 blockers, and beta-blockers. Pure antagonists can prevent or reverse the action of an agonist without producing their own effects on the cell. Some antagonists can be displaced if there is an increased concentration of the agonist; these antagonists are called *competitive*, or *surmountable*, antagonists.[9] Other drugs are noncompetitive agonists that reduce the effect of an agonist through binding with the agonist or preventing the agonist effect.[3]

Receptors can vary in their functions. With constant stimulation of receptors by agonists, desensitization (also known as refractoriness or down-regulation) may result. This results in a decreased response, such as occurs with the use of beta-adrenergic blockers in treating asthma. Receptor malfunction is believed to play a role in such conditions as myasthenia gravis, testicular feminization syndrome, and some forms of insulin-resistant diabetes mellitus.[9] Up-regulation can also occur when there is an increased synthesis of receptors (sensitization).

Some receptors are categorized by how they respond to various agonists and antagonists. Examples are: nicotinic versus muscarinic cholinergic receptors and subtypes of adrenergic blockers (alpha$_1$, alpha$_2$, beta$_1$, beta$_2$).

Other Mechanisms of Drug Action

Some drugs act by mechanisms other than through affecting receptors. Examples are drugs such as chelating agents that "unite" with metals and assist in their removal from the body. Mannitol acts through creating hyperosmolarity in the vascular tree and thereby attracting fluids out of the interstitial space; this increase in vascular volume results in osmotic diuresis. Some drugs act by altering the function of cell membranes by dissolving in them (e.g., general anesthetics, heart muscle depressant drugs, sedative-hypnotics).

PATIENT VARIABLES AFFECTING PHARMACOKINETICS AND PHARMACODYNAMICS

Physiological processes play a major role in the absorption, biotransformation, distribution, and excretion of drugs. Diseases or other factors (such as genetics) that affect these processes can affect drug kinetics and thus variations in drug effects.

The blood flow to and from cells, tissues, and membranes influences the ability of drugs to reach various sites of action and excretion. Drugs are more effectively absorbed from sites that are highly perfused (e.g., muscles). If circulation is impaired, such as in congestive heart failure, hypotension, or shock, absorption may be delayed. Absorption from SC and IM sites can be influenced by factors that alter blood flow, such as exercise, increased external temperature, or vasoconstriction from smoking. The degree of tissue perfusion is one of the patient variables that can affect the half-life of a drug. Tissue perfusion is a function of heart contractility, blood pressure, circulating volume, and the status of the blood vessels.

Pathophysiological factors influencing the usual pH within the various compartments of the body will affect the ability of a drug to pass through the surrounding membrane by affecting the degree of ionization of the drug. Factors affecting gastric emptying can alter the usual absorption of acidic or alkaline drugs; i.e., a delayed gastric emptying may result in greater absorption of acidic drugs and delayed absorption of alkaline drugs. Alterations in the blood pH may cause ionization of drugs and prevent their passage out of the blood to interstitial spaces and cells.

The degree of porousness of membranes can influence the diffusion of drugs. In capillaries the pores are sufficiently large to allow most therapeutic agents to cross. The exception is the cerebral capillaries that form the blood-brain barrier. In the cerebral capillaries, the endothelial junctions are tight or occluded[3] and there are fewer pinocytotic vesicles. Thus the main way for drugs to cross the blood-brain barrier is through their solubility in fat; i.e., fat-soluble drugs pass the blood-brain barrier. Some areas of the brain are not as protected from toxins and certain drugs by the blood-brain barrier, most notably the vomiting center. Other drugs, because of their structural similarity to natural endogenous substances, may be transported by carrier-mediated transport. Pathological conditions can increase the permeability of the blood-brain barrier and expose the brain to undesired drug effects. Inflammation of the meninges and hypoxia are two conditions that may increase the permeability of the blood-brain barrier; when this occurs there is a risk of injury to sensitive brain tissues from drugs or other substances that normally do not cross the barrier.

Protein Binding

Several patient factors may influence the protein binding of drugs. Any condition that decreases the amount of albumin will decrease the availability of binding sites and may cause toxic levels of the unbound portion of highly protein-bound drugs. Patients with malnutrition, liver disease, renal failure, and burns are examples of patients who may have low levels of albumin. Other patients at risk are patients who are NPO for more than 3 days or those who choose not ot eat or cannot eat for more than 3 days (e.g., dental abscess, surgery, etc.). In liver or renal disease, albumin may have a decreased binding capacity for certain drugs (e.g., decreased binding of diazepam in patients with cirrhosis).[2]

Biotransformation

A patient's liver function is a key factor influencing drug biotransformation. Therefore, a patient with liver disease, including cirrhosis, viral or acute drug-induced hepatitis, heavy metal poisoning, porphyria, and hemochromatosis, must receive careful consideration of both the drug and the dosing.[2] An exaggerated pharmacological response resulting from decreased hepatic biotransformation of diazepam, morphine, and tolbutamide may occur in patients with liver dysfunction.[4] This is related to the loss of functioning of Kupffer cells and the inability of the P-450 enzymes to metabolize the drug. Impaired circulation of the blood to the liver, as may occur with cardiac insufficiency or beta-adrenergic blockade, can also decrease the hepatic metabolism of drugs.

Microsomal enzyme levels may be influenced by other drugs the patient is receiving (see Table 3-3). Some drugs inhibit the microsomal enzymes resulting in possible higher serum levels of other drugs usually metabolized under their influence. Cimetidine (Tagamet) is a commonly used prescription and OTC drug capable of inhibiting these enzymes. Inducers of enzymes include drugs as well as other agents such as insecticides, smoking, and alcohol.

Other drugs the patient is receiving may compete for metabolic pathways, with the possibility of toxic effects from the more slowly metabolized drug. An example is the toxic level of dicumarol when given with cimetidine. Alcohol interferes with the metabolism of acetaminophen; this can result in hepatotoxicity and possible liver failure in alcoholics using doses of acetaminophen even in the high therapeutic range (see the discussion in Chap. 11).

Aging

Normal growth and aging affect the ability of the body to handle drugs. As individuals age, there are a variety of physiological changes that affect pharmacokinetics and pharmacodynamics. Decreases in muscle mass and increases in fat in the body occur with normal aging and affect the distribution and storage of water-soluble and fat-soluble drugs.

Hepatic blood flow may be decreased by as much as 50 percent in individuals over 65 years; therefore, these individuals may experience toxicity when given usual doses of first-pass effect drugs. Liver mass and overall metabolic activity decrease with aging.

Decreases in serum albumin and/or binding capacity may result in increased serum levels of the "free" or unbound portion of the protein-bound drugs. When a drug that has protein-binding properties is absorbed, if the albumin levels are low (or change), the drug, taken in its usual dose, may not have enough protein to bind to and be stored for future use. Instead the drug remains in the plasma and can exert toxic effects on tissues, especially the liver and kidneys since the amount of the drug in the circulation is so high. With some drugs such as phenytoin, a decrease in the albumin results in it having increased availability to be biotransformed by the liver. In this case, the enhanced decrease in serum levels could result in the patient having a seizure because of decreased drug levels.

The activity of certain microsomal enzymes decreases with age; this helps to explain why desired drug effects can be achieved with smaller doses in the elderly. Drugs metabolized through Phase II conjugation and those not metabolized under the influence of the microsomal enzymes are not significantly affected by aging.[2] Since the various benzodiazepines show considerable differences in their biotransformation, those used in the elderly need to be carefully selected based on their biotransformation processes.

Renal function generally decreases with increasing age, estimated to be at the rate of 1 percent per year after age 30. Blood-urea-nitrogen (BUN) levels are poor indicators of renal function in the elderly because of the decrease in muscle mass and other variables affecting BUN levels. Serum creatinine levels can be used to estimate creatinine clearance (see Chap. 5) but are less reliable in the elderly.

In addition to the alterations due to normal aging processes, the elderly are more likely to have chronic pathological conditions that may affect drugs. Table 7-1 illustrates alterations caused by aging and by pathological conditions that may affect drug kinetics in the elderly. The elderly also are more likely to be taking other drugs that may influence pharmacokinetics and pharmacodynamics.

Gender

Since women have been largely excluded from much if not most drug research until recently (see Chap. 6), differences in pharmacodynamics and pharmacokinetics related to gender have not been extensively studied. Some data suggest that there is decreased oxidation of certain drugs such as estrogens and benzodiazepines in women.[4] The impact on drug kinetics and dynamics of hormone levels in general and their fluctuations during the menstrual cycle is not known for most drugs. Women have a relatively greater proportion of fat which could impact on the amount of a fat-soluble drug distributed to and stored in fat. Pregnancy status and lactation are major variables to consider because of variations in pharmacokinetics during pregnancy as well as possible deleterious effects on the fetus or the newborn (see Chap. 6).

Circadian Rhythm Variations

Many of the changes in physiological function over the 24-hour day have been determined. Increasingly, the roles of these diurnal fluctuations are being studied as a basis
for variations in responses of patients to a drug depending upon the time of day. Tissue
plasminogen activator (t-PA) has been found to be more effective when given in the late
afternoon. Many individuals have "insulin resistance" in the early morning hours,
resulting in increased blood glucose levels. Adrenocorticosteroid therapy has been
found to cause less adrenal suppression if all or most of the daily dose is given around
8 A.M. rather than in the evening (see Chap. 17 for further explanation).

Diseases

Most diseases have the potential to alter drug kinetics or dynamics. Diseases affecting
the liver, kidney, and circulation are of special concern because of their roles in the metabolism, distribution, and elimination of most drugs.

Liver

Conditions causing decreased blood flow through the liver, such as congestive heart
failure or advanced cirrhosis, may result in reduced clearance and therefore increased
blood levels and possible toxicity of drugs, especially the high first-pass effect drugs
(see Table 3-3). Available liver function tests do not correlate well with impairment of
drug biotransformation by the liver. Measurement of drug serum levels is recommended
in advanced liver disease in order to avoid toxicity.[8]

Renal Excretion

Conditions affecting the renal excretion of a drug include any condition that causes a
decrease in plasma proteins; this could result in increased renal excretion of the portion
of the drug that is unbound. The higher drug concentrations in the ultrafiltrate can damage the tubules. In patients with uremia, acidic by-products may cause the displacement
of drugs from binding sites.

Loss of integrity of the glomerulus sieve such as seen in severe chronic hypertension
allows larger molecules such as protein to enter the loop. This results in proteinuria.
Proteinuria may result in the excretion of protein-bound drugs as they become excreted
along with the protein. This excreted bound drug has not exerted a pharmacological
effect; therefore the patient will receive less effect from the drug dose given.

Decreased blood flow to the kidneys, such as may occur with congestive heart failure or shock, will decrease the excretion of drugs from the kidneys and could result in
a more prolonged half-life and toxicity.

Impaired renal function usually affects the excretion of drugs and therefore a
patient's renal status needs to be carefully assessed both before and during drug therapy.
The degree of decrease in renal function, however, does not entirely predict the rate of
clearance of the drug from plasma because other nonrenal mechanisms may compensate.

Therefore, for many commonly used drugs nomograms have been developed that relate changes in drug elimination (usually expressed in terms of plasma half-life values) to creatinine clearance (a quantitative measure of renal functional status). These nomograms provide a guide for adjusting dosing regimens to the needs of each individual patient.[2] See Chap. 4 for approaches to estimating creatinine clearance from serum creatinine levels. Normal and abnormal values of creatinine clearance are as follows:

Normal: Males: 85 to 125 mL/min; females: 75 to 115 mL/min
Mild renal impairment: 50 to 80 mL/min
Moderate renal impairment: 10 to 50 mL/min
Severe kidney dysfunction: less than 10 mL/min

Some drugs are of particular concern in patients with uremia. Drugs with a narrow benefit/risk ratio such as digitalis or the aminoglycosides should be monitored by more frequent blood level measurements. In patients with decreased renal function there is a greater likelihood of toxic effects from some drugs. Salicylates and other analgesics are more likely to cause gastric ulceration, anticoagulants are more likely to cause bleeding, and drugs affecting potassium levels such as spironolactone may cause hyperkalemia. Aminoglycosides, amphotericin B, and gold may be more toxic to the uremic kidney even in smaller doses.[8(p68)]

GI Tract

Conditions affecting the GI tract may alter the rate and extent of absorption of orally administered drugs. This may occur through increasing or decreasing the gastric emptying time or intestinal transit time, or through alteration of the usual pH.

Cardiovascular Function

Cardiovascular conditions affecting the circulation of the blood and/or the blood components may alter the transport and distribution of drugs. Impaired circulation will decrease absorption from most routes of administration and also may prevent the transport of drugs to the liver for metabolism and to the kidneys for excretion.

Genetics

Pharmacogenetics is a relatively recent area of inquiry for understanding variations in patient responses to drugs. Especially in the area of biotransformation there is ample room for considerable variation in enzymatic processes based upon genetic makeup. All major genetic variations related to drug metabolizing activity are inherited as autosomally recessive traits.[4]

Pharmacogenetic variation can result in (1) altered clearance of drugs resulting in a "functional" overdose" in those individuals unable to metabolize the compound; (2) failure to convert a pro-drug to an active drug; (3) altered pharmacodynamics [e.g., hemolytic anemia secondary to glucose-6-dehydrogenase (G6PD) deficiency]; and (4) idiosyncratic drug reactions such as aplastic anemia or hepatotoxicity.[10]

The rapidity of acetylation is a well-known example of a genetically based difference in the metabolism of drugs. Individuals may be rapid or slow acetylators; about half of the population in North America are estimated to be slow acetylators.[2] A greater proportion of the Asian and Inuit population are rapid acetylators, while many slow acetylators are Caucasians. About 50 percent of African-Americans and whites are slow acetylators, as are 60 to 70 percent of northern Europeans. Only 5 percent of individuals of Asian descent are slow acetylators.[4] Rapid acetylators metabolize the antitubercular drug isoniazid (INH) more rapidly than many Caucasians of northern European ancestry, tend to experience liver side effects rather than the peripheral neuropathy that tends to occur in slow acetylators taking INH, and may require increased or more frequent dosing. Other drugs with genetic variations in acetylation are hydralazine (slow acetylators may be more likely to develop hydralazine-induced lupus erythematosus), procainamide, and sulfasalazine.[3]

A genetic basis for slow hydroxylators has been identified affecting the microsomal enzyme metabolism of drugs such as beta-adrenoceptor blockers, dextromethorphan, phenformin, and tricyclic antidepressants.[2] Individuals who are impaired metabolizers of debrisoquin may experience an increase in adverse effects of encainide, flecainide, metoprolol, and perphenazine.[4]

Genetic alterations can be the basis of some adverse drug reactions. Examples are genetic alterations in G6PD that cause hemolysis when the patient ingests oxidative drugs such as aspirin, and malignant hyperthermia, in which a patient develops a potentially fatal reaction to anesthetics.

Considering the hundreds of enzymes in the human body, there is a great likelihood for a genetic basis for variations in an individual's response to a drug.

CONTEXTUAL VARIABLES AFFECTING PHARMACOKINETICS AND PHARMACODYNAMICS

Some of the variables that may affect a patient's response occur even before the drug reaches the body or the site of absorption.

Variations in Pharmaceutical Preparation and Manufacturing

As drugs are manufactured they are usually mixed with other substances or vehicles that assist in their administration. Legally, a drug preparation must contain the stated amount of the drug; however, the preparation may contain such substances as binders, preservatives, dyes (e.g., tartrazine, or Yellow Dye No. 5), waxes, coatings (e.g., enteric), or other substances included by the manufacturer to promote dissolution and/or absorption. These added ingredients may account for variations in bioavailability among different brands of the same drug or among brand drugs and generic drugs. These additives explain why some patients may have a reaction to one brand of drug but can safely take another brand. Other bases for variation include differences occurring in the formulation or manufacturing of the drug, such as particle size or crystallization. These differences can account for variations in bioavailability among drugs manufactured by different manufacturers. These differences in bioavailability may be of particular concern with drugs with a narrow margin of safety; monitoring of serum levels may be necessary if brands are changed. Clinicians may wish to indicate "no substitution allowed" on prescriptions for drugs with a narrow therapeutic range that are known to vary considerably by brand. *Approved Drug Products with Therapeutic Equivalence Evaluations* is a useful reference that contains FDA standards for bioavailability and interchangeability of various drug products. See Table 3-5.

Some tablets have special coatings that make them easier to swallow. These "added" substances can account for differences in bioavailability as well as possible adverse reactions. Individuals allergic to Yellow Dye No. 5 (tartrazine) may experience allergic reactions when taking a drug preparation containing this dye; they are allergic to the dye and not necessarily to the drug. Patients with an allergy to aspirin may have a cross-sensitivity to tartrazine. Injectable drugs need to be checked carefully for the appropriateness of that particular preparation for the use intended. Preparations of local anesthetics to be used in spinal anesthesia or drugs to be used in the eye need to be checked carefully to be sure that the preparation is labeled explicitly for that route and use.

TABLE 3-5

Examples of Drugs with High Variation in Equivalence

Bioinequivalence	Therapeutic Inequivalence
digoxin	dicumarol
erythromycin	digoxin
hydrochlorothiazide	L-dopa
L-dopa	
phenobarbital	
prednisone	
warfarin	

SOURCE: Godin D: Pharmacokinetics, in Munson PL (ed): *Principles of Pharmacology*. New York: Chapman & Hall, 1995. Used with permission.[2]

Dosage Form

The dosage form, especially for orally administered medications, may alter the rate and extent of absorption (see Table 3-6). Topical drugs may vary in their absorption according to the ingredients used as the base (e.g., as in scopolamine or nitroglycerin patches); certain drugs for intramuscular (e.g., procaine penicillin) or subcutaneous administration

TABLE 3-6

Oral Medication Dosage Forms

Form	Comments
Elixir	Contains alcohol; do not use if patient on disulfiram (Antabuse) therapy.
Syrup	Contains 85% sucrose.
Chewable tablets	For patients with difficulty in swallowing; usually must be chewed or else will not dissolve well in stomach.
Buccal	Not placed under tongue; absorption increased by hot liquids.
Sublingual	Dissolved by saliva.
Effervescent	Reaction helps to dissolve ingredients.
Hard gelatin capsules	Usually contain between 65 and 1000 mg of drug and generally better release, dissolution and absorption than from a tablet.
Soft gelatin capsules	One-piece; contains liquid solution or suspension in vehicle such as mineral oil and glycols surrounded by soft plasticized gelatin shell.
Oral controlled-release preparations	Use various mechanisms to allow slower or continuous absorption; mechanisms include: use of different coatings that dissolve under differing conditions in GI tract, e.g., pH; ion-exchange resins; osmotically actuated (Osmol system). All must be swallowed whole. Potential problem of some of drug components getting trapped or adhering to folds of GI tract leading to localized irritation, obstruction, and/or ulceration. Remnants of some systems may be excreted in stool and do not mean the drug did not dissolve, e.g., sustained-release nifedipine.

SOURCE: Adapted from DiPiro J, Talbert RL, Yee GC (eds): *Pharmacotherapy: A Pathophysiological Approach*. New York: Elsevier, 1997.[11]

(e.g., NPH insulin) have added ingredients intended to slow their rate of absorption from these sites.

Storage

Deterioration of the drug and/or the other substance through either incorrect storage or use beyond the expiration date can result in suboptimal therapeutic effects and/or actual deleterious effects from degraded products. Tetracyclines used after their expiration date may produce Fanconi syndrome in the kidneys.

Correct Use

Other external variables relate to whether the drug gets to the patient correctly. Variables here include degree of accessibility of the drug to the patient (e.g., cost issues), patient compliance (see Chap. 2), medication errors, and errors in proper administration.

Table 3-7 lists pharmacological terms, concepts, and implications.

TABLE 3-7

Pharmacological Terms, Concepts, and Implications

Terms and concepts	Definition	Comments and Implications
Area under the curve (AUC)	When the plasma concentrations of a drug are plotted on a graph, the area under the curve (AUC) reflects the degree of absorption of the drug.	When used in individual patient, can be used as basis for individualized dosing (e.g., cancer chemotherapy).
Bioavailability	Amount of drug in plasma when given a specific route compared to amount in plasma when drug given IV. Example: $$\text{Bioavailability} = \frac{\text{AUC oral}}{\text{AUC IV}}$$	Important when comparing or selecting different brands, brand names versus generic products, drug formulations, or routes.
Bioequivalence	When two related drugs show comparable bioavailability	
Therapeutic equivalence	When two similar drugs have comparable efficacy and safety.	

TABLE 3-7

Pharmacological Terms, Concepts, and Implications (continued)

Terms and concepts	Definition	Comments and Implications
Therapeutic index (TI)	Ratio of dose causing toxicity to dose producing desired therapeutic effect. $$TI = \frac{TD_{50} \text{ or } LD_{50}}{ED_{50}*}$$	In drugs with a low therapeutic index, a small change in bioequivalence is more likely to have therapeutic consequences. These drugs are more likely to require monitoring via serum levels; keeping patient on same brand of medication may be more critical than with other drugs.
Efficacy	Maximum response that a drug can produce.	Two drugs may produce same effect (same efficacy), but if one does this at a lesser dosage, it is more potent than the other.
Potency	Dose of drug necessary to achieve half of the desired therapeutic effect.	See efficacy above.

*TD_{50} = therapeutic dose; LD_{50} = lethal dose (concentration of drug causing death in 50% of subjects); ED_{50} = dose that induces specified clinical effect in 50% of subjects.

SUMMARY

This chapter has discussed the various factors related to the patient, the drug, and the context (P-D-C) that can influence the effects produced by a drug in an individual patient. It also provides a basis for understanding why the same drug might cause different effects at different times in the same patient.

This knowledge is essential for the clinician to use in evaluating patients before and during drug therapy and in the selection of a specific drug, dose, route, etc. Safe and effective drug therapy depends on consideration of many factors. The framework of the patient, the drug, and the context can provide the clinician with a useful approach to consider and analyze all of these complex and interacting variables.

REFERENCES

1. Melmon KL, Morrelli HF, Hoffman BB, Nierenberg D W (eds): *Melmon and Morrelli's Clinical Pharmacology. Basic Principles in Therapeutics,* 3d ed. New York: McGraw-Hill, 1992.

2. Godin D: Pharmacokinetics, in Munson PL (ed): *Principles of Pharmacology.* New York: Chapman & Hall, 1995.

3. Stringer JL: *Basic Concepts in Pharmacology.* New York: McGraw-Hill, 1996.

4. Benet LZ, Kroetz DL, Sheiner LB: Pharmacokinetics, in Hardman JG, Limbird LE (eds): *Goodman & Gilman's The Pharmacological Basis of Therapeutics.* 9th ed. New York: McGraw-Hill, 1996.

4a. Olson J: *Clinical Pharmacology Made Ridiculously Simple.* Miami, FL: MedMaster, 1977.

5. Mycek MA, Harvey RA, Champe PC, et al (eds): *Lippincott's Illustrated Reviews: Pharmacology.* 2d ed. Philadelphia: Lippincott-Raven, 1997.

6. Meyer JM, Rodvold KA: Drug biotransformation by the cytochrome P-450 enzyme system. Medscape (Internet), 1996.

7. Thayer WS: Biotransformation, in DiPalma JR, DiGregorio GJ: *Basic Pharmacology in Medicine,* 3d ed. New York: McGraw-Hill, 1990.

8. DiPalma JR, DiGregorio GJ: *Basic Pharmacology in Medicine,* 3d ed. New York: McGraw-Hill, 1990.

9. Ross EM: Pharmacodynamics, in Hardman JG, Limbird LE (eds): *Goodman & Gilman's The Pharmacological Basis of Therapeutics.* 9th ed. New York: McGraw-Hill, 1996.

10. Nies AS, Spielberg SP: Principles of therapeutics, in Hardman JG, Limbird LE (eds): *Goodman & Gilman's The Pharmacological Basis of Therapeutics,* 9th ed. New York: McGraw-Hill, 1996, p 54.

11. DiPiro J, Talbert RL, Yee GC (eds): *Pharmacotherapy: A Pathophysiological Approach.* New York: Elsevier, 1997.

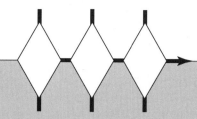

Chapter 4

PATIENT ASSESSMENT AND DRUG THERAPY

Laurel A. Eisenhauer

OVERVIEW

Patient assessment is an essential part of any clinician's role. Assessment is essential for providing a basis for diagnosis; it is also essential for monitoring patient responses and evaluating the outcomes of interventions. An additional and important role of a holistic assessment is to provide an understanding of the patient's lifestyle and psychosocial variables that may affect the ability or willingness of the patient to adhere to a pre-scribed therapeutic regimen. This may influence the choice of therapy, including the specific drug, the dosing schedule, and the route. Assessment also provides data that can be used to guide the selection of nondrug interventions that may either prevent or decrease the need for many drug therapies.

Various frameworks and approaches to patient assessment are available; the use of a "medical" versus a "nursing" approach has long been a source of tension for APNs. Each APN needs to develop a systematic approach to assessment and the recording of assessment data that elicits essential data and allows communication among health team members. This approach should also demonstrate the nursing contribution to care and not focus solely on the "medically" oriented aspects of medical diagnoses and the prescribing of medical interventions.

Regardless of which framework or approach is used, the assessment of the patient for allergies or intolerances to drugs is critical and needs to be determined early and recorded prominently according to agency policies. It is important to assess and seek clarification about responses to current, past, and proposed medications. Some patients may state that they have allergies or are allergic to a drug, but they actually are refer-ring to a side effect such as nausea, diarrhea, or other intolerance. Therefore, it is impor-tant to try to establish the exact medication, the dates, the sequence, and the specific nature of the symptoms. Questions should be asked also about similar drugs with cross-allergies (e.g., penicillins and cephalosporins, aspirin and ibuprofen) and the family history of intolerance or allergies to drugs.

This chapter will present two formats (Functional Health Pattern Assessment[1] and Review of Systems[4]) for obtaining a patient history, illustrating how drug therapy and pharmacological considerations can be elicited and considered for their implications for prescribing or monitoring of drug therapy. Another section will highlight drug effects that may be detected during physical assessment.

A case study illustrating how important information for drug therapy can be derived from the "nursing" data from a Functional Health Pattern Assessment is provided at the end of the chapter. Nurses learning to be APNs or APNs preparing for a prescriptive role need to increase their ability to elicit and interpret patient data in terms of the relevance of these data for drug therapy.

ASSESSMENT OF FUNCTIONAL HEALTH PATTERNS

The Functional Health Patterns (FHPs)[1] provide a useful framework for assessing the myriad of factors that can influence drug response impact on compliance and successful outcomes of drug therapy. The FHPs discussed below incorporate both subjective and objective data. The effects of drug therapy on physical assessment are outlined later in this chapter. Through discussion of each of these 11 patterns, one can see how each pattern may affect drug therapy as well as how drug therapy may impact on that pattern.

1. HEALTH PERCEPTION–HEALTH BELIEF PATTERN:
"Client's perceived pattern of health and well-being and how his or her health is managed."

Impact of Pattern on Drug Therapy

Assessment of this pattern can provide a rich database for planning drug and other therapeutics. It provides insights into the beliefs of the client, current health practices that may affect drug therapy, and resources (or lack of) to enhance health.

Elicitation of beliefs about the nature of health and factors affecting it or the causation of a current illness can provide insights into beliefs about disease causation and how disease should be treated. The use of home remedies is an important area to explore since these may interfere with drug therapy; they also can provide clues to the patient's understanding of health, disease, and treatment. Examples include the use of baking soda as an antacid, the use of Chinese medicines, and the use of herbs. Beliefs about the "yin and yang" or the "hot and cold" basis of disease and the use of opposite treatments may mean that one particular type of medication may not be acceptable while another would be. Use of homeopathy, health foods and other related preparations, and OTC drugs should be determined in order to prevent interactions with current or future drug therapy. The history of the patient's current medications and past drug therapy and responses to drug therapy is essential. This can also serve to detect any "allergies" or intolerances to drugs or any familial responses to drug therapy.

The meaning of drug therapy to patients can reveal whether "taking pills" connotes being ill to an extent that either could enhance or interfere with compliance. This information can be useful in determining motivating factors that can help a patient comply with a regimen.

Questions to elicit patterns of compliance are useful in predicting future compliance; they may also elicit any indications of drug-seeking behavior—seeking drug therapy as the answer for any symptom or illness or, in the extreme, the drug-seeking behavior of addiction. It may be helpful to ask the patient to describe how he or she takes medications, eats meals, manages other therapeutic interventions, and his or her typical daily activities and events. Taking a history of immunizations provides specific information about immunization status and also can provide clues about patient's degree of appropriate management of health status.

The use of alcohol, cigarettes, and drugs is important to determine because of possible interactions with drug therapy. Alcohol as a CNS depressant can interact with many other CNS depressants to produce excessive sedation or even death. It also causes gastric irritation that may compound gastric problems with aspirin (ASA), nonsteroidal anti-inflammatory drugs (NSAIDS), and steroids. Alcohol can affect the microsomal enzymes and therefore the metabolism of many drugs. The impact of chronic alcohol use on liver function also can affect the biotransformation of many drugs.

Cigarette smoking may affect risk factors for complications of oral contraceptives and may be a contraindication. Nicotine can also affect biotransformation of drugs (e.g., theophylline).

Unfortunately, health resources available to the patient may affect the choice of drug therapy. Today health insurance and managed care impact on what drugs can be prescribed. HMO formularies may have only certain drugs that can be prescribed. Medicare, Medicaid, and health insurance plans with coverage for drugs may mandate the use of generic drugs. Most restrict the number of tablets that can be dispensed at any one time, which may impact on the person's ability to go to the pharmacy or otherwise obtain the medication every 30 days. While this does save money in the event that a medication becomes unnecessary, it does require intricate planning for a patient on multiple medications with differing renewal dates. The cost of medications is a factor in patient compliance with the drug therapy. As a rule of thumb, each prescription medication costs about $50 per month. Therefore, an individual on three or four or more medications can have a considerable financial cost, especially if he or she does not have insurance.

Assessment of the patient's home and living situation will show if the patient has family members or other caregivers who can help with management of the drug therapy if necessary. This is of particular importance with drug therapy such as insulin in diabetes or adrenocorticosteroids in Addison's disease where daily administration is necessary and where patients can become incapacitated or severely compromised if they do not receive the required doses. The patient's living situation also needs to be assessed in terms of drug storage and disposal. If children (or grandchildren) are present, there is a need to ensure appropriate storage and use of childproof caps. Availability of a refrigerator is necessary for storage of certain drugs, e.g., suppositories, insulin (preferred storage). Medications can be particularly difficult to manage in individuals who are homeless or living in marginal housing situations.

Impact of Drug Therapy on Pattern

The necessity of taking medication for whatever reason on a daily basis may cause the patient to believe that he or she is ill and dysfunctional. Certain drug side effects may impact upon the patient perception of his or her health and well-being. Psychotropic drugs cause many physical side effects (e.g., dystonias, akathisia, parkinsonism, anticholinergic side effects) that make these patients feel physically ill when the condition being treated is of a psychological or emotional nature. These side effects can interfere with the patient's agreement to continue with the drug therapy. Many antihypertensive drugs can produce side effects that may interfere with the patient's willingness to continue therapy for a condition that often is symptomless. Patients can feel ill from the drug and not from their illness.

Some drugs cause changes in appearance that can affect the patient's body image or self-image. For example, steroids cause moon face, and redistribution of fat to the upper torso. Cancer drugs cause loss of hair and changes in facial appearance.

---

2. NUTRITION-METABOLIC PATTERN:
"Pattern of food and fluid consumption relative to metabolic need and pattern indicators of local nutrient supply."

Impact of Pattern on Drug Therapy

Assessment of physical parameters related to this pattern provides valuable data for drug therapy. The patency of the gag reflex and the ability to swallow obviously impact upon the ability to take oral medications.

The patient's height, weight, and body mass are important for determining drug dosages. Some drugs are prescribed on basis of actual weight while others may be prescribed on the basis of dry weight. Weight loss and weight gain are important to determine in order to evaluate the need for adjustment of drug dosages. The amount of body fat may have implications for the distribution and therefore the dosing of fat-soluble drugs.

The patient's usual dietary pattern and timing of meals will provide data about when drug therapy should be scheduled, e.g., in conjunction with meals or at other times. The use of vitamins or other nutrients or supplements is important to know in terms of usual patterns and potential interactions.

Types of foods usually consumed will provide information about potential interactions with foods, e.g., intake of natural licorice and antihypertensive drugs, intake of certain foods with monoamine oxidase inhibitors (MAOIs) and potential interference of certain foods with anticoagulant therapy.

It is important to assess caffeine intake—not only the caffeine in coffee or tea but also in cola and other beverages, as well as in chocolate. The possible interference of caffeine with medications such as theophylline and sedatives and also its contribution to gastric irritation are of concern.

The amount and type of fluid intake may influence drug effects. Orally administered drugs will not dissolve as rapidly as expected unless given with an adequate amount of fluid. As a general rule, at least a half glass of water is preferred. Fluids other than water may cause interactions or alter gastric pH; the outcome depends on the particular drug. Giving an enteric-coated drug with milk or an antacid may result in the premature dissolution of the enteric coating in the stomach (rather than the alkaline pH of the small intestines), thus causing the gastric irritation or other side effects the enteric coating was meant to avoid.

Growth factors that occur during adolescence, menopause, and aging may indicate the need for adjustments in dosage of certain medications such as insulin or vitamins.

Impact of Drug Therapy on Pattern

Drugs may affect the nutrition-metabolic pattern by altering gastrointestinal function. Drugs, such as those with anticholinergic effects, cause drying of saliva, which can affect the ability to swallow tablets or food; these drugs also delay gastric emptying, which could increase the rate of absorption of acid drugs and delay the onset of action of alkaline drugs.

Drugs that cause nausea and/or vomiting as side effects can seriously affect the metabolic pattern. The cancer chemotherapy drugs are a major example; these drugs also cause stomatitis and mucositis that can severely impact on the patient's readiness to ingest food.

Some drugs may interfere with the absorption of nutrients. For example, the absorption of tetracyclines will be decreased if given with antacids or iron preparations. Thyroid drugs may increase or decrease the patient's general metabolic rate. Insulin and oral agents for diabetes mellitus have an intricate relationship with the amount, type, and timing of food intake.

Malnutrition can affect a patient's response to a wide variety of drugs. The decrease in serum protein (albumin) can result in highly protein-bound drugs having higher than expected levels of "free" drug. Patients with severe malnutrition usually cannot mount an adequate immune response, resulting in possible false-negative results with diagnostic tests such as tuberculin testing that rely on an intact immune response. Immunizations may be less effective.

---

3. ELIMINATION PATTERN: "Patterns of excretory function (bowel, bladder, skin)."

Impact of Pattern on Drug Therapy

Assessment of this pattern is important in order to establish the adequacy of the function of systems that are responsible for the excretion of drugs. In particular, since most drugs are excreted by the kidneys, it is essential to take renal function into account in selecting drugs as well as during the ongoing monitoring of drug therapy.

Renal function can be assessed through a variety of methods. Estimates of creatinine clearance are often used to estimate renal function and to serve as a basis for adjusting drug dosages if necessary. A 24-hour urine specimen can be used. More convenient for general purposes is the estimation of creatinine clearance from the serum creatinine level. (BUN is considered less reliable because it can be affected by a variety of other factors). In the elderly the serum creatinine level is less reliable as an indicator of renal function because of the normal reduction of muscle mass.

The following formula[2] is often used to estimate creatinine clearance:

$$\text{Creatinine clearance} = \frac{(140 - \text{age}) \times \text{lean weight (kg)}}{72 \times \text{serum creatinine}} \times 0.85 \text{ for females}$$

Lean weight is calculated as follows:

For males: 50 kg + 2.3 kg for each inch over 5 feet
For females: 45 kg + 2.3 kg for each inch over 5 feet

Another formula, which does not use weight, is the Jelliffe formula:[3]

$$\text{Creatinine clearance} = \frac{98 - 0.8 (\text{age} - 20)}{\text{serum creatinine}}$$

Drug elimination via the bowel occurs with some drugs. Elimination of drugs from the lungs occurs with alcohol and paraldehyde. Elimination of drugs through the skin often is not appreciated because it is not usually visible. Alcohol is eliminated from the skin. The anti-infective rifampin provides colorful evidence of its excretion by its orange discoloration of tears (it also can discolor contact lenses), perspiration, and urine.

It is important to know the patient's usual pattern of urinary and bowel elimination in the scheduling of diuretics and laxatives.

Impact of Drug Therapy on Pattern

Discoloration of the feces can be caused by drugs such as bismuth and iron. Diarrhea may be caused by superinfection of antibiotic therapy and may indicate adverse effects of antibiotics such as pseudomembranous colitis. Undiluted liquid KCl or large amounts of diet foods containing sorbitol can cause diarrhea by creating hyperosmolarity (diet food syndrome). Constipation can be caused by drugs with anticholinergic effects, calcium channel blockers, opioids, calcium- or aluminum-based antacids, and iron.

Urinary output may be increased directly by diuretics and indirectly by digitalis and other cardiotonics as they improve blood circulation to the kidneys. A patient's bowel and kidney elimination pattern can be also affected by the timing of administration of these drugs, as well as by pharmacokinetic variables. Urine discoloration can be caused by drugs such as phenolphthalein, pyridium, and rifampin, as well as by the dyes in many vitamin preparations.

4. ACTIVITY-EXERCISE PATTERN: "Pattern of exercise, activity, leisure, recreation."

Impact of Pattern on Drug Therapy

The amount and type of physical activity involved in the patient's daily life—either at work or as part of an exercise routine—can influence drug therapy. Assessment of a patient's usual patterns of exercise can provide clues to overall health-related lifestyle as well as detect any extremes. It could reveal the use of muscle-bulking agents and illicit use of anabolic steroids, which could alter drug pharmacokinetics.

Muscular aches and pains from exercise can lead to self-medication with NSAIDs and ASA, which can be the basis for gastric irritation and bleeding or renal dysfunction.

Exercise and insulin, drug, and diet therapy are intricately related in diabetes mellitus. The dosing regimen and planning of meals and snacks in relation to exercise are important.

Knowledge of patient's leisure and recreation preferences may be useful in motivating patients as well as devising diversional activities as might be desired in the management of chronic pain. Leisure activities such as travel or outdoor camping may indicate a need for certain immunizations or preventive drugs (e.g., for hepatitis A and B, tetanus, or malaria).

Impact of Drug Therapy on Pattern

Knowledge of the patient's work role and activities can alert the clinician to possible dangers of sedative side effects of drugs. For example, beta blockers may not be the preferred drug in individuals who participate in rigorous physical activity because of the "braking" effect on cardiac responsiveness.

Drugs may affect the coordination of movement and muscle activity, e.g., antipsychotics producing Parkinson-like changes, dystonias, and akathisias.

5. SLEEP-REST PATTERN: "Patterns of sleep, rest, and relaxation."

Impact of Pattern on Drug Therapy

This pattern is of special significance in determining the effects of circadian rhythm variations on drug therapy. The emerging fields of chronobiology and chronopharmacology are revealing differences in the effects of drugs given at different times of the day and night. The most well known is that of diurnal variation in blood steroid levels.

The peak blood steroid levels in the 24-hour cycle of a person who sleeps at night and is awake during the day occur in the 4 A.M. to 8 P.M. time period. Administration of exogenous pharmacological (above physiological replacement) doses during the early morning provides much less suppression of the hypophysis-pituitary-adrenal (HPA) axis and adrenal cortical function than when doses are given in the evening. An evening dose results in an additional time period of suppression of ACTH and the adrenal cortex and thus increases the probability of adrenal atrophy. If a person is a night worker, his or her diurnal variations may differ and a different dosing schedule may be needed in order to prevent adrenal atrophy.

The adequacy of sleep is best judged by the patient's perception of feeling rested rather than the hours of sleep. If sleep pattern disturbances are detected, careful assessment of environmental factors and of the patient's bedtime routine is necessary before recommending drug therapy. Drugs with CNS stimulating effects need to be given earlier if they are interfering with sleep (e.g., theophylline, Ritalin).

Impact of Drug Therapy on Pattern

Several drugs can affect the sleep pattern, and many of these have psychotropic effects (e.g., antianxiety, antipsychotic). Antidepressants often improve a disturbed sleep pattern (which is a common sign of depression). Alcohol and other CNS depressants can cause sedation and promote the onset of sleep; often, however, the sleep is not restful and may produce undesirable dreams.

CNS stimulants, including caffeine from diet sources as well as from the metabolic breakdown of theophylline, can affect sleep onset. The scheduling of theophylline too close to bedtime should be avoided if it interferes with sleep.

Rebound insomnia and daymares can occur after a patient has been using hypnotics. This is believed to result from the effect of the hypnotic in decreasing REM sleep; abrupt discontinuance of the hypnotic leads to rebound REM. Hypnotics also can affect this pattern through a hangover effect the next day.

---

6. COGNITIVE-PERCEPTUAL PATTERN: "Describes sensory-perceptual and cognitive patterns."

Impact of Pattern on Drug Therapy

Assessment of mental status, hearing and visual acuity, and language and reading skills, as well as learning style preferences, provides data useful in judging the patient's ability to manage his or her therapeutic regimen and how he or she can best be taught.

Short-term memory can be important in the patient's ability to remember to take medications and whether he or she has actually taken a particular dose.

Assessment of sensory pattern will provide data concerning perception and response to pain, either in the past or present.

Impact of Drug Therapy on Pattern

Many drugs can affect cognitive function in addition to CNS depressants, antidepressants, and psychotropics. Ritalin and amphetamines are drugs that enhance cognitive function in adults (and produce calming effects in hyperactive children).

Amnesia can result from many drugs, but of note is the amnesia that can occur with hypnotics with short half-lives (e.g., Halcion) and the intended amnesia from drugs administered as part of conscious sedation or monitored anesthesia care. This amnesia can extend backwards to a period of time prior to administration; therefore, patient teaching done just before a procedure may not be recalled by the patient.

Neuropathy (altered sensations or pain) can result from a variety of drugs such as various cancer chemotherapy agents or isoniazid (INH).

Ototoxicity can result in both hearing loss and damage to the vestibular branch of the eighth cranial nerve. Ataxia, dizziness, and tinnitus may be early signs. Antibiotics (e.g., aminoglycosides) and loop diuretics (e.g., furosemide, bumetanide) are commonly used drugs with this potential effect. Knowledge of a patient's impaired hearing might result in the choice of a different drug rather than risk a further loss of hearing. Assessment of hearing prior to the initiation of drugs with potential ototoxic effects can provide a baseline for evaluating hearing level during and after the course of the drug therapy.

Impaired vision may result from drugs producing mydriasis (e.g., atropine or anticholinergic drugs) or miosis (opiates). Other drugs may produce cataracts, glaucoma, or retinopathy.

---

7. SELF-PERCEPTION–SELF-CONCEPT PATTERN: "Describes self-concept pattern and perceptions of self, image, identity, general sense of worth, general emotional pattern."

Impact of Pattern on Drug Therapy

Patients' perception of themselves as well or ill can depend on their perception of the meaning of drug therapy. Patients with hypertension usually do not experience symptoms and do not see themselves as ill. Being on drug therapy can result in their changing their perception of themselves from being well to being ill; this could result in denial and a subsequent refusal to comply with the prescribed drug therapy.

Some patients do not wish to have others know that they have certain conditions and therefore may not want to take any medications that must be taken at work or school (e.g., patients with epilepsy). This may have implications for the choice of a particular drug or the use of the particular dosing schedule.

Assessment of a patient's emotional pattern and his or her usual ways of responding to life events may indicate the need for psychotropic drug therapy.

Impact of Drug Therapy on Pattern

Physical changes to body appearance, such as those that occur from steroid, cancer chemotherapy, and parkinsonian side effects and the extrapyramidal effects of antipsychotic drugs, can affect a person's body image and sense of self-worth.

Body and head hair can affect a person's image. Alopecia, moon facies, and facial hirsutism can occur with glucocorticosteroids. Local alopecia may occur with the use of birth control pills. Hair growth on the head, face, and/or other areas of the body can be an effect of minoxidil; whether this is desirable or not depends on why the minoxidil is used and where the hirsutism occurs.

Skin color changes also may affect self-image. Birth control pills may produce melasma—the "mask of pregnancy." Quinacrine can cause brown discoloration; yellow skin discoloration may indicate drug-induced jaundice (e.g., from INH or tetracycline). Gold injections and bismuth can cause gray or gray-blue discoloration.[4 (p4–6)]

Mood changes can occur with some drugs; generally any change in hormone levels produces changes in mood and emotional response.

---

8. ROLE-RELATIONSHIP PATTERN: "Pattern of role engagements and relationships, perceptions of major roles and responsibilities in current life situations."

Impact of Pattern on Drug Therapy

Assessment of the patient's family roles and responsibilities can provide an indication of the degree of responsibility taken for his or her own health as well as that of others. Caregiving responsibilities for both children and parents are important to assess in terms of providing expertise in caregiving and also as a source of stress to the patient. Stress and time involved in caregiving for others could result in unintentional noncompliance with therapeutic regimens. It is also important to assess the availability of caregivers for the patient in the event that he or she becomes unable to manage his or her therapeutic regimen. Assessment of family relationships can often provide clues to alcohol or drug abuse in the client and/or family.

Information about work activities can provide data about the potential influence of environmental agents on drug therapy (e.g., contact with insecticides). The location and timing of work activities may have implications for scheduling and administration of medications during work hours. Persons with diabetes and epilepsy, as well as others, may need to take medication routinely at work or school and need to work out the best way to do this in their particular setting.

Impact of Drug Therapy on Pattern

Assessment of occupation and work roles can provide important information for planning drug therapy. It is especially important to determine if any roles and responsibilities require alertness and quick judgment. This is of particular concern when prescribing drugs with sedating effects. Sometimes the sedation produced by many drugs as a side effect usually abates after two or three weeks. Clinicians need to warn patients about this sedation; many occupations require employees to report to their employers whenever they are taking any medications (e.g., bus drivers, pilots, etc.). All patients should be warned not to drive a car or operate any dangerous machinery until these effects have been determined or have abated.

---

9. SEXUALITY-REPRODUCTIVE PATTERN: "Patterns of satisfaction or dissatisfaction with sexuality; describes reproductive pattern."

Impact of Pattern on Drug Therapy

It is important to assess any methods of fertility control used (birth control drugs or drugs to enhance fertilization). Some women may forget to mention oral contraceptives as a medication unless specifically asked about this because they do not necessarily think of these drugs as medications. Knowledge of current reproductive status and methods of birth control is essential in order to determine the risk of any medication to a fetus at the present or in the future. The use of breastfeeding is important data in order to determine potential effects of a drug on a breastfeeding infant.

It is important to establish future reproductive intentions before initiating chemotherapy or other drug therapy that may affect male sperm production or female egg maturation. Some individuals may wish to arrange to preserve their sperm, ova, or fertilized ova for their future use before initiating certain drug therapies.

A drug used during pregnancy must be carefully chosen, balancing the risks and benefits to both the mother and fetus in light of what is known about a drug's teratogenicity (see Chap. 6).

Impact of Drug Therapy on Pattern

A number of drugs can affect sexual function (e.g., impotence, difficulty in achieving orgasm). Sexual dysfunction is a not uncommon side effect of several types of antihypertensive drugs; patients may be reluctant to discuss this problem or may not realize its possible relationship to the drug therapy.

Other drugs (e.g., antipsychotics) can alter a woman's menstrual cycle. Certain drugs may interfere with the effectiveness of oral contraceptives (e.g., antibiotics), necessitating the use of alternate methods of birth control during drug therapy. Secondary sex characteristics can be altered by adrenocorticosteroids and sex hormones (e.g., androgens given to women or estrogens to men). A prostaglandin analogue (misoprostol) used to prevent gastric ulceration in patients on NSAIDs can cause uterine contractions and could precipitate a miscarriage in a pregnant woman.

10. COPING–STRESS TOLERANCE PATTERN: "General coping pattern and effectiveness of the pattern in terms of stress tolerance."

Impact of Pattern on Drug Therapy

Assessment of the ways in which the patient usually handles stress can provide clues to possible self-medication with alcohol or other drugs (licit or illicit) to help handle stress.

Drug therapy itself should be assessed as a possible stressor—the degree to which it produces stress on the patient and the extent to which the patient is able to handle this stress. This may provide clues to the need to simplify drug regimens, especially in cases of polypharmacy, in which drugs are added to the regimen to deal with the side effects of another drug, often leading to a multiplicity of often unnecessary drugs.

Impact of Drug Therapy on Pattern

Antianxiety agents and other psychotropics obviously can alter emotional responses and reactions to stress.

Any drug causing sedation can interfere with a patient's immediate response to stress and ability to react to it. This can be a positive or negative effect, depending upon the situation and the intent of the drug therapy.

Adrenergic blockers block the effects of the sympathetic nervous system on target tissues and therefore alter many of the physiological reactions to stress; this is the basis for their use in treating hypertension as well as stage fright.

11. VALUE-BELIEF PATTERN: "Patterns of values, goals, or beliefs (including spiritual) that guide choices or decisions."

Impact of Pattern on Drug Therapy

Careful and sensitive assessment of this pattern can provide insights into patients' beliefs about the meaning of health, suffering, and illness, the causation of illness, and what will help or cure them. This information can help in designing an effective regimen that the patient will adhere to.

Certain religious beliefs and practices may affect a person's willingness to take certain medications. A Catholic may refuse to take oral contraceptives; a Jehovah's Witness may refuse a drug based on blood products; and an orthodox Jew may decline the use of insulin derived from pork.

The beliefs elicited in this pattern are closely related to the first pattern (health perception—health belief) providing a full circle of the patterns and demonstrating their interactive nature.

Impact of Drug Therapy on Pattern

A patient receiving drug therapy causing severe side effects may find this a challenge to his or her beliefs and expectations that the drug therapy will restore health. Long-term drug therapy, especially when the regimen is complex, may further test a patient's confidence in medical therapy as well as his or her beliefs about quality of life.

ASSESSMENT USING REVIEW OF SYSTEMS APPROACH

Another approach to obtaining information relevant to drug therapy is to use the review of systems (Table 4-1). Since this focuses primarily on physiological variables, psychosocial variables and family history are additional categories that also need to be assessed.

DRUG THERAPY AND PHYSICAL ASSESSMENT

Physical assessment is an integral part of any encounter of the clinician and the patient. The extent and focus of physical assessment depend on the circumstances. A brief and focused assessment may be done when monitoring specific aspects of a patient's ongoing drug and other therapy or when investigating a specific complaint. A general overall assessment is used in order to evaluate overall health status.

The drug therapy that a patient is receiving may impact on the findings of the physical assessment. The purpose of this section is to highlight the effects of commonly used drugs on physical examination findings. Some of these effects are interferences, i.e., they are drug side effects that might lead to a confused or perhaps erroneous or dangerous conclusion if the clinician does not realize that the effects were from the drug therapy. Not all of these effects are necessarily benign; many require some type of follow-up as to whether they are affecting the patient's quality of life or functioning or need to be treated to prevent further damage.

TABLE 4-1

Drug History: A Review of Systems Approach

Organ System	Symptoms	Drugs
General	Fever, fatigue, weight change, pain	Narcotic and non-narcotic analgesics, antibiotics, antipyretics
Mental status	Nervousness, sadness, insomnia, hallucinations, irritability, tension	Antidepressants, anti-psychotics, hypnotics, anxiolytics, stimulants
Integument	Rashes, dryness, itching, hair loss, dandruff	Antibiotics, antifungals, corticosteroids, anti-dandruff-antiseborrheics, anesthetics/antipruritics, cytotoxics, antivirals, anti-infestation agents, antiseptics/disinfectants
Head/face	Dizziness, fainting, seizures, headache	Antivertigo drugs, analgesics, anticonvulsants
Eyes	Redness, poor eyesight, pain, blurring, discharge, glaucoma, cataracts	Glaucoma drugs, mydriatics, cycloplegics, topical antibiotics, corticosteroids
Ears	Hearing loss, tinnitus, earache, discharge, excessive wax	Topical anti-infectives, ceruminolytics
Nose/sinuses	Colds, runny nose, hay fever, sinus problems	Antihistamines, cough and cold medicines, antiallergy drugs, nasal decongestants, topical corticosteroids
Mouth/pharynx	Sore throat, gum soreness or bleeding, dental problems, mouth ulcers, hoarseness	Antibiotics, cough and cold medicines, antihistamines, local anesthetics, decongestants, antiallergy drugs
Neck	Swollen lymph nodes, goiter, swollen glands, neck pain	Antithyroid drugs, thyroid hormones, antibiotics, analgesics
Chest/lungs	Dyspnea, wheezing, cough, asthma, bronchitis, emphysema, pneumonia, tuberculosis, hemoptysis	Beta-adrenergics, antibiotics, bronchodilators, corticosteroids, antihistamines, anticholinergics, antimycobacterial drugs, antitussives, expectorants

TABLE 4-1

Drug History: A Review of Systems Approach (continued)

Organ System	Symptoms	Drugs
Cardiovascular	Chest pain, hypertension, heart attacks, heart murmur, paroxysmal nocturnal dyspnea, orthopnea, palpitations, intermittent claudication, orthostatic hypotension	Beta-adrenergic blocking drugs, calcium channel blockers, angiotensin-converting enzyme inhibitors, antianginal drugs, antiarrythmic drugs, cardiac glycosides, antihypertensives, antihyperlipidemic agents, diuretics, anticoagulants, hemorrheologic agents, antiplatelets, thrombolytics
Abdomen	Swallowing problem, heartburn, diarrhea, constipation, nausea/vomiting, pain, vomiting blood, blood in stool, hemorrhoids, ascites, change in bowel habits	Antacids, H_2 blockers, laxatives, hemorrhoidal preparations, sucralfate, proton pump inhibitors, cholinergic drugs, antidiarrheal agents, anticholinergic/antispasmodic drugs
Urinary	Dysuria, frequency, urgency, pain, nocturia, dribbling, incontinence, polydipsia, bleeding, urinary retention, stones	Diuretics, antidiuretic hormone, potassium supplements, electrolyte supplements, anticholinergics, tricyclic antidepressant drugs, alpha-adrenergic drugs, cholinergic drugs, urolithiasic drugs
Genital-reproductive	*Female:* vaginal discharge, itching, menstrual problems, venereal diseases, hot flashes, premenstrual tension	Anticandidial products, birth control pills, hormone shots, estrogen replacement, progestins, topical antifungal agents, nonsteroidal anti-inflammatory drugs
	Male: itching, discharge, sores, testicular pain/swelling, poor libido	Antibiotics, hormones

TABLE 4-1

Drug History: A Review of Systems Approach (continued)

Organ System	Symptoms	Drugs
Musculoskeletal	Joint swelling, pain, deformities, redness, stiffness, limit of movement, gout, arthritis, backache, muscle cramps	Nonsteroidal anti-inflammatory drugs, immunosuppressants, hypouricemics
Neurologic	Fainting, blackouts, seizures, local weakness, numbness, tremors, tingling, walking problems, muscle wasting, spasm, stiffness, vertigo	Anticonvulsants, muscle relaxants, anticoagulants, antiparkinson agents, anticholinergics, antihistamines, antivertigo, antiemetics
Endocrine	Thyroid problems, diabetes mellitus, diabetes insipidus, Addison/Cushing disease	Adrenocortical hormones, thyroid hormones, insulin, oral hypoglycemic drugs, androgenic agents, estrogens

SOURCE: Reprinted by permission from *Physical Assessment: A Guide for Evaluating Drug Therapy*, by R. Leon Longe, Pharm.D. and Jon C. Calvert, M.D., Ph.D., edited by Lloyd Y. Young, Pharm.D., published by Applied Therapeutics, Inc., Vancouver, Washington, © 1994.

Since drugs can cause so many different adverse effects and may actually cause disease, it is sometimes difficult to make a clear distinction between interferences or inconvenient side effects and signs of actual *adverse* effects caused by a drug. Adverse effects of drugs and the approaches to monitoring them are discussed in Chap. 5.

Overall General Assessment

Observing the patient as he or she walks into a room can give clues to ataxia and other gait disturbances that may be a result of such drugs as ototoxics (e.g., antibiotics, loop diuretics), tardive dyskinesia (antipsychotics), or peripheral neuropathy (e.g., INH).

As the clinician begins to interact with the patient, clues to mental status and the mental and physical ability to follow directions can be assessed as the examination progresses.

Facies

Masklike: may indicate pseudoparkinsonism from antipsychotics
Cushingoid moon face, buffalo hump, trunkal fat deposits: may indicate the patient is on steroid therapy
Smacking of lips, gyrations of tongue, grimacing: may indicate tardive dyskinesia

Skin

Skin eruptions are commonly caused by drugs and may indicate allergic responses. Drug therapy should always be considered as a possible cause of any skin eruption.

Discoloration of skin:
    Dark hyperpigmentation: chlorpromazine
    Jaundice: may be from drug-induced liver damage or from drug-induced cholestasis (phenothiazines, INH, tetracycline)
    Brown: quinacrine
    Gray: deposition of metallic salts such as silver, gold, and bismuth

Hair:

Alopecia: steroids, male hormones (male pattern baldness), cancer chemotherapy
Patches of hair growth: minoxidil, oral contraceptives
Pigmentation ("melasma of pregnancy"): oral contraceptives
Dryness: anticholinergics, other drugs with anticholinergic side effects (e.g., psychotropics)
Bruising: anticoagulants, aspirin, steroids, any drugs causing bone marrow depression (antibiotics, cancer chemotherapy)
Thinning, striae, and darkening of skin: steroids
Scarring, needle tracks: cue to drug abuse
Contact dermatitis: from direct skin contact with drug or chemicals (e.g., aminoglycosides)
Acne: suggests changes in sex hormone levels
Livedo reticularis (reddish-blue netlike pattern)[1] amantadine
Yellow or orange stain on soles or palms: isotretinoin, rifampin, or excessive ingestion of foods rich in carotene
Red neck syndrome or red man syndrome; rapid infusion of vancomycin or codeine
Darkening of nails: cancer chemotherapy
Oncholysis: tetracycline, doxorubicin, captopril
Tophi: thiazides (from increased uric acid causing deposits in skin)

Eyes/Vision

Exophthalmos and lid edema: steroids
Dryness of eyes: anticholinergics, sympathomimetics
Corneal deposits: from heavy metals such as gold and silver
Lens deposits: from use of phenothiazine
Cataracts: steroids, drugs given to treat gallstones
Primary-angle closure: glaucoma can be induced by atropine-like drugs; ibuprofen; prolonged topical steroid therapy can increase intraoptical pressure
Retinopathy: antimalarials, phenothiazines
Blurred vision: anticholinergics, certain antihistamines and certain antibiotics
Mydriasis (enlarged pupils): from atropine or other drugs given locally for purpose of causing mydriasis (as before eye exam) or as side effect of atropine or other drugs with atropine-like anticholinergic side effects

Miosis (pinpoint pupils): opioid drugs; exposure to drugs with cholinergic effects, e.g., pilocarpine, bethanechol, neostygmine, physostigmine

Impairment of night vision: pilocarpine

Nystagmus: hydantoin (Dilantin)

Toxic ambylopia: digitalis preparations, high doses of nicotinic acid

Diplopia: acetophenazine, oral contraceptives

Color disturbances: may occur as result of digitalis therapy (yellow scotomotor); ethambutol may cause loss of green vision

Ears/Hearing

Drugs may affect either or both branches of the eighth cranial nerve (acoustic or vestibular), affecting hearing and/or vestibular function. It is important to assess in a patient receiving an ototoxic drug that is excreted by the kidneys: Ototoxic drugs include aminoglycoside antibiotics (e.g., streptomycin, gentamycin, kanamycin), loop diuretics (e.g., furosemide, bumetanide, ethacrynic acid); vancomycin (even if only topical administration), chloroquine, quinine, quinidine, and phenylbutazone.

Drug effects on the vestibular function can be assessed through Romberg's test; finger-to-nose test. Ataxia and imbalances are early signs of vestibular dysfunction. The clinician also should check for nystagmus. If the patient is taking antiemetics or a drug with an antiemetic side effects, this could interfere with the testing of vestibular function.

Vital Signs

Blood pressure (orthostatic hypotension): antihypertensives, diuretics

Increased blood pressure: drugs causing sodium and fluid retention; beta blockers blunt or prevent the reflex tachycardia normally present on standing[4]

Nose

Inflamed nasal membranes: cocaine use, neosynephrine, high levels of female sex hormones

Rhinitis medicamentosus (dry red nasal mucosa): abuse of decongestants

Mouth

Bleeding gums: anticoagulants

Blue-black gum margins: bismuth therapy

Overgrowth of gums (gingival hyperplasia): hydantoin, excessive oral contraceptives

Dry mouth: anticholinergics

Stomatitis: cancer chemotherapy

Candida: anti-infective or immunosuppressive therapy

Hairy tongue: overgrowth of fungi from antibiotic therapy

Discoloration of teeth: tetracycline, liquid iron preparations

Taste:

　　Metallic taste: oral hypoglycemics

　　Garlic taste: dimethyl sulfoxide (DMSO)

　　Partial or total loss of taste: penicillamine

　　Taste disturbances: lithium, certain TB drugs

Lymph Nodes

Generalized enlargement: can occur from mediastinal effects of hydantoins, PAS, or phenylbutazone

Breasts

Gynecomastia: cimetidine, adrenocorticosteroids, androgens, cardiac glycosides, oral contraceptives, vincristine, reserpine, INH, phenothiazines, spironolactone, marijuana, antihypertensives, tranquilizers, antidepressants, amphetamines

Galactorrhea: psychotropic medications, oral contraceptives, morphine, heroin, metoclopramide

Cardiac

Many drugs cause cardiac effects detectable by physical examination. Most of these are adverse effects of the drugs or extensions of their pharmacological effects (e.g., slowing of heart rate from digitalis glycosides or beta-adrenergic blockers).

Respiratory

Cough: ACE inhibitors

Beta blockers, especially those that are considered to be noncardiac-selective can produce wheezing and other indications of bronchial constriction

Wheezing and other signs and symptoms of asthma: allergic response triggered by drug therapy

Abdomen

Epigastric distress can be a result of reflux of drugs from the stomach into the lower esophagus. This can occur as a result of swallowing a pill or tablet and lying down immediately. The patient should be taught not to lie down for at least a half hour after taking drugs. Epigastric distress can also result from any drugs causing gastric irritation. Nausea, vomiting, and diarrhea can be an indication of a reaction to almost any drug. Bleeding from the upper GI tract can be the result of use of ASA, NSAIDs, steroid therapy, or anticoagulant therapy.

Examination of the liver should be done routinely on all patients on oral contraceptive therapy because of the potential development of liver tumors. Jaundice may be the result of drug-induced liver damage (e.g., INH, PAS, chlorpromazine) or cholestasis (e.g., Elavil, chloramphenicol thiazides, thorazine). Observe for scratching from pruritus caused by jaundice. It may be necessary to use a different type of lighting since fluorescent lighting will not reveal excessive bile pigmentation in the skin.

Bowel sounds may be decreased by anticholinergic drugs, opioid drugs, or any drug causing hypokalemia (e.g., thiazide or loop diuretics). Hyperactive bowels sounds and diarrhea may be the results of superinfection from broad-spectrum antibiotics. Redness from scratching in the anal area may be due to pruritis ani caused by breakdown products of tetracyclines.

Kidney/Bladder

Hematuria: crystallization from sulfa drugs

Smoky bloody urine: may indicate low grade hematuria

Distended bladder: possible side effect of anticholinergic drugs (constriction of urinary sphincter)

Extremities

Edema: beta blockers, lithium

Neurological

Drug-related cerebellar toxicity: alcohol, phenytoin

Tardive dyskinesia: antipsychotic drugs

Dystonias, akathesia extrapyramidal side effects, parkinsonian syndrome: antipsychotics

Peripheral neuropathy (drug-induced neuropathy usually expresses itself as palsies, paresthesia, or fasciculations): can be caused by many antibacterial and antitubercular agents and antidepressants such as MAOIs and tricyclic antidepressants; a decrease in Achilles' tendon reflex may indicate the beginning of peripheral neuropathy.

CASE ANALYSIS: DRUG THERAPY AND PATIENT DATA INTERRELATIONSHIPS

The following case analysis is intended to illustrate how assessment data can be used in planning, monitoring, and evaluating current and future drug therapy. The case uses the Functional Health Pattern approach; it is missing some data that are relevant. Before reading the analysis following the case, the reader may wish to first analyze the case by circling or underlining information relevant to drug therapy or by adding data to be elicited from the patient.

CASE

C. G. (Adapted from a case by Kathleen McWha)

Demographic/Personal Information

Initials: C. G. Age: 53 years. Current residence: Massachusetts. Place of birth: Rhode Island. Marital status: single. Highest grade achieved: college graduate. Vocational status: floral manager. Medical diagnoses: hypertension, hypercholesterolemia, post-CVA.

History of Present Illness

Spring (5 years ago): Sought medical attention because writing became smaller and was unable to arrange flowers with left hand. Client knew what to do but physically could not perform the actions. Blood pressure at that time: 225/120.

Was hospitalized with diagnosis of CVA and placed on Tenoretic 50 mg PO daily and Klor-Con 1 tab PO daily.

Fall (5 years ago): Joined health club. Complained of numbness of mouth. Hospitalized with diagnosis of TIA post-CVA. Placed on IV therapy with potassium for 2 days. Discharged on Tenoretic 50 mg PO daily and Klor-Con 10 1 tab PO daily. BP stable at 130/76.

Past 4 years: Regular primary care clinic visits every 6 months.

Three months ago: medication changed to Tenormin 100 mg PO daily, niacin 3000 mg PO tid; and Bufferin 500 mg daily. Continues with regular primary care visits every 6 months.

Functional Health Pattern Assessment

Health Perception–Health Belief Pattern: Maintains medication regimen. No known variables preventing health maintenance at this time. No colds within the past year. Walks 4 miles daily for exercise. Smokes one-half pack of cigarettes daily and drinks socially. Unable to define specific illness. Seeks health care for alteration in perceived health status.

Nutrition–Metabolic Pattern: Eats 3 meals daily. Maintains a "fat-free" low-cholesterol diet of 2200 k-cal daily. Eats red meat 2 times per month. Drinks 5 glasses of water and 2 cups of coffee daily. No weight loss or gain, or loss of height. Appetite is good. No food or eating discomfort or swallowing difficulty. No skin lesions; skin is dry. Heals well. Last cholesterol: 252.

Elimination Pattern: Daily bowel elimination. No discomfort. Brown soft stool. No incontinence or laxative use. No elimination problems. Control good. Urine clear, without odor.

Activity–Exercise Pattern: States he has sufficient energy for desired activity. Regular walking 4 miles daily. Hobbies include: swimming, vacation, boating, dancing, cooking, and arranging flowers.

Sleep-Rest Pattern: Generally rested and ready for activities after sleep. No sleep onset problems. Does not use aids. Does not take rests or relaxation periods except for vacations and days off.

Cognitive-Perceptual Pattern. No hearing difficulties. Does not use hearing aid. Wears glasses for decreased vision in right eye. Short-term memory loss. At times unable to locate car in parking lot. No difficulty in learning.

Self-Perception—Self-Concept Pattern: Client states "most times I am well and feel good about myself." Client states that the following residual effects from his illness do not present a problem to him: If he is quiet and there is a sudden noise, he has no control over his left hand and his arm will fly to the side; weakness on left side when lifting; and handwriting is not as neat.

Role-Relationship Pattern: Client lives with 80-year-old mother who is independent in ADL. Their relationship is good. His mother depends on him to drive her to doctor's appointments, shopping, and household maintenance. Client states, "I have quality friends to socialize with." He enjoys his work and relates well to his co-workers.

> *Sexuality–Reproductive Pattern*: Client states that he has no problems and is not involved.
>
> *Coping–Stress Tolerance Pattern*: There have been no major changes in client's life during past year. Client states, "I have family members and close friends available when I need to talk things over, and a network of support is available to me. There are no big problems."
>
> *Value-Belief Pattern*: Client states, "I generally get what I want out of life and am looking forward to my niece's wedding. Religion is a big part of my life."

Screening Examination

Well-groomed, neat, and clean appearance. Oral and mucous membrane is pink and intact with no lesions. Client has natural teeth, no dentures, and no missing teeth. Hearing is good. Wears glasses. Pulse: 70 regular rhythm and strong. Respirations: 24, deep regular rhythm. No abnormal breath sounds. BP: 126/70. T: 99 PO.

Hand grasp is weaker on the left side. Can pick up pencil. Writes, eats, and places flowers with left hand; cuts and performs other activities with right hand.

Skin is dry. No color changes or lesions. Gait is normal. Posture is good, and there are no absent body parts.

Functional ability: full self-care. Weight: 184 lbs. Height: 5 ft, 6.5 in. Oriented to time, place, and person. Able to grasp ideas and questions clearly. Speaks English. Speech and voice pattern are clear. Eye contact is present with normal attention span.

Analysis of Case C.G. *by Amy Borden*

Demographic/Personal Information

Age is a factor in deciding which drug to prescribe because of the potential impact of the physiological changes of aging on drug kinetics and dynamics. Marital status is important, because a partner may be included in teaching about the drug, side effects, and toxic effects. The educational level is a factor to consider in the method of teaching about the drug, the depth of detail of information taught, and the simple and technical language used. The medical diagnosis is important in deciding the drug therapy and results desired. It is indicated that the patient had hypertension post-CVA: therefore, an antihypertensive is indicated. The hypercholesteremia is important, since it may be a contributing factor to atherosclerosis, which is a risk factor for cardiovascular accident (CVA) and hypertension (HTN).

Missing information from the nursing history is a complete review of the symptoms, past medical history, current drug therapy, or OTC medications used. These are very important pieces of information, because Tenoretic should be used cautiously with patients with asthma (even though it contains Tenormin, a cardioselective B_1 receptor blocker, it may also affect B_2 receptors in the respiratory tract). Tenoretic is metabolized in the liver and is excreted by the kidneys, so it should be used cautiously if a patient has liver or kidney dysfunction, and the dosage may need to be reduced. Since Tenoretic causes a reduced heart rate, it is contraindicated in patients with bradycardia. The pulse is especially important to monitor throughout therapy. Also, the patient's *allergies* are not identified.

It is important to identify the patient's allergies because hypersensitivity to sulfonamide drugs may be predictive of possible hypersensitivity to Tenoretic. In addition, the history should include any history of anaphylactic reactions to a variety of allergens because they have a more severe reaction on repeated challenge, either accidental, diagnostic or therapeutic. While taking a beta blocker, a patient may be unresponsive to the usual dose of epinephrine used to treat the allergic reaction.

Also missing are the other medications (OTC drugs too), which are important since drug interactions could occur. A complete baseline blood profile is missing, such as CBC, electrolytes, BUN and creatinine, glucose, and liver enzymes. These values need to be monitored because Tenoretic is a combination of atenolol (the beta blocker) and chlorthalidone (the thiazide derivative). The chlorthalidone component can cause and increase loss of water, potassium, magnesium, and sodium, the most important of these being potassium and magnesium. The Tenormin component may contribute to hypoglycemia or hyperglycemia.

The information taught to the patient is missing, and the patient's understanding of side effects, adverse reactions, and potential electrolyte imbalances is not presented. This can be vital because a toxic reaction or adverse reaction could be detected early, and medical intervention should be initiated before permanent problems occur. (Adverse effects include difficulty breathing, cold hands or feet, mental depression, skin rash, swelling of the ankles, feet, or legs, slow pulse, headache, dizziness, nausea or vomiting, diarrhea, unusual tiredness or weakness, disturbed sleep, decreased sexual ability, and hypotension.)

The history of the present illness is too brief, with no indication of the cause of CVA (hemorrhagic, embolic, thrombolytic) and no information about any similar previous events. Missing is information on the suddenness of the episode or if a headache was experienced, and the complete neurologic exam is missing. The drug treatment is markedly different if there is an infarct versus hemorrhage or embolus. If there is an infarct, anticoagulants may be indicated; if there is a hemorrhage, medication to control hypertension and diuretics to control intracranial pressure may be indicated initially. If an embolus is present, pursuit of the source, possibly cardiac, may indicate the need for an antiarrhythmic.

The physical symptoms are important, and any residual deficits should be indicated because they may impact upon the patient's ability to understand the drug therapy and his ability to take the medication as prescribed.

It is important to know that he was prescribed Klor-Con daily, yet when admitted with numbness of the mouth and a diagnosis of TIA, his K+ level must have been low because of reported IV potassium administration. This brings into question whether or not he was taking his medication as prescribed; if he wasn't, this may have contributed to having TIA and hypokalemia. Missing data, again, are the other electrolyte levels and the complete vital sign report (especially heart rate).

In October of 1990 his medication was changed to Tenormin 100 mg daily (therefore, the diuretic component of Tenoretic is no longer a concern, and there is no further need for Klor-Con supplements) with the niacin 3000 mg ordered. This suggests a continued problem with hypercholesterolemia, since niacin causes a decreased plasma cholesterol and triglycerol. The lab data are missing, such as the cholesterol level and ratio of HDL to LDL. The Bufferin is important because it could be prescribed to decrease the flushing that is a common side effect of niacin therapy, or it may be used for its anticoagulant properties. Missing is the review of symptoms, lab values, and vital signs at each entry of clinic visits.

Health Perception–Health Belief Pattern

The importance of maintaining the medication regime is highlighted because treatment with blockers must never be stopped quickly, since rapid withdrawal may precipitate cardiac arrhythmias. One factor that could be considered is whether the Tenormin is contributing to the hypercholesterolemia, because one adverse effect of the drug is that triglycerol levels may increase. It is important that he walks 4 miles daily for exercise because exercise is important in cardiovascular conditioning and in reducing high blood pressure. The fact that he smokes a half a pack of cigarettes daily is significant, because it is a serious risk factor for HTN and needs to be addressed with the patient. The nicotine could also interact with his beta blocker and cause adverse effects. Missing information is the amount of alcohol consumed while taking atenolol. It is of concern that he is "unable to define specific illness," because his HTN has had serious consequences, and he is taking a medication with potentially serious side effects and adverse reactions. There needs to be more information as to whether a residual cognitive impairment is the cause of his lack of awareness or denial or is due to a lack of exposure to the information. It is also noted that he "seeks health care for alterations in perceived health status;" if he is unaware of the specifics of his illness and drug therapy, it could mean that he seeks health care too late. He needs to understand fully the potential adverse reactions of his drug therapy and which of these indicate the need to seek medical advice. He should be monitoring his pulse at home and notifying the health care provider if his pulse slows to 50 bpm or slower, even if he is feeling well. (This could prevent the potential adverse reaction of cardiac failure due to Tenormin.)

Nutrition-Metabolic Pattern

It is important that he is following a reduced-fat and low-cholesterol diet, because this will help to reduce his cholesterol level and he may no longer need the niacin therapy in the future. Missing are the nutritive values of his meals (the report only states "three meals daily"), with information about his vitamin, mineral, daily supplement intake. His plasma proteins should be drawn, because the protein binding of the drug may be reduced if he is protein-deficient. His hematocrit level would indicate whether he is getting sufficient iron, since fish and poultry are high in protein, but lower in iron than red meat. It is not mentioned whether or not he is on a low-sodium diet; a low-sodium diet could help to lower his BP. This diet combined with exercise, a decrease in alcohol intake, cessation of smoking, weight loss, and stress reduction could decrease his need for drug therapy, or possible require a decreased dose of Tenormin. His coffee consumption is important, because caffeine is a drug that could interfere with the drug therapy. It is highlighted that he has had no weight loss or gain; this could affect the dosage of medication required (if he had a significant change in weight) and could indicate CHF if a sudden weight gain occurs. He should monitor his own intake and output and weigh himself daily, with the awareness of this serious potential adverse reaction.

"Appetite is good" also indicates that anorexia and nausea are side effects not experienced. "No food or eating discomfort" or "swallowing difficulty" is important, because potential side effects are agranulocytosis, weakness, aching, sore throat, laryngospasm, and dry mouth. "No skin lesions and healing capacity is good" is important, because it suggests that the patient has good nutritional status and is not experiencing adverse effects from Bufferin, such as bleeding problems. The last cholesterol level of 252 is important because it indicates that it is still elevated (greater than 200), but missing data are the baseline level and HDL/LDL ratio. This is important in determining whether or not the niacin therapy and low-cholesterol diet have been beneficial. There should be information about when he takes his medication in relation to his meals, since it is absorbed best when taken one hour before meals, or at bedtime.

Elimination Pattern

It is important to note that his bowel movements are normal with soft, brown stool because this indicates that he is not having the potential adverse reaction to Tenormin of diarrhea or constipation, or to the Bufferin of GI bleeding. Testing the stool for occult blood would be beneficial to indicate GI bleeding. Also, a side effect of niacin is gastric disturbances, which are not apparent.

Activity-Exercise Pattern

Since he says that "he has sufficient energy for desired activity," this indicates that he is not having the side effects of tiredness, fatigue, lethargy, or depression from Tenormin. It also supports that he is getting sufficient kilocalories for activities on his low-fat, 2200-calorie diet. His "regular walking 4 miles/a day" indicates that he is constantly getting cardiovascular exercise, which is good for lowering BP, and has the energy and motivation to be active in his health care.

Sleep-Rest Pattern

It is important that he reports that he feels "generally rested" and has no trouble with onset of sleep, because a side effect of Tenormin could be insomnia, or drowsiness, which he does not report having. It is noted that he does "not rest or take relaxation periods"; such periods might contribute to stress reduction as a component of reducing BP, and this might not be recognized by the patient. Missing data are the number of hours spent sleeping per night and the amount of dreaming experienced. Tenormin can cause increased dreaming as a side effect.

Cognitive-Perceptual Pattern

"Wears glasses for decreased vision in right eye" is significant, because this could be a deficit from the CVA, or an unrelated problem, and also could impact his ability to take his medication. His eye exam should be noted, and whether or not this impairment impacts his functioning. "Short-term loss" is important; details are missing about whether this is a deficit related to the CVA, or if it is new in onset. If new, it could be due to ischemia to the cerebrum and needs to be investigated.

Having a short-term memory loss could impact his ability to recognize signs of adverse drug reactions or to remember whether he took his daily dose. He could either inadvertently abruptly stop his medication, which could cause heart failure, or could overdose and become toxic, and not remember that his symptoms are serious. "Sometimes things make me angry and annoyed" seems to contradict his statement that his life is not affected by the residual effects of his CVA. More details need to be included about what "things" make him angry, because he could possibly be having adverse reactions to his medications that he hasn't identified, and these can be addressed.

Role-Relationship Pattern

Missing are more specifics about the work that he does, because this could be significant in the management of his drug therapy (whether he works irregular hours and doesn't consistently take his medication, and if he has health benefits and has any trouble obtaining his medications).

Sexuality-Reproductive Pattern

The client should be more specifically asked if he is experiencing impotence or diminished libido, because these are side effects of Tenormin, and are also side effects of HTN.

Coping–Stress Tolerance Pattern

It is noted that he has family and close friends for support, which is often a factor in success with maintaining stress reduction and medical therapy. Missing data are what his significant others' roles are in assisting him with the lifestyle to decrease risk factors, and how aware they are of his hypertension and medication effects.

Value-Belief Pattern

There is nothing about whether the patient believes that the drug therapy is effective, or anything about his beliefs about preventive care, such as alterations in lifestyle (stopping smoking, decrease in ETOH, exercise, diet, stress reduction). This could impact his future need for Tenormin and niacin because often BP medication does not have to be forever, especially when lifestyle changes can drastically lower BP. Also, his perception about when to seek medical attention could seriously impact the chances of another CVA or hypertensive episode.

Screening Examination

It is important that his pulse is 70, regular rhythm and strong, respirations are 24, deep and regular, and BP is 126/70. This is evidence that the drug therapy has been effective, without causing adverse reactions (such as bradycardia and respiratory bronchospastic effects). There seems to be no change in his functional ability, with the residual left-handed weakness apparent earlier.

It is important that his gait is normal since an adverse reaction to Tenormin is dizziness, vertigo, and ataxia. Missing from the report is orthostatic BP, which is important because beta blockers can cause postural hypotension. Also missing is whether or not he has any pain, such as headaches or leg pain, which also could be due to the beta blocker.

His weight of 184 lb and height of 5 ft 6 in. are significant in evaluating his drug dosages, and also in whether it is recommended that he lose weight. This seems to be much more than the ideal body weight for a man his height, unless he is very muscular (a triceps skinfold test could make the data more complete). Weight loss, if necessary, could impact his future need for BP medication.

A more thorough neurological exam would be beneficial, with the results of a tool such as the minimental status examination (MMSE) to evaluate his ability to "grasp ideas clearly." All systems could potentially be affected adversely by his drug regime. Therefore, a thorough systems examination, especially cardiac and pulmonary, should be done. Tests such as a baseline EKG, chest X-ray, electrolytes, and complete blood cell count levels would add more information about adverse reactions.

REFERENCES

1. Gordon M: *Nursing Diagnosis*. St. Louis: Mosby, 1994.
2. Cockcroft DW, Gault MH: Prediction of creatinine clearance from serum creatinine. *Nephron* 16:31, 1976.
3. Jelliffe RW: Creatinine clearance: Bedside estimate. *Ann Intern Med* 79:604, 1973.
4. Longe RL, Calvert JC: *Physical Assessment: A Guide for Evaluating Drug Therapy*. Vancouver, WA: Applied Therapeutics, 1994.

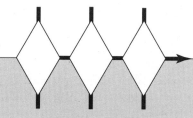

Chapter 5

MONITORING AND EVALUATION OF DRUG THERAPY: THERAPEUTIC EFFECTIVENESS, SIDE EFFECTS, AND INTERACTIONS

Laurel A. Eisenhauer

EVALUATING DRUG EFFECTIVENESS

Once a patient is taking a prescribed drug, the clinician must monitor for effectiveness as well as for the development of side effects. The clinician also needs to continue to evaluate the patient for changes in his or her condition that might affect drug pharmacokinetics or pharmacodynamics.

In order to evaluate effectiveness of a drug, the therapeutic goals and the goals of the drug therapy must be clear. The clinician, in conjunction with the client, needs to establish goals. For example: Is the drug therapy intended to control a symptom or is it intended to cure a disease?

The outcomes of drug therapy need to be stated in measurable terms. In some conditions certain markers are used as the outcome measure instead of the direct measurement of the degree of control of a disease. Surrogate measures themselves do not indicate the benefit to the patients but are thought to correlate with them and lead to a clinical benefit.[1] Examples include blood pressure for hypertension or arteriosclerosis; blood glucose for control of diabetes mellitus, viral load measures in HIV-infected patients, or peak expiratory flow rate (PEFR) for evaluating degree of control of asthma.

Assessing for drug effectiveness is an integral part of ongoing professional judgment and also can prevent any unnecessary exposure of a patient to adverse effects of a drug. Continuing a drug when it is no longer necessary for control of the condition for which it is prescribed, e.g., antibiotics taken beyond the point of control of an infection and prolonged or unnecessary use of adrenocorticosteroids after control of allergic response or remission of a condition such as arthritis, can cause adverse effects.

The effects of some types of drugs can be evaluated only through subjective measures such as patient reports. Visual analogue scales for patients to rate their level of pain or nausea have been useful both in clinical practice and in research to establish the degree of effectiveness of therapeutic regimens.

MONITORING FOR COMPLIANCE/ ADHERENCE TO DRUG AND THERAPEUTIC REGIMEN

Various techniques have been proposed and studied to determine whether or not patients take medications as prescribed. Some of these techniques are frequency of refills and/or requests for new prescriptions, actual counts of pills, and special containers or devices that record the number of times and/or actual time that a drug container has been opened.

Usually, the most effective approach is to simply ask the patient. Questioning is usually more effective if directed toward how he or she takes the medications rather than directly asking, "Do you take your medications?" Especially with patients on multiple drugs, it is very helpful to ask them to bring in all the medications they are taking from all prescribers and any OTC medicines and herbs. Patients sometimes have to be specifically asked or reminded to include oral contraceptives, vitamin pills, or herbal preparations since they may not think of them as "medications."

MONITORING SERUM LEVELS OF DRUGS

Monitoring of serum levels of a drug is used primarily to determine the need for dosage adjustment. Because of the wide variations in therapeutic responses to a drug dose, drug serum levels rarely reflect the efficacy of a drug in a particular patient.

Serum levels have become increasingly available for more drugs; however, in practice they usually are used only for drugs with a low therapeutic index, that is, where there is a narrow range between the effective and toxic serum levels (e.g., lithium, digoxin, theophylline, phenytoin, aminoglycosides). Serum levels should not be obtained just because the test is available. Assays also may be helpful in helping to determine if noncompliance is the basis for therapeutic failures (see Table 5-1). Monitoring of drug serum levels may also be useful when factors that may affect normal pharmacokinetics are present, such as drug interactions or liver or kidney disease.

The timing of measurement of drug serum levels is of concern in ensuring that the value obtained will provide meaningful and accurate information for adjusting doses. Serum monitoring is of most help when trying to determine the need to adjust the dose. For most drugs, taking the sample just before the next dose (trough level) provides the

TABLE 5-1

Criteria for Assaying Drugs in Blood, Serum, or Plasma

1. There must be a demonstrated relationship between the concentration of the drug in the plasma and the eventual therapeutic effect that is desired and/or the toxic effect that must be avoided.
2. There should be substantial interpatient variability in the disposition of the drug (and small intrapatient variation). Otherwise, concentrations of drug in plasma could be predicted from dose alone.
3. It should be difficult to monitor intended or unintended effects of the drug. Whenever clinical effects or minor toxicity are measured easily (e.g., the effect of a drug on blood pressure), such assessments should be preferred in the decision to make any necessary adjustment of dosage of drug.
4. The concentrations of drug required to produce therapeutic effects should be close to the value that causes substantial toxicity.

SOURCE: Nies and Spielberg.[2]

most accurate data. If the serum level is within the therapeutic range, the patient can be considered to be receiving therapeutic doses. Taking serum levels too soon after administration may result in a level that seems higher that it actually is because the drug may not yet have distributed from the blood to the other body tissues. If done too soon after a dose, the serum level obtained may not reflect total absorption of the drug (will be falsely "low") or may reflect the first surge of distribution when the drug is more concentrated in the blood before it further distributes to other organs and tissues (will be falsely "high").

RULE OF THUMB: Measure drug serum levels well after the previous dose or just before the next planned dose (exceptions would be drugs that are virtually totally eliminated between doses).[3]

RULE OF THUMB: Since a toxic drug could produce deleterious effects before the next dose, a useful rule of thumb is to take the first sample after two half-lives. If this is above 90 percent of level expected eventually, then the dosage rate should be halved and then another sample obtained after two half-lives. If the concentration remains too high, the dose would again be halved.[3]

Appendix B provides information on the therapeutic range, peak time of acting, and toxic levels of several drugs. Data to be provided to the laboratory along with the serum sample include drug name, daily dosage, route of administration, time administered, time when blood sample was obtained, and age of patient.

MONITORING FOR
ADVERSE EFFECTS

No drug available today has only one effect; therefore, all drugs have side effects. (With future forms of drugs, such as with use of monoclonal antibodies, the targeting or specificity of drug effects on particular tissues may become possible.) Therefore, the clinician needs to monitor for drug side effects as well as for the intended therapeutic effect.

Definitions

Various terms are used to describe drug side effects. A *side effect* is any effect other than the intended therapeutic effect; the intended therapeutic effect depends on a particular condition for which it is prescribed and the expected therapeutic outcome. The same drug effect may be either an intended therapeutic effect or a side effect in different patients, depending on the intended outcome. Sometimes this will vary according to the dose (e.g., 1 tsp or 4 cc of milk of magnesia for antacid effect versus an ounce or 30 cc for a laxative effect) or the route (e.g., diazoxide given PO for hypoglycemia versus IV diazoxide for treatment of acute hypertension).

Differences in terminology to describe side effects usually reflect degrees of the alteration produced. In some references, *side effects* are considered to be expected effects and are treated only if they are bothersome to the patient or cause noncompliance.

The terms *adverse reactions* or *adverse drug effects* usually reflect that a drug produces serious effects. Definitions of adverse drug effects vary (Table 5-2). These definitions exclude overdosage from suicide or accidental exposure or failure of the drug to have the intended effect.

TABLE 5-2

Definitions of Adverse Drug Reactions or Adverse Drug Effects

- Any response to a drug which is noxious and unintended, and which occurs at doses normally used in man for prophylaxis, diagnosis, or therapy of disease, or for the modification of physiological function.[4]
- Any response to a drug which is noxious and unintended, and that occurs at doses used in humans for prophylaxis, diagnosis, or therapy, excluding failure to accomplish the intended purpose.[5]
- Any drug-induced noxious change in a patient's condition that occurs at normal dosages and that (1) requires treatment, (2) indicates decrease or cessation of therapy with the drug, or (3) suggests that future therapy with the drug poses an unusual risk to the patient.[6]

Adverse events reported to FDA, however, include events beyond these definitions, such as:[6]

1. Overdosage, either accidental or intentional
2. Drug abuse
3. Withdrawal of drug
4. Any significant adverse events occurring from failure of expected pharmacological action

The FDA MedWatch program considers a reportable serious adverse event (of drugs or medical devices) when the patient outcome is death, is life-threatening, requires hospitalization, results in disability or a congenital anomaly, or is a reaction requiring intervention to prevent permanent impairment or damage.

Toxic effects is a term used to refer to adverse effects from too much of the drug, i.e., too high a dose or too high levels in the blood or other body tissues.

A useful reference in sorting out relative importance of symptoms reflecting side effects is the *USP Dispensing Information* (Volume I For Health Professionals and Volume II for Patients).[6a] Signs and symptoms are categorized as to whether they only need medical attention if they are bothersome to the patient versus those indicating the need for immediate medical attention.

Incidence

Side effects of drugs are not completely known at the time that a drug has been approved by the FDA. Only 3000 to 5000 patients may have been studied at that time; clinical trials usually have specific inclusion and exclusion criteria so that patients with certain other diseases or conditions and other drug therapy are not included. Clinical trials can usually detect adverse effects that have an incidence greater than 1:1000.[7] In order to detect an adverse effect with an incidence of 1:10,000, a minimum of 30,000 patients would need to be studied.[8] Clinical trials typically study patient exposure to a drug for less than a year.[9] Therefore, adverse effects from chronic use of the drug will not appear until after the drug is used widely and for long periods of time.

As the drug becomes more widely used by more and more patients, side effects with low incidences will appear, as will side effects that may result from alterations in pharmacokinetics and pharmacodynamics. With the increasing ethnic diversity of the population there is the increasing likelihood of genetic variations in drug response. Until recently women and the elderly (who account for a major percentage of drugs used) have not been systematically included in clinical trials. Therefore, a patient may have a side effect that is not reported in the package insert (which is based on the clinical trial data at the time of approval of a new drug) or in drug references.

Rare drug side effects are difficult to ascertain during the premarketing studies. In order to detect a side effect that occurs at the rate of 1 in 3300, a study would have to include at least 10,000 patients who are receiving the drug; also, the side effect can be attributed to the drug only if it does not occur spontaneously in the control group. If the adverse event does occur spontaneously in the control group, a substantially greater number of patients and controls must be followed to establish the drug as the cause of the event.[10] Some adverse drug effects and interactions are less likely to occur during clinical trial because of the inclusion and exclusion criteria; patients with various pathophysiologies and other concurrent medications may be excluded from clinical trials but become part of the population that receives the drug when it is approved.

Serious adverse effects of drugs may take years to be widely recognized. For example, with oral contraceptives, it took 3 years for pulmonary embolism and 5 years for myocardial infarction to be widely recognized.[11]

Clinicians need to monitor the clinical literature for newly emerging side effects. Knowing about the typical side effects of a new drug can guide the clinician in monitoring for possible side effects.

Reporting Adverse Drug Effects

Once a drug is released as a new drug by the FDA, there is no requirement that side effects be reported by clinicians. However, both manufacturers and the FDA have initiated measures to encourage the reporting of suspected adverse effects of medications (drugs or biologics), medical devices, special nutritional products, and other products regulated by the FDA. The MedWatch program provides a mechanism for the voluntary reporting of suspected problems; it is not necessary to have definitively established that the drug has caused the effect. The patient's name is held in strict confidence; the name of the person reporting the problem may be provided to the product's manufacturer unless requested otherwise.

A copy of the MedWatch form is in the Appendixes. It also can be found in the *Physicians Desk Reference* (PDR), *FDA Drug Bulletin*, *AMA Drug Evaluations*, and other references. The forms also can be obtained 24 hours a day, 7 days a week, by calling 800-FDA-1088.

Most hospitals have a system for reporting adverse drug events since this is a requirement for Joint Commission on Accreditation of Health Organization (JCAHO) accreditation. Clinicians need to be aware of policies and procedures within their practice settings related to adverse drug events as well as medication errors.

Establishing Adverse Effect of a Drug

It is not always clear when a sign or symptom is caused by a drug. Table 5-3 provides criteria for establishing that an adverse effect is caused by a particular drug. Rechallenge (administering the drug again to see if the effect occurs) is not usually feasible or in some cases would be unethical because of the potential danger posed to the patient.

Incidence of Adverse Drug Effects

There are various estimates of the incidence of adverse effects of drugs. Generally they are considered to be underreported. When clinicians encounter an unexpected outcome, they often fail to consider a drug-induced basis but rather tend to assume that the event

TABLE 5-3

General Criteria for Establishing That an Adverse Effect Is Caused by a Drug the Patient Is Taking

- Is the temporal sequence from the administration of the drug to the onset of the untoward event appropriate?
- Is the untoward event in keeping with a known pharmacological effect or adverse effects of the drug?
- Is the patient's illness or nonpharmacologic therapy sufficient to account for the event?
- What happens when the drug is discontinued?
- What happens when the patient resumes the drug, either accidentally or intentionally?

SOURCE: Karch and Lasagna.[5,12]

is related to the disease process or other non-drug-related factors.[13] Adverse reactions to drugs are the most common cause of iatrogenic disease.[14] Some useful figures to illustrate the scope of the problem of adverse drug effects are shown in Table 5-4.

There have been several studies on the incidence of drug-related adverse effects in hospitalized patients.[15–17] Up to 15 percent of hospitalized patients may have at least one adverse drug reaction.[18]

Data concerning the incidence of adverse drug reactions in the ambulatory setting are more limited. Estimates vary over the range of 3 to 41 percent but with variations in the criteria and methodology used.[6] Lower estimates tend to occur in studies where data are collected from physicians, higher estimates appear in studies where patients are surveyed.[19] As patients continue to spend less and less time in the hospital, it can be expected that many more adverse reactions will occur more often in the home or ambulatory care settings. Nurses at all levels of practice must be alert to the possibility of

TABLE 5-4

Statistics on Adverse Drug Reactions

- 3 to 5 percent of all hospitalizations (300,000 hospitalizations annually in the United States) can be attributed to adverse drug reactions.
- Once hospitalized, patients have about a 30 percent chance of an untoward event related to drug therapy; the risk attributable to each course of drug therapy is about 5 percent.
- The chance of a life-threatening drug reaction is about 3 percent per patient in the hospital and 0.4 percent per each course of therapy.

SOURCE: Jick.[17]

TABLE 5-5

Potential for Adverse Drug Reactions with Increasing Number of Medications

- 6 percent when two drugs are taken together
- 50 percent when five drugs are taken together
- 100 percent when eight or more medications are taken together

SOURCE: Shaughnessay.[21]

patients developing adverse drug reactions; families and other caregivers need to be taught the signs and symptoms that indicate the need for immediate medical attention.

Patients at Risk

Although all patients have some degree of risk of adverse drug effects, certain groups of patients or those in certain situations may be more likely to experience them. These include children and the elderly because of variations in ability to metabolize and eliminate many drugs. Women have been reported to have a higher percentage of adverse drug reactions than men, about 40 to 60 percent.[6] Some of the increased risk in women may be related to alterations in pharmacokinetics that can occur during menarche, pregnancy, delivery, lactation, and menopause. Patients with HIV infection have a higher incidence of adverse drug reactions; impairment of their capacity to clear drugs and metabolites, severe immunosuppression, and the development of drug-specific antibodies contribute to this.[20]

Other bases for increased risk are prior adverse drug reactions or a history of allergic disease, and multiple medications. Various studies have reported that elderly patients in both hospital and ambulatory settings take an average of 3 to 8 drugs. Table 5-5 illustrates the increased risks with increases in the number of medications taken.

MONITORING FOR ADVERSE DRUG REACTIONS

A complete and thorough assessment is needed to detect possible adverse drug effects. Prescribers need to be alert for anticipated adverse drug effects as well as able to consider the drug therapy as a possible etiology for development of new patient symptomatology, especially in the elderly or others on multiple drugs. The consideration of drug effect as an etiology for diseases or symptoms should be part of the clinician's differential diagnosis.[9]

Ongoing patient evaluation should be done to detect changes in organ or system function, especially the development of pathophysiological changes that could affect pharmacokinetics and pharmacodynamics.

TABLE 5-6

Adverse Drug Effects Commonly Monitored through Laboratory Testing

- Thiazide and loop diuretics: potassium levels for hypokalemia
- Coumadin: prothrombin time for bleeding
- Clozepin: WBC and differential for agranulocytosis
- Cancer chemotherapy: blood counts for neutropenia and thrombocytopenia

Clinicians also need to be aware that with many drugs high doses may result in a plateau of effectiveness; increasing the dose may result in an increase in the incidence and severity of adverse drug effects without any concurrent increase in benefit.[9]

Laboratory Testing for Monitoring Drug Effects

Laboratory tests often are used to monitor for the presence and/or extent of drug side effects (see Table 5-6). The costs of these need to be incorporated into the cost-benefit analysis; the impact on the patient of the need to have the test done should also be considered.

Diagnostic tests themselves may be affected by drugs the patient is taking—either by causing a diagnostic interference or by producing false-negative or false-positive results (or falsely high or low). Another concern in evaluating laboratory tests is determining if a value is caused by the drug and if so whether it reflects actual change and damage in physiological function. Most drug references provide information about interferences with common laboratory tests.

INTERVENTIONS TO ASSIST PATIENTS IN COPING WITH DRUG SIDE EFFECTS

Nurses can have an extremely important role in assisting patients in coping with drug side effects. Through this often unacknowledged role, the nurse plays a major role in assisting the patient to remain on the prescribed regimen. Drug side effects can be the basis for noncompliance and may be a result of intelligent noncompliance.[22] In particular, the role of oncology nurses is of special note; a considerable amount of nursing research has been done on nurses' effectiveness in the management of the side effects of cancer chemotherapy and in the control of symptoms such as pain and nausea.[23] Table 5-7 includes some nursing interventions to reduce the impact of some drug side effects.

(Text resumes on page 134)

TABLE 5-7

Drug-Related Side Effects

Drug-Related Side Effects	Monitor for:	Examples of Drugs Involved	Comments/Nursing Implications
Anticholinergic or Atropine-like Side Effects	Blurred vision, dry mouth, decreased GI motility, constipation, decreased perspiration, heat intolerance/fever, difficulty in initiating void	Anticholinergics (e.g., atropine), antipsychotics, antidepressants (tricyclics), antianxiety agents	Have patient chew gum or use no- or low-calorie candy to combat mouth dryness. Ensure adequate intake of fluids and bulk in diet. Monitor urinary and bowel elimination. Warn patient about blurred vision, need to avoid being in hot environment, and need to avoid use of other OTC drugs with anticholinergic effects (e.g., cold remedies, sleep remedies). Monitor elderly or others receiving multiple drugs with anticholinergic effects for development of anticholinergic syndrome.
Gynecomastia	Enlargement and/or soreness of breasts in men or women	Cimetidine, estrogens	Assess patient
Hematological Disorders			
Aplastic anemia	Fatigue, weakness, stomatitis, easy bruising, petechiae, purpura, bleeding, infection	Antihistamines, chloramphenicol, chloroquine, chlorothiazide, indomethacin, antidiabetics, oxyphenbutazone, phenothiazines, phenytoin, propylthiouracil, quinidine, sulfonamides	With pancytopenia, a decrease in RBC, WBC, and thrombocytes occurs. Reverse isolation may be necessary. Early withdrawal of offending drug may allow reversal of aplastic anemia. May be treated with antithymocyte globulin, corticosteroids, or bone marrow transplant if necessary.

Agranulocytosis	Sore throat, fever, malaise, weakness, chills, granulocytes <2000/mm^3	Acetaminophen, aspirin, β-lactam antibiotics, benzodiazepines, captopril, chloramphenicol, chlorpropamide, cimetidine, desipramine, ethacrynic acid, gentamycin, ibuprofen, indomethacin, isoniazid, levodopa, meprobamate, methyldopa, phenothiazine, phenylbutazone, phenytoin, propranolol, rifampin, streptomycin, sulfa drugs, thiazides, tolbutamide	Symptoms usually occur within 7-14 days after initial drug exposure. Advise patients to report symptoms immediately. Protect patient from sources of infection.
Neutropenia	Polymorphonuclear neutrophil count (PMN) below 1500/µL (1.5 × 10 − 9/L)	Antibiotics, phenothiazines, phenytoin, sulfonamides, cancer chemotherapy agents	Drug-induced neutropenia almost always resolves with withdrawal of drug, usually within 6 weeks.[25]
Hemolytic anemia	Weakness, orthostatic hypotension, headache, tinnitus, pallor, decreased hematocrit, renal failure; positive direct Coombs test	Acetaminophen, cephalosporins, chlorpromazine, hydrochlorothiazide, ibuprofen, isoniazid, levodopa, methadone, methyldopa, penicillin, probenecid, procainamide, quinidine, sulfa drugs, streptomycin, tetracycline, triamterene	Monitor for symptoms; assist patient to conserve energy if fatigued.

(continued)

TABLE 5-7

Drug-Related Side Effects (continued)

Drug-Related Side Effects	Monitor for:	Examples of Drugs Involved	Comments/Nursing Implications
Glucose-6-phosphate-dehydrogenase (G6PD) deficiency	Decreased hemoglobin and hematocrit, hemoglobin-uria, jaundice	Ascorbic acid, aspirin, benzocaine, chloram-phenicol, chloroquine, ciprofloxacin, dapsone, diazoxide, menadiol, methylene blue, naladixic acid, nitrofurantoin, nitro-furazone, phenazopyri-dine, primaquine, sulfa-pyridine, sulfisoxazole, also naphthalene (moth balls) and fava beans	G6PD deficiency occurs in about 13% of African-American males, 3% of African-American females, and in some ethnic groups of Mediterranean ancestry. Patients should avoid oxidative medications and foods (e.g., fava beans); patients need to be taught to carefully read list of ingredients when pur-chasing OTC drugs.
Thrombocytopenia	Bruising, epistaxis, pete-chiae, bleeding, decrease in platelets (below 100,000/μL, hematuria, hemoptysis, guaiac positive stool	Aspirin, cephalothin, chlorothiazide, cimetidine, desipramine, diazepam, digitoxin, furosemide, heparin, isoniazid, mor-phine, penicillin, phenyl-butazone, phenytoin, quinidine, sulfisoxazole, trimethoprim	Assess patient for risk factors, e.g., anticoag-ulant therapy, NSAID use, peptic ulcer, severe hypertension, uterine fibroids, or age >75 years. Protect patient from causing bruis-ing or injury, e.g., careful cleaning of teeth, use of electric razor, avoiding sharp objects or dangerous activities. Monitor for signs of internal and external bleeding, e.g., guaiac stools, retinal hemorrhages, neurological assessment, postural blood pressures, hema-turia, mucosal bleeding.

Liver Disorders/Hepatotoxicity

	Alteration in effects/toxicity of any drugs, nausea, vomiting, upper abdominal pain or fullness, darkening of urine, pruritus, bruising or bleeding, jaundice; alteration in prothrombin time, liver enzymes, serum bilirubin; BSP or indocyanine green excretion tests may be used to evaluate hepatic clearance; liver biopsy/scan may be used	Cytotoxicity: isoniazid, methyldopa, phenytoin	Since many drugs are biotransformed by the liver, any decrease in liver function can result in increased drug availability (therefore toxicity) or decrease in drug availability; risk of hepatotoxicity and of death from hepatotoxicity is higher in those over 78 years. Patients receiving drugs that have potential to produce hepatotoxicity should be counseled to avoid use of alcohol. Adjust dosage based on degree of decrease in clearance and prolongation of drug half-life.
Cholestasis	Often asymptomatic; mild to moderate increase in serum bilirubin	Androgens, captopril, chlorpromazine, erythromycin estolate and ethylsuccinate, estrogens, phenothiazines, sulfonamides, sulfonylureas	
Centrilobular necrosis	Elevations in serum transaminases	Acetaminophen, drugs cleared by cytochrome P-450 system, halothane	Antidote for acetaminophen overdose is acetylcysteine (140mg/kg q 4–6h for 42–72h). Liver damage from halothane occurs after exposure to it more than once.
Steatonecrosis	Hepatomegaly; symptoms similar to those of alcohol cirrhosis	Alcohol, tetracyclines, valproic acid	

(continued)

TABLE 5-7

Drug-Related Side Effects (continued)

Drug-Related Side Effects	Monitor for:	Examples of Drugs Involved	Comments/Nursing Implications
Toxic hepatitis		Toxic hepatitis: aspirin, halothane, ketoconazole, nitrofurantoin; chronic active hepatitis: dantrolene, isoniazid, methyldopa, nitrofurantoin	Onset of symptoms may be delayed as much as a week. INH hepatotoxicity occurs in 10–20% of patients on long-term therapy and has greater risk for patients over 35.
Hypersensitivity reactions (hepatocellular and/or cholestatic)	Fever, rash, arthritis, eosinophilia, hemolytic anemia; granulomas within liver upon biopsy, elevated serum bilirubin	Sulfonamides, penicillin, oxacillin, chlorpromazine, nitrofurantoin, long-term estrogen therapy	Hepatocellular cholestatic jaundice from chlorpromazine usually begins in first four weeks but may be delayed several months.
Oculotoxicity			
Alterations in oculomotor function	Nystagmus, oculogyric crisis, strabismus, and ocular weakness and paralysis	Anticonvulsants (e.g., phenytoin and phenobarbital), antipsychotics (e.g., phenothiazine, and butyropherones), corticosteroids, nalidixic acid, ethanol, vincristine	
Alterations in tear secretion	Decrease in tear secretion	Drugs with anticholinergic effects/side effects, sedative hypnotics (e.g., barbiturates), amiodarone, some beta blockers, antihistamines, busulfan, cyclophosphamide, isotretinoin, thiazide diuretics	Use of artificial tears may be indicated.

Condition	Symptoms	Drugs	Comments
	Hypersecretion	Drugs with cholinergic effects, doxorubicin, 5-fluorouracil, methotrexate	
Allergic conjunctivitis/keratoconjunctivitis	Redness and irritation of eye	Allopurinol, chloral hydrate, phenytoin, NSAIDs, sulfa drugs, quinidine, antineoplastic agents, isotretinoin, injectable gold salts	
Conjunctival deposits	Located in conjunctival cysts; color may vary from unpigmented to black	Amiodarone, phenothiazines, tetracyclines (long-term therapy), gold salts, iron supplements, quinoline derivatives, penicillamine	Usually have little clinical significance unless patient is concerned for cosmetic reasons.
Corneal deposits	Decreased corneal sensation, glare, blurred vision, photophobia, halos around light	Antimalarials (e.g., chloroquine and hydroxychloroquine), chlorpromazine, phenothiazine, other antipsychotics, prolonged tetracycline therapy	Usually dose-related; not usually necessary to discontinue drug; usually disappears 3–12 months after drug is discontinued. Use of artificial tears may help to prevent or reduce severity of deposits.
Cataracts	Decreased vision	Phenothiazines	Phenothiazine-induced cataracts are believed to be a photosensitivity reaction, rarely produce symptoms, and usually are slowly reversible after drug is discontinued.

(continued)

TABLE 5-7

Drug-Related Side Effects (continued)

Drug-Related Side Effects	Monitor for:	Examples of Drugs Involved	Comments/Nursing Implications
Cataracts (cont.)		Corticosteroids (systemic or topical to eye)	Incidence estimated to 5–96% of patients receiving corticosteroid therapy and may be related to dose and duration of therapy. Patients on long-term steroid therapy should have regular ophthalmic examinations.
		Allopurinol, bisulfan, chlorambucil, mitotane	
Retinopathy	Blurred vision, altered color vision, scotomas (blind spots), decreased night vision	Phenothiazines (esp. thioridazine), chlorpromazine, antimalarials (e.g., chloroquine), clofazimine, chemotherapeutic agents	Baseline and periodic assessment of retina should be done when patients are receiving these drugs. Thioridazine effect is dose-dependent (>800–1200 mg/d). Chloroquine effects are similar to that produced by aging process; can produce "bulls-eye retinopathy" (increased macular granular pigmentation surrounded by alternating concentric rings of hypo- and hyperpigmented retinal epithelium). Baseline exam and follow-up exam q 4–6 months during therapy. Use of dark sunglasses and drug holidays during summer months may help to limit toxicity.
		Nifedipine, cardiac glycosides (e.g., digoxin)	May produce transient decrease in acuity and visual field defects. Visual disturbances, especially altered color vision, result from digitalis toxicity.

Optic neuropathy	Blurred vision, scotomas, constricted visual fields, altered color vision, edema or hyperemia of optic disk	Deferoxamine, ethambutol, isoniazid (INH), chloramphenicol, minoxidil, antineoplastic agents, amiodarone, barbiturates, corticosteroids, metronidazole, propoxyphene (high doses) sulfonylureas and other sulfa derivatives, tamoxifen	Baseline exam needed; patient should be told to report immediately any decrease in visual acuity, blind spots, trouble in reading, or abnormal color vision. Peripheral neuropathy may precede optic neuropathy.
Ototoxicity	Cochlear signs: tinnitus, hearing loss; vestibular signs: vertigo, lightheadedness, headaches, whirling sensation, ataxia, nystagmus, nausea and vomiting, cold sweats, audiograms at 250–8000 Hz.	Antibiotics (e.g., aminoglycosides, erythromycins, vancomycin, tetracyclines), antimalarials (e.g., quinine and chloroquine), deferoxamine, NSAIDs (e.g., aspirin, indomethacin); loop diuretics (e.g., furosemide, ethacrynic acid, bumetanide); antitumor agents (e.g., cisplatin)	Ototoxicity may affect the cochlea and/or vestibular function. Ototoxicity is defined as an increase in auditory threshold of 15–20 dB. Audiometric monitoring in patients receiving ototoxic drugs includes establishing baseline levels, serial audiometry during therapy, and audiometry after drug is discontinued. Vestibular symptoms usually occur when the patient moves. Risk factors for increased incidence of drug-induced ototoxicity: dehydration, fever, increased drug levels, and/or prolonged exposure of inner ear to the drug, concomitant use of more than one ototoxic drug, noise exposure, preexisting hearing loss, bacteremia, heredity, prior exposure to ototoxic agents, and old age.

(continued)

TABLE 5-7

Drug-Related Side Effects *(continued)*

Drug-Related Side Effects	Monitor for:	Examples of Drugs Involved	Comments/Nursing Implications
Renal Disorders/Nephropathy			
	Proteinuria, enzymuria, oliguria, increase in serum creatinine and blood urea nitrogen, decrease in creatinine clearance, fluid and electrolyte disturbances		Excretion of other drugs may be affected. Dosage of many drugs in patients with impaired renal function probably will need to be adjusted, usually on basis of creatinine clearance. Dosage guidelines based on creatinine clearance can be found in package insert accompanying drug.
Acute tubular necrosis		Aminoglycosides, radiographic contrast media, cisplatin, amphotericin B	Glomerular filtration rate decreases in 5–20% of patients treated with aminoglycosides
Glomerulonephritis		NSAIDs, chronic use of heroin, parenteral gold therapy	

| Nephritis | Fever, hematuria, pyuria, proteinuria, oliguria, maculopapular rash, eosinophilia; renal biopsy or imaging may be needed | Methicillin, NSAIDs | Acute allergic interstitial nephritis causes about 8% of acute renal failures. Onset of symptoms with methicillin usually occurs 2–44 days after initiation of therapy. Onset with NSAID may be delayed for 5 months from initiation of therapy. Nephrogenic diabetes insipidus (polyuria from impaired ability to concentrate the urine) occurs in 20–70% of patients receiving lithium. Mild renal insufficiency may occur in 10% of patients on long-term lithium therapy and could result in severe renal insufficiency and end-stage renal failure. To prevent renal insufficiency, advise each patient of the importance of monitoring serum lithium levels, avoiding dehydration, and maintaining sodium intake in diet. |

(continued)

TABLE 5-7

Drug-Related Side Effects (continued)

Drug-Related Side Effects	Monitor for:	Examples of Drugs Involved	Comments/Nursing Implications
Necrosis	Inability to concentrate urine, proteinuria, pyuria, hypertension, decrease in creatinine clearance	Analgesics (e.g., phenacetin), combinations of analgesics	Although sales of phenacetin and combination analgesics have been restricted in U.S., other combinations of analgesics are available without prescription. Patients, especially those with renal disease or on long-term use should be advised to avoid the use of combination products and to decrease the use of any of the analgesics as much as possible.
Obstructive nephropathy (renal tubules, nephrolithiasis)	Hematuria, oliguria/anuria, flank pain	Chemotherapeutic agents, sulfonamides, ascorbic acid (massive doses), triamterene	Acute acid nephropathy can occur after chemotherapy for hematologic malignancies; prevent by pretreatment, hydration, alkalinization of urine to pH 7, and administration of allopurinol. Ensure adequate fluid intake to provide excretion of 1500 mL/day of urine.

Respiratory Disorders

Asthma/bronchospasm	Bronchospasm often associated with rhinorrhea, flushing of head and neck, and conjunctivitis	Aspirin, beta blockers, NSAIDs, contrast media, sulfites (preservatives in food and wine), tartrazine (FD+C Yellow Dye No. 5)	Careful history of sensitivity or intolerance to any drugs, foods, and cosmetics should be done on all patients. There may be cross-reactivity between aspirin and other anti-inflammatory drugs. Aspirin sensitivity occurs in 4–20% of all asthmatics and 14–23% of

			those with nasal polyps. Bronchospasms may be severe and life-threatening. Be sure emergency drugs such as corticosteroids and epinephrine are immediately available.
Pulmonary edema	Persistent cough, rales, tachypnea, tachycardia, hypoxemia, cyanosis, blood-tinged sputum	Narcotic analgesics	Symptoms may occur within minutes of IV administration or up to 2 hours after oral administration.
Pulmonary fibrosis	Chills, fever, malaise, cough, dyspnea, rales, inspiratory crackles, changes in chest X-rays and pulmonary function tests (e.g., abnormal diffusion capacity followed by decreased vital capacity)	Antineoplastic agents (e.g., bleomycin, busulfan, carmustine, cyclophosphamide, methotrexate), amiodarone, gold salts	

Sexual Dysfunction

| | Decrease in libido, impotence, priapism, inability to achieve orgasm | Antipsychotics, antidepressants, antihypertensive agents, androgens, estrogens, beta blockers, thiazide diuretics | Assess carefully for presence of sexual dysfunction and concerns of patient and sexual partner. Consider that the sexual dysfunction may be caused by the underlying condition being treated. |

(continued)

TABLE 5-7

Drug-Related Side Effects (continued)

Drug-Related Side Effects	Monitor for:	Examples of Drugs Involved	Comments/Nursing Implications
Skin Diseases			
Maculopapular eruptions	Flat or raised reddened lesions, often starting on trunk or in areas of pressure of trauma; usually symmetrical; fever	Allopurinol, barbiturates, carbamazepine, chloramphenicol, erythromycin, ethionamide, gold salts, hydantoin, ibuprofen, isoniazid, nitrofurantoin, penicillins, penicillamine, phenothiazines, piroxicam, rifampin, streptomycin, sulfonamides, sulindac, tetracyclines, tolmetin	Careful history of prior use of medications is needed. Early eruption appears within 2–3 days of drug administration. Late reaction may occur about 9 days after exposure. Rash usually fades a few days after drug is discontinued. Recurrence may present as more serious and extensive exfoliative reactions. Have patient wear Medic-Alert and advise of need to avoid the drug in the future.
Urticaria	Pruritic erythematous wheals (hives)	Aspirin, gold, heparin, ibuprofen, indomethacin, iodinated radiocontrast media, naproxen, opiates, penicillins, sulfonamides, sulindac, tartrazine, tolmetin	May be first indication of anaphylaxis—have emergency drugs available; monitor patient. Immediate reaction within minutes to hours of drug exposure. Accelerated reaction within 12–36 hours after exposure; late reaction within 8–12 days after exposure. Usually resolves within 1–3 days after drug has been discontinued; advise patient to avoid heat or hot bath or showers and scratching skin.

Fixed drug eruption	Erythematous round or oval lesions up to 20 cm in diameter often on lips or genitalia; with time color turns to a dusky red or violaceous hue; itching, burning sensation, feeling of warmth	Barbiturates, dapsone, digitalis, diphenhydramine, disulfiram, erythromycin, gold, hydralazine, ibuprofen, metronidazole, phenothiazines, phenylbutazone, quinidine, sulfonamides, sulindac, tetracycline, trimethoprim	Healing usually occurs after 7–10 days. Patient should be told not to take drug again since extensive bullous lesions may occur.
Photosensitivity	Similar to sunburn, erythema, edema, papules, plaque-like urticarial lesions; appears on areas of skin receiving greatest exposure to sunlight	Amiodarone, carbamazepine, furosemide, naproxen, oral contraceptives, phenothiazines, phenylbutazone, quinidine, sulfonamides, sulfonylureas, sulindac, tetracyclines, thiazides	Phototoxic reaction occurs on first exposure to sun. Photoallergic reaction requires sensitization period. Advise patient to avoid sun and/or use sunscreens; however, sunscreens may produce their own photosensitivity.
Hyperpigmentation	Color changes in skin: brown, black-brown, blue-black, gray, violet gray, bluish, depending on drug	Amiodarone, antimalarials, antineoplastics (busulfan bleomycin, doxorubicin), heavy metals (e.g., mercury, silver, bismuth, gold), phenothiazines, oral contraceptives, tetracyclines	Region involved depends on drugs. Usually fades with decreased sun exposure but does not completely disappear.

(continued)

TABLE 5-7

Drug-Related Side Effects (continued)

Drug-Related Side Effects	Monitor for:	Examples of Drugs Involved	Comments/Nursing Implications
Erythema multiforme	Initial 1–10 cm erythematous round macule, then enlarging into plaques or concentric rings of erythema; usually on hands, feet, limbs, face, and mucous membranes	Barbiturates, carbamazepine, diflunisal, hydantoins, ibuprofens, penicillins	Treated symptomatically, lesions usually begin to resolve in 4–5 days. Monitor patient for progression to more severe form (see Stevens-Johnson syndrome below).
Stevens-Johnson syndrome (SJS)	Severe form of erythema multiforme with high fever, arthralgias, myalgias, vomiting, diarrhea, extensive mucosal and conjunctival edema, erosions, skin lesions may have large bullae and areas of denudation	Phenylbutazone, propranolol, quinine, salicylates, sulfonamides, sulfonylureas, sulindac, thiazides, antibiotics	Healing usually occurs within six weeks. Complications include blindness, pneumonia, dehydration, esophagitis, death.
Toxic epidermal necrolysis (TEN)	Macular lesion with burning sensation that enlarges over the body; may form flaccid bullae and/or massive detachment of the epidermis	Allopurinol, barbiturates, chloramphenicol, hydantoins, ibuprofen, indomethacin, penicillins, penicilliamine, phenylbutazone, quinine, sulfonamides, sulindac, tolmetin	Protect skin from rubbing off; avoid infection to skin; monitor for fluid and electrolyte imbalance septicemia, corneal ulceration, erosion of mucous membranes. May also affect internal organs. Mortality is about 3% within 3–4 days of acute episode.

Sleep Pattern Disturbances

	Drug withdrawal insomnia, insomnia, dreams, nightmares	Hypnotics, benzodiazepines	Abrupt discontinuation of hypnotics after chronic use can result in an increase in REM sleep to as much as 40% of sleep time. REM sleep may have frightening dreams or nightmares. Patients should be tapered off the hypnotic gradually, and should be counseled that dreams may increase for a while. Hypnotics should be used only for short-term insomnia.
Insomnia	Inability or difficulty in initiating or maintaining sleep.	CNS stimulants (e.g., amphetamines), xanthines (e.g., caffeine, theophylline)	Avoid giving within 6 hours of bedtime. Avoid use of caffeine in coffee, tea, colas, chocolate.
Sedation/excessive sleeping		CNS depressants, psychotropic agents (e.g., antianxiety drugs, antipsychotics, antidepressants)	Sedation usually occurs in early stage of use. Patients may become tolerant to this effect. Caution patient to avoid driving, use of dangerous machinery, or any activities requiring alertness. Judgment and rapid motor response; patients should avoid use of alcohol or other drugs causing sedation or CNS depression.

SOURCE: Selected information based on or adapted from information in DiPiro JT et al: *Pharmacotherapy: A Pathophysiological Approach*. New York: Elsevier, 1997, and Herfindal ET, Gourley DR: *Textbook of Therapeutics. Drug and Disease Management*, 6th ed. Baltimore: Williams & Wilkins, 1996.

TYPES OF DRUG SIDE EFFECTS

Drug side effects have been characterized as being either type A or type B. Type A adverse drug reactions are extensions of the pharmacologic actions of either the drug or its metabolities. About 70 to 80 percent of drug reactions are of this type; they often are predictable and may be preventable. They are usually detected during clinical trials.

Type B adverse drug reactions are unpredictable and based primarily on patient variables rather than on drug characteristics. They are the most life-threatening and a major cause of important adverse drug reactions. They usually occur independent of drug dose or route of administration; they usually do not occur until after 5 days of therapy (except for anaphylaxis), and most occur by the twelfth week of therapy. However, there is no maximum time for them to occur and some may occur even after the drug is discontinued. Type B adverse effects include idiosyncratic reactions, allergic or immunologic reactions, and carcinogenic/teratogenic effects.[9]

Another kind of adverse reaction to a drug is one that occurs when the drug is withdrawn, such as occurs with discontinuation of narcotics or steroids.[6]

Drugs can produce a wide variety of adverse effects. Those more commonly directly associated with drug therapy are discussed here. Additional side effects are delineated in Table 5-7.

Liver

Although hepatic injury is a relatively small proportion of all adverse drug effects, drugs are responsible for 2 to 5 percent of hospital admissions for jaundice in the United States. A careful history of medication use for the past three months should be taken on any patient with liver disease.[6] An estimated 20 to 30 percent of cases of hepatic failure may be drug-induced.[24]

Acute hepatic injury from drugs may be from damage to hepatocytes (cytotoxic), from arrested bile flow (cholestasis), or a combination. The incidence of acute liver damage that is drug-related is estimated to be about 10 percent overall but increases to 50 percent of cases in patients over 50 years.[25] Cholestasis often resembles extrahepatic obstructive jaundice with pruritus, jaundice, pale stools, and dark urine as the main manifestations. Serum bilirubin levels are increased in all cases of drug-induced cholestasis, but usually are less than 170 µmol/L (normal 2 to 17 µmol/L).[26]

Serum enzyme levels may indicate hepatic damage, but do not always occur in certain types of hepatic injury or may be delayed or erratic. At the present time there is no quantitative predictive test that can be reliably used as a guide for adjusting drug dosing in hepatic dysfunction. For drugs excreted primarily by the kidney, no adjustment in dosage is necessary unless the drug is highly protein-bound, in which case a patient with low serum albumin may need a dosage decrease. If a drug is primarily metabolized or excreted by the liver, the clinician needs to use the degree of prolongation of half-life and the degree of decrease in drug clearance as a guide to dosing.[27]

Patients with chronic liver disease often have low serum albumin and ascites, resulting in larger volume of distribution; this can result in a prolonged half-life and the resulting need to administer the drug less often. The lower binding to albumin results in some drugs being distributed in greater amounts to the tissues and can be the basis for increased encephalopathy, especially from analgesic and sedative drugs.[27]

RULES OF THUMB: Generally, in a patient with liver dysfunction resulting in decreased clearance of a drug metabolized or excreted by the liver, the dosage of drug should be decreased by about the same percentage as the decrease in the clearance of the drug.

Monitor the patient closely for both therapeutic effects and adverse effects through close observation as well as plasma levels.

If possible choose drugs with a short half-life and a wide margin of safety.

Avoid the use of oral administration of drugs with high first-pass effects.

If possible choose drugs metabolized through glucoronidation in the liver since this produces metabolites that are pharmacologically inactive.[27]

Kidney

Toxicity to the kidney is of importance not only for its effects on the organ itself but also for the effects of decreased renal function on the excretion of most drugs. Therefore, renal function needs to be assessed prior to initiating therapy (see formulas in Chap. 4) as well as throughout the course of drug therapy, especially when nephrotoxic drugs are prescribed. Observations should also be directed toward toxic effects that might indicate the decline in excretion of drugs usually eliminated via the kidney.

Drug references and package inserts provide nomograms for dosage adjustments necessary when there is a decease in renal function. Renal failure is considered to occur if serum creatinine ≥ 150 µmol/L, creatinine clearance ≤ 50 mL/min, or urea nitrogen ≥ 17 µmol/L.[25]

Laboratory tests for renal failure need to be interpreted in light of the characteristics of the individual patient and the changes in these values within the individual. For example, a doubling of the serum creatinine over a six-month period could indicate renal insufficiency even though the values may not be much higher than the upper limits of "normal."[25]

Analgesic nephropathy was initially thought to be caused only by phenacetin but other analgesics such as aspirin, acetaminophen, antipyrine, and aminopyrine have been implicated. Pathologies that may occur are interstitial nephritis and papillary necrosis. Indications of the latter include fever, flank pain, hematuria, and nocturia; these symptoms mimic those caused by kidney stones.[6] NSAIDs can produce reversible renal effects in some patients. These effects are believed to be related to the inhibition of prostaglandin. Patients should be monitored for decreased urine output, increase in weight (reflecting sodium and fluid retention), and rapidly rising serum BUN and creatinine levels. Patients at high risk are elderly patients with cirrhosis, congestive heart failure, preexisting renal disease, and volume depletion.[6] The concurrent administration of other nephrotoxic drugs also increases risk.

Other drugs that cause renal damage include aminoglycoside antibiotics (estimate of 10 to 20 percent of patients treated), radiocontrast agents, and cancer chemotherapeutic agents. Drugs may cause crystallization (acyclovir, methotrexate, sulfonamides) or stones (acetazolamide, allopurinol, triamterene). Fanconi syndrome (proximal tubular damage) can be caused by outdated or degraded tetracyclines.[6]

Allergic Responses

Drug allergies may result from the drug or sometimes may be caused by other ingredients in the drug formulation such as tartrazine (Yellow Dye No. 5). Many drug preparations, as well as foods, have this dye added during the manufacturing process. It can cause allergies in some individuals; persons with an allergy to aspirin may have a higher incidence of allergy to tartrazine. A useful reference that contains information about product ingredients such as tartrazine is *Drug Facts and Comparisons* (see Chap. 1). Tables 5-8 and 5-9 cover types of hypersensitivity reactions and predisposing factors for allergic reactions.

TABLE 5-8

Types of hypersensitivity reactions

I. Immediate, anaphylactic, IgE-mediated
   Examples: anaphylaxis,* extrinsic allergic asthma, seasonal allergic rhinitis, some cases of urticaria
II. Cytoxic
   Examples: Coombs-positive hemolytic anemia, antibody-induced thrombocytopenia
III. From deposition of circulating antibody-antigen complexes in vessels or tissues
   Examples: serum sickness from serum, drugs, or viral hepatitis antigen, systemic lupus erythematosus, rheumatoid arthritis (may be preceded by type I, IgE-mediated response); symptoms of urticaria, fever, arthralgia, and lymphadenopathy 7 to 21 days after exposure
IV. Cell-mediated, delayed, or tuberculin type from sensitization of lymphocytes after contact with antigen
   Examples: contact dermatitis, allograft rejection

*A reaction that resembles anaphylaxis but is not immune-mediated is called an anaphylactoid reaction.
SOURCE: Beringer and Middleton[28] and Glazener.[6]

TABLE 5-9

Predisposing Factors for Allergic Reactions

Age: older > younger
Sex: females > males
Genetic factors: e.g., slow acetylators are more likely to develop indications of
   systemic lupus erythematosus when given procainamide or hydralazine.
Associated illnesses: e.g., higher incidence of maculopapular rash from ampicillin in patients with Epstein-Barr infections (e.g., infectious mononucleosis), lymphocytic leukemia, or gout. (Certain AIDS patients may have high
   incidence of adverse reactions to drugs (e.g., skin rash from sulfonamides)
   and higher incidence of skin eruptions with amoxicillin-clavulanate therapy.
Previous drug administration: previous history of allergic reaction to drug or
   one that is immunochemically similar.
Drug-related factors: dose, frequency of exposure, and route of administration
   may affect likelihood of allergic response. Topical route has the greatest risk
   of producing sensitization; the oral route has the least risk. IV administration
   to an already allergic patient poses greatest risk of an allergic response.

SOURCE: Beringer and Middleton.[28]

For a true immune response to occur, the patient must have had prior exposure to a
drug. However, allergic responses may occur without this condition appearing to have
been met; one situation in which this can occur is when a patient has been exposed to
antibiotics through the ingestion of meat (e.g., chicken or beef) in which these animals
have been treated with antibiotics before slaughter. This is a major concern in the development of drug resistance but also can be a problem in sensitizing people to antibiotics
and later producing allergic responses. A detailed drug history is important in determining if a reaction is an allergy. An important first step is to carefully clarify a
patient's response to questions about previous allergic reactions. Often patients say they
have had a drug allergy when they mean that they did not tolerate it well (e.g., had upset
stomach or diarrhea). Sometimes, even when a patient did experience an allergic
response to drugs, it may have been related to other ingredients (e.g., sulfite, dyes) in a
particular preparation or brand; therefore, the dates when the allergy occurred (since
some drugs have been reformulated or are now available in a purer form) and the particular brand (if known) could be valuable information.

Drug fever can be the result of an allergic reaction but it also can be caused by the
release of cellular contents such as occurs with cancer chemotherapeutic agents. Other
drugs may raise body temperature by increasing metabolism (e.g., thyroid), interfering
with heat regulation (e.g., atropine and other drugs with anticholinergic effects that decrease perspiration), or causing idiosyncratic syndromes such as malignant hyperthermia
from general anesthetics and other drugs, and neuroleptic malignant syndrome from

some of the psychotropic agents. Fever can also result from drug effects on the CNS regulatory center (e.g., phenothiazines). Some drugs such as bleomycin and amphotericin B have a direct pyrogenic effect. Fever associated with a hypersensitivity reaction can occur within hours of administration but typically occurs between day 7 and 10 of therapy. Usually a fever associated with a drug will disappear within 48 hours after the drug is discontinued.[29]

Blood

Blood dyscrasias may result from a wide variety of drugs; drugs may affect all three blood components or only one of the components (e.g., anemia, thrombocytopenia, agranulocytosis-neutropenia). About 5 percent of adverse drug reactions are blood dyscrasias. The following definitions are used in the discussion:[30]

Leukopenia: total WBC count < 3000/mm³
Granulocytopenia: granulocyte count including eosinophils and basophils < 1500/mm³
Neutropenia: neutrophil-segmented polymorphonucleocytes < 1500/mm³
Agranulocytosis: severe form of neutropenia with total granulocyte count < 500/mm³

Aplastic anemia is a severe and often fatal blood dyscrasia; it often is unpredictable in that in some patients it is not related to the dose or the length of the drug therapy. Although rare, an estimated one-third to two-third of cases are related to drug therapy.[30a] Chloramphenicol is a drug that can cause aplastic anemia; this drug was once widely used but has had much more selective use since it was determined that it can produce a type of fatal aplastic anemia that is not dose-related and is probably related to a genetic variation in the patient. It does produce also a dose-related aplastic anemia that occurs when serum concentrations reach 25 µg/mL or higher.[6] A careful risk-benefit analysis must be done before prescribing chloramphenicol.

Hemolytic anemia can result from a genetic enzyme deficiency known as glucose-6-phosphatase-dehydrogenase (G6PD) deficiency. Persons with this genetic defect experience hemolysis of their red blood cells when they ingest oxidative drugs and foods. The erythrocytes of these individuals are relatively resistant to *Plasmodium falciparum*, which causes malaria; thus, there is a higher incidence of G6PD deficiency in individuals whose genetic heritage comes from areas of the world where malaria was or is endemic.[31] Females usually have a less severe form. Persons of African heritage or from ethnic groups from around the Mediterranean area may have this genetic defect. The Mediterranean type results in more severe lysis of red blood cells than does the African type. About 10 percent of African-Americans have G6PD deficiency and as many as 50 percent of people of southern European ancestry (especially Greeks, Sardinian Italians, and Kurdish Jews) have G6PD deficiency.[30]

Symptoms experienced depend on the extent of the destruction of the red blood cells and include fatigue, hyperbilirubinemia, urobilinogenuria, decreased hemoglobin, increased indirect serum bilirubin, and abdominal or back pain. The urine may test positive for blood in the urine, but this only reflects the presence of hemoglobin; red blood cells would not be present.[30]

Examples of drugs to be avoided in persons with G6PD deficiency include, acetanilid, chloroquine, dapsone, doxorubicin, furazolidone, methylene blue, nalidixic acid, nitrofurantoin, phenazopyridine, phenylhydrazine, primaquine, quinine, sulfacetamide, sulfamethoxazole, sulfanilamide, and sulfapyridine. Also, ingestion of fava beans (also known as broad beans) should be avoided.

In addition to discontinuing the offending drug, treatment would consist of providing adequate hydration to prevent or decrease renal toxicity that can occur from the effect of hemoglobin on the tubules.

Hemolytic anemia also may result from an immune response to the drug or one of its metabolites. Examples of drugs that can cause this are penicillin, quinidine, and methyldopa.

Coagulation

Drug effects on coagulation and bleeding include the reversible effects of NSAIDs and aspirin's irreversible inhibition of platelet function (a single dose of aspirin can irreversibly affect platelets for 7 to 10 days). In a normal individual aspirin prolongs the bleeding time by a factor of 1.5 to 2, but significant bleeding is not common.[32] Some antibiotics such as valproic acid, high doses of penicillin, and certain cephalosporins may also affect platelet function and cause prolonged bleeding.

Thrombocytopenia

Thrombocytopenia (platelet count less than $100,000/mm^3$) can result from suppression of bone marrow or through destruction of platelets. Some drugs known to cause thrombocytopenia are alcohol, quinine, quinidine, and thiazide diuretics. If the thrombocytopenia is mild there may be no symptoms; purpura, petechiae, and hemorrhagic oral bullae may be early signs. Heparin also produces thrombocytopenia even when used in heparin flushes. It usually occurs after 6 to 12 days of therapy and usually resolves 4 to 7 days after heparin is discontinued.[30]

Neutropenia

Neutropenia can result from bone marrow suppression or an immune response. Agranulocytosis is responsible for about 26 percent of drug-related deaths and has a mortality rate of about 30 percent.[30] Signs and symptoms include the development of infections; however, some of the usual signs may be absent. A sore throat may be an indication of leukopenia.

Several antibiotics (e.g., cephalosporins, penicillin) and phenothiazines may cause neutropenia. The neutropenia usually occurs after 2 weeks of therapy; with phenothiazine neutropenia usually would not occur later than 10 weeks of therapy. The antipsychotic agent clozepin may cause a life-threatening agranulocytosis. Patients on clozapine need to have a baseline WBC and differential and then weekly WBC counts during therapy and for 4 weeks after therapy.

Discontinuation of the offending drug is necessary. Other implications for management are in Table 5-7. The discussion of blood dyscrasias in Chap. 20 on the management of chemotherapy-induced side effects also includes additional information applicable to managing blood dyscrasias.

Skin

Medications should be considered as a potential cause of almost any skin eruption; skin disorders are the most common drug-related adverse reactions. Skin responses to drugs may be isolated to the skin or may reflect serious systemic involvement; they are usually considered to be hypersensitivity reactions. About 5 percent of hospitalizations in dermatology departments are attributed to drugs.[25]

The most common skin reactions from drugs are pruritus, urticaria, and maculopapular eruptions; these account for about 80 percent of drug-related skin reactions.[25] Table 5-7 includes further information about specific drug-related skin reactions.

SUMMARY

Monitoring patient responses to drug therapy is an integral part of the nursing role; it becomes even more important when the APN assumes responsibility for prescribing drugs. Drug effects and side effects need to be carefully evaluated and documented and changes in the drug regimen made as indicated by these evaluations.

REFERENCES

1. Temple R: Trends in pharmaceutical development. *Drug Information J* 27:355–366, 1993.
2. Nies AS, Spielberg SP: Principles of therapeutics, in Hardman JG, Limbird LE (eds): *Goodman & Gilman's The Pharmacological Basis of Therapeutics,* 9th ed. New York: McGraw-Hill, 1996.
3. Benet LZ, Kroetz DL, Sheiner LB: Pharmacokinetics, in Hardman JG, Limbird LE (eds). *Goodman & Gilman's The Pharmacological Basis of Therapeutics*, 9th ed. New York: McGraw-Hill, 1996.
4. World Health Organization: *Requirements for Adverse Drug Reaction Reporting.* Geneva, Switzerland: The Organization, 1975.
5. Karch FF, Lasagna L: Adverse drug reactions: A critical review. *JAMA* 234:1236–1241, 1975.
6. Glazener FS: Adverse drug reactions, in Melmon KL, Morelli HF, Hoffman BB, Nierenberg DW (eds): *Melmon and Morelli's Clinical Pharmacology: Basic Principles in Therapeutics,* 3d ed. New York: McGraw-Hill, 1992.
6a. *USP Dispensing Information* (Volume I for Health Professionals and Volume II for Patients). (Annual.) Rockville, MD: U.S. Pharmacopeia.
7. Norrby SR, Lietman PS: Safety and tolerability of fluoroquinolones. *Drugs 1993* 45 (Suppl 3): 59–64, 1993.
8. Lewis JA: Post-marketing surveillance: How many patients? *Trends Pharmacol Sci* 2: 93–94, 1981.
9. Goldman, SA, Kennedy DL, Lieberman RL: *Clinical Therapeutics and the Recognition of Drug-Induced Disease: A MedWatch Continuing Education Article.* Rockville, MD: Staff College, Center for Drug Evaluation and Research, Food and Drug Administration, 1995.
10. Strom BL, Tugwell P: Pharmacoepidemiology: Current status, prospects, and problems. *Ann Intern Med* 113:179–181, 1990.
11. Venning, GR: Identification of adverse reactions to new drugs II: How were 18 important adverse reactions discovered and with what delays. *Br Med J* 286:365–368, 1983.

12. Karch FE, Lasagna L: Toward the operational identification of adverse drug reactions. *Clin Pharmacol Ther* 21:247–254, 1977.

13. Kessler DA: The FDA's new MedWatch program. A role of NPs and PAs. *Clinician Reviews* 63,64,70, 1993.

14. Leape LL, Brennan TA, Laird N, et al: The nature of adverse events in hospitalized patients. Results of the Harvard medical practice study II. *New Engl J Med* 324:377–384, 1991.

15. Schimmel EM: The hazards of hospitalization. *Ann Int Med* 60:100–110, 1964.

16. Steel K, Gertman PM, Crescenzi C, Anderson J: Iatrogenic illness on a general medical service at a university hospital. *New Engl J Med* 13:200–204, 1973.

17. Jick H. Adverse drug reactions: The magnitude of the problem. *J Allergy Clin Immunol* 74:555–557, 1984.

18. Stafford CT: Adverse drug reactions. *Med Times* 116:311–342, 1988.

19. Schneider JK, Mion LC, Frengley JD: Adverse drug reactions in an elderly outpatient population. *Am J Hosp Pharm* 49:90–96, 1992.

20. Schroeder DJ, Barone JA: Adverse drug reactions and drug-induced diseases, in Herfindal ET, Gourley DR (eds): *Textbook of Therapeutics: Drugs and Disease Management*, 6th ed. Baltimore: Williams & Wilkins, 1996.

21. Shaughnessay AF: Common drug reactions in the elderly. *Emerg Med* 24:21–32, 1992.

22. Michaud PL: *Independent older persons managing medications at home: A grounded theory.* Unpublished doctoral dissertation, Boston College, May 1996.

23. Smith MC, Holcombe JK, Stullenbarger E: A meta-analysis of intervention effectiveness for symptom management in oncology nursing research. *Oncol Nurs Forum* 21(7):1201–1210, 1994.

24. Zimmerman JH: *Hepatotoxicity: Adverse Effects of Drugs and Other Chemicals on the Liver.* New York: Appleton-Century-Crofts, 1978.

25. Benichou C (ed): *Adverse Drug Reactions. A Practical Guide to Diagnosis and Management.* New York: Wiley, 1994.

26. Jim, LK, Gee JP: Adverse effects of drugs on the liver, in Young LY. Koda-Kimble MA (eds): *Applied Therapeutics: The Clinical Use of Drugs,* 6th ed. Vancouver, WA: Applied Therapeutics, 1995.

27. Hoyumpa AM, Schenker S: Influence of liver disease on the disposition and elimination of drugs, in Schiff L, Schiff ER (eds): *Diseases of the Liver,* 7th ed. Philadelphia: Lippincott, 1993, vol I.

28. Beringer PM, Middleton RK: Anaphylaxis and drug allergies, in Young LY, Koda-Kimble MA (eds): *Applied Therapeutics: The Clinical Use of Drugs*, 6th ed. Vancouver, WA: Applied Therapeutics, 1995.

29. Hofland SL: Drug fever: Is your patient's fever drug-related? *Crit Care Nurse* 5(4): 29–34, 1985.

30. Peterson CW: Drug-induced blood disorders, in Young LY, Koda-Kimble MA (eds): *Applied Therapeutics: The Clinical Use of Drugs,* 6th ed. Vancouver, WA: Applied Therapeutics, 1995.

30a. Vincent PC: Drug-induced aplastic anemia and agranulocytosis: Incidence and mechanisms. *Drugs* 31:52–63, 1986.

31. Meyer UA: Drugs in special patient groups: Clinical importance of genetics in drug effects, in Melmon KL, Morrelli HF, Hoffman BB, Nierenberg DW (eds): *Melmon and Morelli's Clinical Pharmacology. Basic Principles in Therapeutics,* 3d ed. New York: McGraw-Hill, 1992.

32. Noguchi JK, Stephens M: Coagulation disorders, in Herfindal ET, Gourley DR (eds): *Textbook of Therapeutics: Drugs and Disease Management,* 6th ed. Baltimore: Williams & Wilkins, 1996.

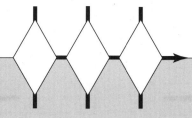

Chapter 6

DRUG THERAPY IN SPECIFIC POPULATIONS: ISSUES IN PREGNANCY AND LACTATION

Laurel A. Eisenhauer

OVERVIEW

A clinician in a primary care setting caring for a patient population that includes women of childbearing age needs to be aware of the issues and principles related to the use of drugs during pregnancy and during lactation. The purpose of this chapter is to provide an overview that alerts the primary care clinician to these issues and concerns; however, consultation with or referral to a specialist in maternity and/or the use of books, references, and other information sources specifically concerned with these problems and issues is appropriate.

Resources

Briggs GG: *Drugs in Pregnancy and Lactation: A Reference Guide to Fetal and Neonatal Risk*. Baltimore: Williams & Wilkins, 1994.

Friedman JM, Polifka JG: *The Effects of Drugs on the Fetus and Nursing Infant: A Handbook for Health Care Professionals*. Baltimore: Johns Hopkins, 1996.

Shepard TH: *Catalog of Teratogenic Agents*, 7th ed. Baltimore: Johns Hopkins, 1992. (Material extracted from TERIS database.)

TERIS: Database that assists health professionals in assessing risk of possible teratogenic effects. (http://weber.u washington. edu:80/in terisweb/tens/)

PREVENTIVE MEASURES

Since a woman may not realize that she is pregnant for a period of time during which she may be using prescribed or OTC medications, patient counseling about the appropriate use of any medication is valuable in the primary prevention of teratogenic effects. Advice concerning the correct use of the various types of birth control methods and their relative degree of effectiveness is also essential. For women on oral contraceptives, alternate forms of birth control may be necessary when certain other medications such as antibiotics are used (see Chap. 9).

Other general health-promoting measures should be encouraged as preparation for future pregnancy. Promotion of safe sex practices and treatment of sexually transmitted conditions are essential to preventing infections in the fetus or infant as well as helping to ensure a full-term pregnancy.

Women of child-bearing potential who are capable of becoming pregnant are advised to take at least 0.4 mg of folic acid daily in order to prevent neural tube defects.[1] Most regular multivitamin preparations contain at least this amount; patients should be advised to check labels carefully to be sure this amount is included. However, no more than 0.8 mg daily should be taken without medical supervision.

Alcohol use is of concern for its potential effects on the fetus (see below). Substance abuse with cocaine, opiates, etc., obviously can have deleterious effects on the fetus and newborn as well as affecting the overall health of the mother.

In women who have acute or chronic medical conditions requiring the use of medications, a risk-benefit analysis must be done in order to evaluate the relative danger to the mother and to the fetus, including consideration of the harmful effects of an untreated condition in the mother on the well-being of the fetus. Untreated asthma, for example, can result in decreased oxygenation to the fetus.

USE OF DRUGS DURING PREGNANCY

Pregnant women take an average of 3 medications and as many as 15 drugs during pregnancy. An estimated 35 to 100 percent of pregnant women have taken some kind of drug during pregnancy; 40 percent have taken drugs during the first trimester.[2]

Any drug given during pregnancy has the potential to produce adverse effects on the fetus. Teratogens are drugs (or other agents, e.g., environmental contaminants) that cause abnormal growth and development in the fetus. Major structural teratogenic effects occur at the rate of 2 to 4 percent in the United States.[3]

Only about 30 drugs are proven teratogens. The percentage of defects believed to be caused by drugs, metabolites, and chemicals is estimated to be about 3 percent. Genetic influences are believed to account for up to 20 percent.[2]

Establishing that a drug causes a birth defect is not easy since experimental studies in humans are not ethically feasible; therefore, case reports and animal studies are used. However, animal studies do not always predict tetratogenicity in humans.[3]

The FDA Pregnancy Categories (Table 6-1) are useful to the clinician in evaluating the teratogenicity of a drug. However, since only drugs marketed after December 1983 were required to have this categorization, many drugs currently available do not

TABLE 6-1

FDA Pregnancy Categories

A. *Controlled studies show no risk.* Adequate, well-controlled studies in pregnant women have failed to demonstrate risk to the fetus.

B. *No evidence of risk in humans.* Either animal findings show risk, but human findings do not, or if no adequate human studies have been done, animal findings are negative.

C. *Risk cannot be ruled out.* Human studies are lacking, and animal studies are either positive for fetal risk, or lacking as well. However, potential benefits may justify the potential risk.

D. *Positive evidence of risk.* Investigational or postmarketing data show risk to the fetus. Nevertheless, potential benefits may outweigh the potential risk.

X. *Contraindicated in pregnancy.* Studies in animals or humans or investigational or postmarketing reports have shown fetal risk that clearly outweighs any possible benefit to the patient.

have a classification.[3] Therefore, the clinician needs to review the research literature and/or other references and databases focusing on teratogenicity.

When a drug is used during the pregnancy is a factor in whether the drug causes an effect on the fetus and what type of effect.

Day 1 through days 12 to 15: may not have any effect because other cells can continue to develop even if some cells are affected by a drug

Days 18 to 60: period of organogenesis

First 3 months: most critical for malformations

Eight weeks to birth: drug effects on brain may produce functional and behavioral defects

Some teratogenic effects may not develop until long after birth. Examples of postnatal teratogenicity are the potential carcinogenic effects of DES that develop after puberty in exposed daughters and the behavioral alterations from alcohol exposure in utero.

Drugs Crossing the Placenta

Most drugs will pass through the placenta, with fat-soluble drugs, drugs of low molecular weight (less than 400), low protein-binding drugs, or highly nonionized drugs passing more readily. Because the concentration of blood proteins is less in the fetus than in the mother, there may be relatively more "free" drug that can affect the fetus. Drug metabolism in the fetal liver does occur, but this function is not fully developed. Drug excretion by the fetus is slower and occurs primarily via the fetal liver and placenta. A variety of other factors such as the amount of placental metabolism and maternal and fetal blood flow will affect the extent of transfer across the placenta. Some drugs may be present in the serum of the fetus in concentrations above that in the mother; the concentration of other drugs may be half that of the mother.[3]

As the time for delivery approaches, there is concern for the potential impact of a drug on the labor and delivery process. For example, the use of aspirin can prolong bleeding and a drug given predelivery can affect fetal functioning during delivery and during the neonatal period (e.g., opioid analgesics, magnesium sulfate).

Drugs for Chronic or Acute Conditions during Pregnancy

Pregnancy-Induced Alterations in Pharmacokinetics and Pharmacodynamics

As the pregnancy progresses, various changes occur in the woman's physiology that affect drug therapy.

The mother's blood volume increases, with as much as a 40 to 50 percent increase in the fluid portion of the blood that could result in decreased plasma concentrations of some drugs. Serum proteins may be 1 to 1.5 g lower, resulting in increased "free" levels of highly protein bound drugs. Renal blood flow increases by 30 percent and glomerular filtration rate (GFR) by 50 percent; this results in an increased rate of excretion of drugs via glomerular filtration. Serum creatinine, urea, and uric acid levels are decreased.[3]

Decreased GI motility and acidity contribute to the development of constipation and may delay the fecal excretion of some drugs. The nausea and vomiting of pregnancy may decrease absorption of drugs from the GI tract.

Drug metabolism may vary during the course of the pregnancy; there probably is no significant effect on plasma clearance in healthy women.

Drug Therapy for Conditions Occurring as a Result of Pregnancy

In most situations the treatment of conditions arising from pregnancy (such as pregnancy-induced hypertension and gestational diabetes) will be treated by obstetrical specialists. The following is intended to provide an overview for the primary care clinician.

Nausea and Vomiting of Pregnancy

Nausea occurs in up to 90 percent of pregnant women; nausea and vomiting occur in about 55 to 80 percent. This usually occurs in the third to seventh week of pregnancy but can last into the second and third trimesters. Conservative measures should be used first, e.g., small frequent meals, high-carbohydrate meals, high-protein snacks, crackers, and accupressure wristbands. Drugs therapy may be required if the mother's health becomes at risk. Most commonly used is meclizine PO or dimenhydrinate orally, IM, or IV.

Heartburn

Nonpharmacologic measures are recommended (e.g., avoidance of spicy meals, small frequent meals, elevation of head of bed). Antacids (not sodium bicarbonate) can be used, but H_2 blockers and prokinetics are not recommended.

Constipation

Assess the patient's use of OTC drugs, especially aluminum- or calcium-containing laxatives. It is preferable to use bulk-forming cathartics. Stimulants or other strong laxatives should be avoided during pregnancy since they may stimulate uterine contractions. Mineral oil should not be used because of its interference with absorption of fat-soluble vitamins.

Drug Therapy for Preexisting Conditions

The ongoing treatment of serious conditions needs to continue during pregnancy. Ideally, nonpharmacological measures can be used in place of drug therapy. However, in other conditions drug therapy must continue. The woman needs to be aware of the risks and be counseled about prenatal testing.

Asthma

Asthma is variable as to whether pregnancy improves, worsens, or has no effect on the mother during pregnancy. It may worsen near the end of the first trimester; usually the mother's condition returns to prepregnancy levels within 3 months postpartum.[3] Risk to the fetus from uncontrolled asthma must be weighed against teratogenic drug effects.

Terbutaline is used as a tocolytic; therefore, when it is used to treat asthma, it may need to be withdrawn before the time for labor. Theophylline does not appear to cause teratogenicity but can cause adverse effects on the fetus or newborn, such as cardiac arrhythmias, tachycardia, jitteriness, hypoglycemia, vomiting, and feeding difficulty.[2]

Hypertension

Hypertension that is preexisting, as well as that which occurs during the pregnancy, needs to be carefully treated in order to prevent maternal and perinatal morbidity and mortality. Hypertension arising during pregnancy can range from transitory hypertension to preeclampsia or eclampsia. The latter needs to be treated by specialists.

In chronic hypertension, methyldopa usually is used; although it readily crosses the placenta, it produces only rare adverse effects in newborns or in the longer term neonate. Its effects have been studied for up to 7.5 years of age. Hydralazine has been used, but ACE inhibitors are not recommended.

The use of diuretics is controversial because of the effects on the volume status of the patient, which could lead to decreased perfusion of the placenta and uterus.[2] Thiazides have produced decreased birth weight and increased perinatal prematurity, hypoglycemia, fluid and electrolyte imbalances, and thrombocytopenia. Thiazides are not considered first-line agents,[2] but some clinicians say to continue with them if used prior to pregnancy and if they continue to maintain adequate control of blood pressure.

Epilepsy

Women treated with antiepileptic medications have more than a 90 percent chance of having a normal child, but their risk of having a child with major congenital malformations is two to three times that of nonepileptic women.[2] This increased risk is caused by both teratogenic effects of medications as well as from the impact of the mother's disease on the fetus. About a quarter of patients experience a lessening of control of epilepsy, which can result in seizures that can cause hypoxia and acidosis, which in turn can produce adverse effects in the fetus.[2]

Antiepileptic drug therapy is usually necessary when the benefits to the mother and the fetus outweigh the possible adverse effects to the fetus from exposure to these drugs. The issue then becomes one of selecting the antiepileptic drug that has the least risk; the use of a single agent at the lowest possible dose is generally the goal. Valproic acid is teratogenic; phenytoin may be teratogenic and may produce the fetal hydantoin syndrome. It may also cause a deficiency in fetal vitamin K–dependent clotting factors, resulting in serious and sometimes fatal hemorrhage in the newborn.[2]

Because of the many changes in pharmacokinetics occurring during therapy, serum levels need to be monitored during pregnancy and to at least the sixth week postpartum.[2]

Diabetes Mellitus

Diabetic women have a three times greater risk of having children with congenital abnormalities than nondiabetic women; risk is increased further if the diabetes is poorly controlled or when the woman also has other underlying diseases.

The goal is to achieve normal levels of blood glucose and to avoid wide fluctuations in blood glucose levels. Variations can occur due to the pregnancy. The mother may experience hypoglycemia in the first 24 weeks of pregnancy when the fetus acquires its nutrients from the mother; therefore, less insulin may be needed. However, the need for insulin increases in the second and third trimesters because of increases in diabetogenic placental hormones. After delivery insulin needs return to prepregnancy levels.[2] Oral hypoglycemic agents are not recommended since they may induce insulin secretion by the fetal pancreas and lead to fetal hypoglycemia. Usually, regular and NPH insulins are used if insulin is necessary during pregnancy.

Anticoagulation Therapy

Anticoagulation therapy may be necessary in pregnant women either because of the hypercoagulable state of pregnancy resulting in thromboembolic disorders or because of other conditions of the mother (e.g., valvular heart prostheses). The anticoagulant of choice is heparin since it does not cross the placenta. Coumarin anticoagulants are not used because they do cross the placenta and are well-known teratogenics.

DRUG THERAPY DURING LACTATION

Breastfeeding produces many well-known benefits to the infant as well as to the mother-infant bond. Concerns about drug therapy when a woman is breastfeeding center around the potential effects of drugs and drug metabolites secreted in the milk. These can be harmful to the infant because of the immaturity of physiological function (liver biotransformation, hepatic excretion, renal excretion) to handle drugs. The metabolites can also be harmful. Whether a drug or metabolite passes into the milk depends on the content of the milk (e.g. water versus fat), the pH of milk and the pKa of the drug or metabolite; and the water versus fat solubility and degree of protein binding of the drug or metabolite. Another variable is the amount of milk (and therefore whatever drug is in it) that the infant ingests.[2]

Although there are many listings of drugs that should not be used during breastfeeding, these lists are not complete or may not include newly released drugs; therefore, the absence of a drug from such a list does not necessarily indicate that it is safe to use. Drugs that are definitely contraindicated include amphetamines, bromocriptine, cocaine, cyclophosphamide, cyclosporine, doxorubicin, ergotamine, heroin, lithium, marijuana, methotrexate, phencyclidine, and phenindione.

For short-term treatment of an acute time-limited condition requiring drug therapy in the mother, it might be possible for breast milk to be pumped, stored, and used to feed the infant during the drug therapy. Another option that might be possible is to time the administration of needed drugs to avoid their being at peak levels when the mother is nursing; the mother would nurse immediately before taking the drug, which if possible would be at a time when the infant will not be eating again soon (e.g., before sleeping at night or time for a long nap).

Another area of concern is the impact of drug therapy on milk production. Drugs decreasing milk production include androgens, bromocryptine, cloniphene, ergot alkaloids, levodopa, MAO inhibitors, pyridoxine (high dose), sympathomimetics, and thiazide diuretics. Milk production might be increased by drugs that decrease the prolactin inhibitory factor such as amoxapine, antipsychotics, cimetidine, metoclopramide, methyldopa and reserpine.[3]

Table 6-2 summarizes suggested drug therapies for episodic conditions during pregnancy.

TABLE 6-2

Drug Therapy for Episodic Conditions during Breastfeeding

If possible conditions should be treated by nonpharmacologic measures. The following are general guidelines.

Common Cold

It is best to not treat symptoms; usually they are tolerable. If they are treated, use single-entity products rather than preparations with multiple ingredients. Avoid the use of cough medicines containing alcohol. The use of iodides (e.g., SSKI as an expectorant) is contraindicated because they may produce goiters in the fetus.

Antibiotics

Do not use chloramphenicol, isoniazid, or tetracyclines. Penicillins, cephalosporins, and erythromycin usually are acceptable. For metronidazole, use a single 2-g dose and pump breasts (and discard breast milk) for 24 to 48 hours before resuming breastfeeding.

Laxatives

Use bulk-forming laxatives with no systemic absorption. Avoid all others because they have the potential for being absorbed systemically by the mother; observe the infant for diarrhea.

Analgesics

Occasional use usually is acceptable; chronic use of narcotics can cause CNS depression, sedation, and dependence in the infant. ASA at antiarthritic doses can affect infants' prothrombin time; acetaminophen is preferable to ASA.

Alcohol

Occasional moderate use probably is not harmful. Excess or chronic use can result in CNS depression, sedation, and abnormal growth.

Caffeine

Moderate use (one or two cups of caffeine-containing beverages a day) is acceptable unless infant experiences irritability and sleeplessness.

Nicotine

Nicotine slows milk production and may cause nausea, vomiting, diarrhea, restlessness, and tachycardia in the infant.

SOURCE: McCombs.[3]

SUMMARY

The use of drugs during pregnancy and lactation requires consideration of the needs of both the mother and the fetus or infant. The mother needs to be informed of the risks and benefits of any therapy and assisted in deciding on whether or not to use a drug. The APN in primary care can aid patients in making these decisions through referral and collaboration with obstetrical specialists.

REFERENCES

1.   Committee on Genetics of the American Academy of Pediatrics: Folic acid for the prevention of neural tube defects. *Pediatrics* 92:493–494, 1993.
2.   McQueen KD: Drugs in pregnancy and lactation, in Herfindal ET, Gorley DR (eds): *Textbook of Therapeutics: Drug and Disease Management*, 6th ed. Baltimore, MD: Williams & Wilkins, 1996, pp 1775–1796.
3.   McCombs J: Therapeutic considerations in pregnancy and lactation, in DiPiro JT, Talbert RL, Yee GC, et al (eds): *Pharmacotherapy. A Pathophysiological Approach*, 3d ed. Stamford, CT: Appleton & Lange, 1997.

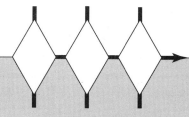

Chapter 7

CLINICAL ISSUES IN SPECIFIC POPULATIONS: DRUG THERAPY IN ELDERLY PATIENTS

Laurel A. Eisenhauer

OVERVIEW

Older patients present a challenge to the clinician. Changes in physiologic function resulting from the normal aging process, as well as the increased incidence of chronic conditions, create a complex situation that must be considered by the clinician in order to provide appropriate care and drug therapy and to avoid the dangers of polypharmacy. Psychosocial variables and cognitive changes may also impact on the elderly person's ability to manage his or her medications safely.

Older persons use more than 200 million drug prescriptions, amounting to $15 billion annually, which is a fourfold greater per capita expenditure than found in younger individuals. About 30 percent of all prescription medications are taken by elderly persons, currently about 12 percent of the population. One study of the urban elderly showed that the average for each person was 2.3 prescribed medications; the drugs used with the highest frequency were vitamins, diuretics, and NSAIDs.[1] About three-fourths of elderly persons living in the community take at least one prescription and about two-thirds take at least one OTC medication.[2] In one study of the elderly about 14 percent of the urban elderly and 27 percent of the rural elderly were found to use four or more OTC drugs daily; almost 35 percent used six or more medications.[3]

In an estimated two-thirds of physician office visits by elderly clients, one or more new prescription drugs are prescribed; it is estimated that 50 percent of these prescriptions will not have their desired therapeutic effect due to a variety of reasons ranging from too high or too low a dosage to not getting the prescription filled.[4]

EFFECTS OF PHYSIOLOGIC AGING AND CONCURRENT DRUG THERAPY

As individuals develop from birth and age, they become increasingly more complex and individualized. Therefore, the elderly as a group have a wide variation in physiological characteristics. Certain alterations in physiologic function, however, do occur to varying degrees in each individual and must be carefully evaluated in prescribing and monitoring medications. These are discussed in Chap. 3.

In addition, the elderly also tend to have acute and chronic conditions that may impact on pharmacokinetics and pharmacodynamics. Since many of these conditions are treated with drug therapy, the impact of the concurrent drug therapy with a newly prescribed drug needs to be carefully considered by the clinician.

Table 7-1 illustrates some of the alterations caused by the aging process and by pathologic conditions and/or other concurrent drug therapies that may impact on drug response in the elderly. Table 7-2 illustrates the drugs that require special consideration if they are used on the elderly.

TABLE 7-1

Effects of Aging and Concurrent Conditions or Drug Therapy on Drug Response

Physiologic Changes of Aging	Effects on Drug Therapy	Examples of Pathologic Conditions or Drugs Affecting Drug Therapy
Decreased GI motility; decreased gastric acidity	Possible decreased or delayed absorption of acidic drugs; decrease in peak effect	Anchlorhydria, malabsorption, diarrhea, gastric ulcers, pyloric obstruction or stenosis, pancreatitis, hypothyroidism, diabetic gastroparesis; antacids, H_2 blockers, proton pump inhibitors
Decrease in GI absorption surface of up to 20%	Effect on drug absorption believed to be minimal but possibly could decrease extent of absorption	

TABLE 7-1

Effects of Aging and Concurrent Conditions or Drug Therapy on Drug Response (continued)

Physiologic Changes of Aging	Effects on Drug Therapy	Examples of Pathologic Conditions or Drugs Affecting Drug Therapy
Dry mouth and secretions (xerostomia)	Difficulty in swallowing drugs	Dehydration
Decreased liver blood flow; decreased liver mass; decrease in microsomal enzymes	Delayed and decreased metabolism of certain drugs	Congestive heart failure, hepatic insufficiency, fever, malignancy
Decreased lipid content in skin	Possible decrease in absorption of transdermal medications	
Increase in body fat (from 18 to 36% in men and 33 to 45% in women); decrease in body water	Possible increased toxicity of water-soluble drugs; more prolonged and possible increased effects of fat-soluble drugs	Obesity, dehydration, diuretic drug therapy
Decrease in serum proteins	Possible increased effect/toxicity of highly protein bound drug; increased possibility of interactions of two or more highly protein bound drugs	Malnutrition, burns, liver disease
Decrease in renal mass, blood flow, and glomerular filtration rate (decline of 50% between age 20 and 90, average of 35%)	Possible increased serum levels/toxicity of drugs excreted renally	Renal insufficiency, CHF hypovolemia, NSAIDs use, use of drugs excreted via kidneys

TABLE 7-1

Effects of Aging and Concurrent Conditions or Drug Therapy on Drug Response (continued)

Physiologic Changes of Aging	Effects on Drug Therapy	Examples of Pathologic Conditions or Drugs Affecting Drug Therapy
Changes in sensitivity of certain drug receptors	Increase in drug effects, e.g., anticholinergics, antihistamines, barbiturates (paradoxical excitation), benzodiazepines, digitalis, warfarin Decrease in drug effects, e.g., amphetamines, beta blockers, quinidine	
Visual and hearing changes	Interference with learning and/or safe administration of medications	Anticholinergic (vision) Loop diuretics, certain antibiotics (e.g., aminoglycosides) (hearing)

TABLE 7-2

Drugs Requiring Special Considerations for Use in Elderly

1. Drugs expected to be widely used in the elderly
2. Drugs that affect or are affected by biologic homeostatic mechanisms that may be deficient in the elderly (e.g., CV system)
3. Drugs that act in the CNS
4. Drugs with a low therapeutic-to-safety ratio that:
   a. Are excreted largely by kidney
   b. Are subject to a large first-pass-effect
   c. Are metabolized by oxidative mechanisms
   d. Generate significant metabolites
   e. Are highly protein bound

SOURCE: Abrams. [5]

ADVERSE DRUG REACTIONS AND IATROGENESIS

Elderly persons are more likely to have more adverse drug reactions because of drug-drug interactions, polypharmacy, and noncompliance. As many as two-thirds of the elderly in the community may have at least one drug-drug reaction or drug-alcohol combination associated with a possible adverse reaction.[6] Adverse drug reactions account for a significant number of hospital admissions of the elderly; as many as 28 percent of hospital admissions were drug-related—11 percent related to noncompliance and 17 percent for adverse drug reactions.

Iatrogenic risks are often related to age, number of drugs taken, and complexity of current illnesses.[7] The potential for adverse drug reactions increases with increasing number of medications: a risk of 6 percent when two drugs are taken together, 50 percent when five drugs are taken together, and 100 percent when eight or more medications are taken together.[8] Elderly women have more adverse drug effects than men, probably due to their use of a greater number of medications than men. Multiple medication use by elderly patients is believed to be related to an estimated 51 percent of deaths and 32,000 hip fractures annually.[9]

Drug therapy for the elderly requires the clinician to make careful assessments of the individual patient's physiological and phychosocial status and of the necessity for drug therapy.

Types of Adverse Effects

Adverse drug reactions may not be recognized as such because their symptoms may be similar to pathophysiological conditions such as cerebral ischemia, MI, or sepsis.[10] Interferences with the activities of daily living may provide clues to adverse drug reactions in the elderly.

The following questions may help to determine if the symptom is drug-related.[11]

1. Is the observed symptom one that is known to be a possible side effect of one or another drug that the client takes?
2. Did the observed symptom develop shortly after the addition of a new drug to the regimen or a dosage increase for an existing drug in the regimen?
3. Did the observed symptom subside when a drug was reintroduced or the dosage increased?
4. Did the symptom reappear when a drug was reintroduced or the dosage increased?
5. What other factors might have led to or contributed to the observed symptom?
6. Has the client had a similar symptom in the past in response to this drug or another one?

Cognitive impairment (e.g., delirium, dementia, depression) can be caused by a variety of medications. Even in healthy individuals, the CNS is very sensitive to chemical imbalances from anticholinergic effects of many prescription and OTC medications.[12] (See the discussion of anticholinergic syndrome below.)

Cognitive changes can interfere with the patients' abilities to manage their medication regimen as well as posing additional dangers to their level of functioning and quality of life. These changes can also interfere with the clinician's ability to assess symptomatology of the patient if he or she is unable to describe symptoms such as the location or degree of any pain experienced, to request PRN medications, or to describe side effects or changes in their well-being. Exhibits 7-1 and 7-2 summarize information related to medication induced cognitive changes.[12a]

Anticholinergic Syndrome

The use of drugs with anticholinergic effects presents a particular problem with the elderly. Studies have shown that 30 to 60 percent of elderly daily receive drugs with anticholinergic activity; between 9 and 32 percent simultaneously take two or more anticholinergic drugs.[13]

Many of these anticholinergic effects—both central and peripheral—can aggravate other conditions being experienced by the elderly. Central anticholinergic effects include agitation, disorientation, poor attention, confusion, hallucinations, and psychosis. Peripheral effects are constipation, urinary retention, inhibition of sweating, decreased salivary and bronchial secretions, tachycardia, and mydriasis.[11] Constipation can be caused by or aggravated by the effects of anticholinergic drugs. Individuals with BPH or other strictures of the urinary urethra may experience increased difficulty in initiating urine flow. Dryness of the mouth and eyes may also be increased; dryness of the mouth can slow the absorption of sublingual medications and may affect the ability to swallow oral preparations. Visual disturbances may be caused by the effects on the eye. Effects on the pulse may alter cardiovascular drug effects and/or lead to cardiovascular drug therapy.

Anticholinergic effects of atropine in the usual order of appearance with increasing atropine dosage are bradycardia, dry mouth, decreased sweating, tachycardia, dilated pupils, blurred near vision, decreased intestinal peristalsis, dysphasia, dysphagia, urinary retention, hyperthermia/flushing, ataxia, hallucinations, delirium, and coma. An aid for remembering anticholinergic effects is as follows:[11]

Dry as a bone	Inhibition of secretions
Red as a beet	Flushing related to absence of sweating
Hot as a hare	Temperature elevation from absence of sweating
Blind as a bat	Cycloplegia and mydriasis
Mad as a hatter	Mental confusion and delirium

Drugs with anticholinergic effects are not only those classified as such (i.e., atropine) but also other drugs with anticholinergic side effects such as antidepressants, antihistamines, antiparkinson agents, antipsychotics, and quinidine. Therefore, the clinician needs to check each drug prescribed or being considered for prescribing for its anticholinergic profile; certain drugs within a pharmacological classification may differ in the severity of their anticholinergic effects. This may serve as a basis for the selection of a different drug within that group that would have less anticholinergic effect.

EXHIBIT 7-1

Underlying Mechanisms of Medication-induced Mental Changes

Mechanism of Action	Medication Examples
Anticholinergic interactions	Atropine; scopolamine; antihistamines; antipsychotics; antidepressants; antispasmodics; antiparkinsonian agents
Decreased cerebral blood flow	Antihypertensives; antipsychotics
Depression of respiratory center	Central nervous system depressants
Fluid and electrolyte alterations	Diuretics; alcohol; laxatives
Altered thermoregulation	Alcohol; psychotropics; narcotics
Acidosis	Diuretics; alcohol; nicotinic acid
Hypoglycemia	Hypoglycemics; alcohol; propranolol
Hormonal disturbances	Thyroid extract; corticosteroids

SOURCE: Miller CA: *Nursing Care of Older Adults: Theory and Practice*, 2d ed. Philadelphia: Lippincott, 1995. Used with permission.[12a]

EXHIBIT 7-2

Adverse Medication Effects as a Cause of Depression

Types of Medications	Examples
Histamine blockers	Cimetidine; ranitidine
Cardiac medications and antihypertensives	Digoxin; procainamide; reserpine; hydralazine; propranolol; methyldopa; guanethidine; clonidine
Central nervous system depressants, antianxiety agents, antipsychotics	Alcohol, haloperidol, benzodiazepines, meprobamate, flurazepam, barbiturates, fluphenazine
Antiparkinson agents	Levodopa; amantadine
Steroids	Corticosteroids; estrogen; progesterone
Analgesics, nonsteroidal anti-inflammatory drugs	Narcotics; ibuprofen; sulindac; indomethacin
Antineoplastic agents	Asparaginase; tamoxifen

SOURCE: Miller CA: *Nursing Care of Older Adults: Theory and Practice*, 2d ed. Philadelphia: Lippincott, 1995. Used with permission.[12a]

PREVENTION OF ADVERSE DRUG EFFECTS IN THE ELDERLY

Prevention of adverse drug effects in the elderly is done through appropriate prescribing, especially the avoidance of polypharmacy. Accurate diagnosis and establishment of a clear need for drug therapy rather than the use of nonpharmacological approaches are essential. Drug therapy should only be used if it is clear that there is a specific diagnosis or clearly documented symptom or condition to be treated. Treatment of the adverse effects of one drug by prescribing another should be avoided; often overlooked unfortunately is the possibility that a presenting sign or symptom is the result of the person's drug regimen. Since the patient may be treated by more than one prescriber, it is important to obtain a complete history of all drugs prescribed. Also, a careful history of the use of OTC preparations and home remedies or the use of alternative medicine is necessary. The use of alcohol should be assessed carefully.

Once it is determined that the drug therapy is necessary, careful consideration must be given to those variables that can affect the pharmacokinetics and pharmacodynamics of drug therapy (Table 7-1). For most drugs, it is important to evaluate the adequacy of the patient's renal and hepatic function. Dosing of most drugs generally should start low and with a longer time interval between doses. The dose can be increased and the interval adjusted if necessary as the patient's response is monitored. When possible, the use of a once-a-day dose should be chosen to avoid problems with compliance. Ongoing monitoring and evaluation of the drug regimen for both effectiveness, adverse effects, and the development of pathophysiology that can alter pharmacological responses, as well as patient compliance, are essential.

Appropriate versus Inappropriate Prescribing Practices

Increased adverse reactions in the elderly also may be due to inappropriate prescribing practices. "Appropriate prescribing may be defined as the selection of a medication and instruction for its use that agree with accepted medical standards. These standards are derived from manufacturer and FDA labeling guidelines, standard medication references, and interpretation of the scientific literature by drug therapy experts."[14]

In a study of nursing home residents, 40 percent received inappropriate medication orders and 7 percent of all prescriptions were inappropriate. Inappropriate prescriptions included drugs that should be avoided in the elderly (with highest incidence for long-acting benzodiazepines, persantine, propoxyphene), drugs with duration limitation (e.g., histamine blockers, short-acting benzodiazepines, oral antibiotics), or drugs with dosage limitations (iron supplements, histamine blockers, antipsychotic agents).[15]

A study of elderly outpatients in a VA clinic showed substantially appropriate prescribing in patients on multiple medications. The areas indicating need for improvement were more exact and more practical directions and the use of less expensive drugs. The study also found that drugs with a high risk for side effects were prescribed more appropriately than those with a low risk.[14]

Appropriate Use of Psychotropics in the Elderly

Inappropriate use of medications in the institutionalized elderly, especially as it may constitute chemical restraint, is an important ethical, clinical, and regulatory concern. The Omnibus Budget Reconciliation Act of 1987 (OBRA 87) established guidelines for the appropriate use of psychotropic drugs in long-term care facilities. These guidelines obviously impact most on NP prescribing for patients in nursing homes and other long-term care facilities; the clinicians practicing in these settings need to review the full regulations and the policies and procedures in place for compliance in that particular setting. The guidelines also provide guidance to other clinicians prescribing for the elderly. Similar regulations and monitoring of prescribing patterns and drug use may also occur as a result of drug use review (DUR) programs mandated by the 1990 OBRA (see Chap. 1).

OBRA REGULATIONS AND INTERPRETIVE GUIDELINES

Some of the provisions of the OBRA 87 regulations and interpretive guidelines are discussed below.[16]

Chemical Restraint

"The resident has the right to be free from any physical or chemical restraints imposed for purposes of discipline or convenience, and not required to treat the resident's medical symptoms."

Unnecessary Drugs

"Any drug when used in excessive dose (including duplicate therapy); or for excessive duration; or without adequate monitoring; or without adequate indications for its use; or in the presence of adverse consequences which indicate the dose should be reduced or discontinued; or any combination of the reasons above."

Use of Antipsychotic Drugs

Based on a comprehensive assessment of a resident, the facility must ensure that:

Residents who have not used antipsychotic drugs are not given these drugs unless antipsychotic drug therapy is necessary to treat a specific condition; as diagnosed and documented in the clinical record.

Residents who use antipsychotic drugs receive gradual dose reductions, drug holidays, or behavioral programming, unless clinically contraindicated, in an effort to discontinue these drugs.

PRN doses of neuroleptics are not to be used more than twice in a 7-day period without further assessment and is to be done only for the purpose of titrating dosage for optimal response or for management of unexpected behaviors that are otherwise unmanageable.

Conditions that are considered to be inappropriate as the sole basis for the use of antipsychotic drugs are wandering, poor self-care, restlessness, impaired memory, anxiety, depression (without psychotic features), insomnia, unsociability, indifference to surroundings, fidgeting, nervousness, uncooperativeness, or agitated behaviors which do not represent danger to the resident or others.

Long-acting benzodiazepines should not be used unless there has been an attempt to use a shorter-acting drug; they should not be used unless evidence exists that other possible reasons for residents' distress have been considered and ruled out; their use results in maintenance or improvement in the resident's functional status; daily use is less than 4 continuous months unless an attempt at a *gradual* dose reduction is unsuccessful; and their use is less than, or equal to, the following total *daily* doses unless higher doses (as evidenced by the resident's response and/or the resident's clinical record) are necessary for the maintenance or improvement in the resident's functional status. Daily doses of long-acting benzodiazepines are as follows:

Generic Name	Brand Name	Daily Oral Dosage for Elderly Residents
Chlordiazepoxide	Librium	20 mg
Clorazepate	Tranxene	15 mg
Clonazepam	Klonopin	1.5 mg
Diazepam	Valium	5 mg
Flurazepam	Dalmane	15 mg
Prazepam	Centrax	15 mg
Quazepam	Doral	7.5mg

Use of Short-Acting Benzodiazepines and Other Anxiolytics

OBRA 87 also regulated the use of short-acting benzodiazepines and other anxiolytics in patients in long-term care facilities.

Use of the listed (below) anxiolytic drugs for purposes other than sleep induction would only occur when: evidence exists that other possible reasons for the resident's distress have been considered and ruled out; use results in a maintenance or improvement in the resident's functional status; daily use (at any dose) is less than 4 continuous months unless an attempt at gradual dose reduction is unsuccessful; use is for one the following indications as defined by DSM-III or subsequent editions: generalized anxiety disorder; organic mental syndromes (including dementia) with associated states which are quantitatively and objectively documented and which constitute sources of distress or dysfunction of the resident or represent danger to the resident or others; panic disorder; symptomatic anxiety that occurs in residents with another diagnosed psychiatric disorder (e.g., depression, adjustment disorder); and use is equal to or less than following listed total *daily* doses, unless higher doses (as evidenced by the resident response and/or the resident's functional status).

Daily use dose of both long- and short-term-acting benzodiazepines should be limited to less than 4 continuous months unless an attempt at gradual dose reduction is unsuccessful; dose reductions should be considered after 4 months.

Generic Name	Brand Name	Daily Oral Dosage for Elderly Residents
Short-Acting Benzodiazepines		
Alprazolam	Xanax	0.75 mg
Halazepam	Paxipam	40 mg
Lorazepam	Ativan	2 mg
Oxazepam	Serax	30 mg
Other Anxiolytics		
Buspirone	BuSpar	30 mg
Chloral hydrate	Many brands	40 mg
Diphenhydramine	Benadryl	50 mg
Hydroxyzine	Atarax, Vistaril	50 mg

The following questions in Table 7-3 can guide the clinician in reviewing appropriateness of drug use and compliance with OBRA 87 regulations:

TABLE 7-3

Evaluating Appropriate Drug Use

1. Is the drug indicated for treatment of a specific condition documented in the medical record (e.g., an established or working diagnosis for which the drug is approved)?
2. Is the condition sufficiently problematic to require treatment?
3. Are there alternative treatments?
4. Will nonpharmacologic interventions supplant the need for the drug or complement drug therapy?

(continued)

TABLE 7-3

Evaluating Appropriate Drug Use (continued)

5. Has informed consent for prescription been obtained from the patient or legally determined surrogate decision maker?
6. Is the prescription likely to be effective as determined by the objective measurement of signs or symptoms expressed in the physician's preset goal for therapy?
7. How long should the drug be used before attempting to titrate downward or discontinue it? Will this be done after some set time or upon some change in the resident's condition?
8. Is the medication prescribed appropriately? Is there duplication? Are the dose and timing correct? Are there potential real drug-drug, drug-disease, or drug-nutritional interactions?
9. Is there adequate monitoring for common serious side effects (e.g., periodic blood levels, functional and mental status tests, movement disorder scales)?[2]
10. If side effects are present, are the negative effects of treatment outweighed by the positive aspects (e.g., improving, maintaining, or slowing decline of resident function or alleviating suffering)?

SOURCE: Smith.[16]

COMPLIANCE

Compliance and general strategies are discussed in Chap. 2. The clinician needs to focus on compliance and appropriate management of drug therapy by elderly patients and/or their caregivers in the home. In a retrospective study of 7247 outpatients, for 12 months patients formerly on digoxin were without digoxin or any other common alternative CHF drug for an average of 111 of the 365 days of follow-up. Only 10 percent filled enough prescriptions to have daily CHF medication. Compliance rates were found to be higher in patients over 85 years of age, women, those taking multiple medications, and those with hospital or nursing home stays before the initiation of therapy.[17]

The higher number of drugs usually prescribed for the elderly makes the regimen more complex. Cognitive changes in the elderly from the aging process, pathophysiology, or drug therapy need to be carefully assessed (initially and on an ongoing basis) in order to determine if the patient is able to understand and remember instructions. Physical limitations may affect their ability to open medication vials and packaging or to administer certain types of medications.

Various levels of cognitive skills and levels of physical skills, depending on the drug and route of administration, can be described as follows:[18]

Ability to read and comprehend main label (prescription)
Ability to read and comprehend the auxiliary labels (e.g., warnings)
Manual dexterity (open vials, remove correct number of tablets, recap medication)

In a small study of frail elderly, more than 50 percent of both Hispanic and Anglo patients reported difficulty in reading drug labels that were written in English.[19]

In a study of 178 older adults, forgetting was the most common reason for missing a medication; however, this was not found to be related to medication regimen complexity; the number of different medications and the total of number of pills to be consumed daily were important contributors to the medication complexity scores.[20]

Major factors found to be related to noncompliance are a poor relationship with the health care professional and declining cognitive function.[21]

Some research has been done to develop measures to predict patients' capacity to comply with medications. The Regimen Adherence Capacity Tests (RACT) have been studies to determine their validity. As part of this research, it was found that while the Folstein MMSE correlated fairly well with the RACT scores, it had less than desirable sensitivity and specificity and therefore would not be a good surrogate test for predicting capacity to comply.[18]

Michaud found that community-dwelling elders engaged in intelligent noncompliance when they encountered side effects that were bothersome or which they felt the prescriber did not address.[22]

Measures to help the elderly manage their medications correctly include simplification of regimen by decreasing to the extent possible the number of drugs and the number of pills to be taken in a day and prescribing medications to be taken at mealtime or in conjunction with other specific daily activities (before brushing teeth at night or before leaving for daily activity (e.g., exercise, card playing) unless contraindicated. When prescribing drugs in relation to meals it is important to determine if the patient does indeed have three meals a day and when he or she eats in order to be sure the medication will be taken at the intended time interval.

Careful instruction should be given, providing written instructions in the language and at the reading level the patient can understand); an audiotape could be used for patients with visual impairments. Instructions should include what adverse effects should be reported and to whom as well as what to do if a dose is missed. If possible, a family member or home caregiver should also receive instructions.

Encouraging patients to obtain all of their medications (prescription and OTC) from the same pharmacy will help the pharmacist to monitor all of the patients' medication use. Prescribers can ask that prescribed drugs be dispensed without the childproof packaging. However, one needs to consider possible dangers to children who might visit the patients' home.

Determine any financial restraints that may impact on the ability of the patient to actually obtain the medication. Some patients also may experience difficulty in physically obtaining the prescriptions, especially if they are on multiple medications with frequent and different dates for refill.

Periodically conduct a total "brown bag" assessment of all medications: ask the patients to bring in all medications they have in their possession at home, including

OTC preparations. These can be checked for outdated preparations, unused/unfinished prescriptions, and overlap or duplication of medications.

HEALTH CARE FRAUD

Health care fraud is an increasing problem; the elderly are more likely to be susceptible to claims of unproven remedies because many elderly have chronic conditions such as arthritis and cancer that are often the target of unproven remedies. Unproven remedies pose two major dangers: from the preparation itself, which may be impure, toxic, and/or incompatible with the patient and his or her ongoing therapy; and delay in or rejection of accurate diagnosis and treatment.[23]

Clinicians need to be able to answer questions patients may have about various health products advertised in the media. They can provide guidelines to patients about how to evaluate claims. Red flags are celebrity endorsements, inadequate labeling, claims that the product works by secret formula, and promotion of the treatment only in the back pages of magazines, over the phone, by direct mail, in newspaper ads in the format of news stories, or 30-minute commercials in talk show format. Other clues are claims that a product is all natural, that it does not list contents, is effective for a wide variety of disorders (e.g., cancer, arthritis, and sexual dysfunction), has no warnings about side effects, or that it works immediately or completely, making visits to the doctor unnecessary.

SUMMARY

The elderly can receive considerable benefit from the many drugs available today that can cure or control diseases and improve longevity and the quality of life. However, the elderly also pose special challenges to the prescribing clinician to provide the appropriate type and dose of medication that optimizes the intended therapeutic effects and avoids or reduces the many potential adverse outcomes of drug therapy that can result from the aging process and other unique characteristics of each individual elderly person.

REFERENCES

1. Hershman DL, Simonoff PA, Frishman WH, et al: Drug utilization in the old old and how it relates to self-perceived health and all-cause mortality: Results from the Bronx Aging Study. *J Am Geriatr Soc* 43:356–360, 1995.
2. Fillenbaum GG, Hanlon JT, Corder EH, et al: Prescription and nonprescription drug use among Black and White community-residing elderly. *Am J Public Health* 83(11):1577–1582, 1993.
3. Stuck AE, Beers MH, Steiner A, et al: Inappropriate medication use in community-residing older persons. *Arch Intern Med* 154(19):2195–2200, 1994.
4. American Medical Association Council on Scientific Affairs: American Medical Association White Paper on Elderly Health: Report of the Council on Scientific Affairs. *Arch Intern Med* 150:2459–2472, 1990.

5. Abrams WB: Development of drugs for use by the elderly; in Moore SR, Teal W (eds): *Geriatric Drug Use—Clinical and Social Perspectives*. New York: Pergamon, 1985, pp 200–205.

6. Pollow RL, Stoller EP, Forster LE, Duniho TS: Drug combinations and potential risk of adverse drug reactions among community-dwelling elderly. *Nurs Res* 43(1):44–49, 1994.

7. Vernon GM: Medication iatrogenesis in the elderly: Common, yet preventable. *Nurse Pract* 19(6):27–28, 1995. Letter.

8. Shaughnessay AF: Common drug reactions in the elderly. *Emerg Med* 24:21–32, 1992.

9. Pelligrino RM: Rx for medication safety. *Office Nurse* 4 (July/August): 6–13, 1991.

10. Ruiz JG, Lowenthal DT: *Geriatric Pharmacology*, in Munson PL (ed): *Principles of Pharmacology*. New York: Chapman & Hall, 1995.

11. Swonger AK, Burbank PM: *Drug Therapy and the Elderly*. Boston: Jones and Bartlett, 1995.

12. Miller CA: Medications that may cause cognitive impairment in older adults. *Geriatr Nurs* 16(1):47, 1995.

12a. Miller CA: *Nursing Care of Older Adults: Theory and Practice*, 2d ed. Philadelphia: Lippincott, 1995.

13. Pepper G: Monitoring the effects of anticholinergic drugs, in Chenitz W, Stone C, Takano J, Salisbury SA: *Clinical Gerontological Nursing. A Guide to Advanced Practice*. Philadelphia: Saunders, 1991, pp 377–389.

14. Schmader K, Hanlon JT, Weinberger M, et al: Appropriateness of medication prescribing in ambulatory elderly patients. *J Am Geriatr Soc* 42:1241–1247, 1994.

15. Beers MH, Ouslander JG, Fingold SF, et al: Inappropriate medication prescribing in skilled-nursing facilities. *Ann Int Med* 117:684–689, 1992.

16. Smith DA: Evaluating appropriate drug use, in *OBRA/HCFA Guidelines. Psychotropics in Long Term Care Facilities*. Columbia, MD: American Medical Directors Association, p 9.

17. Monane M, Bohn RL, Gurwitz JH, et al: Noncompliance with congestive heart failure therapy in elderly. *Arch Intern Med* 154(4):433–437, 1994.

18. Fitten LJ, Coleman L, Siembieda DW, et al: Assessment of capacity to comply with medication regimens in older patients. *J Am Geriatr Soc* 43:361–367, 1995.

19. Lile JL, Hoffman R: Medication-taking by the frail elderly in two ethnic groups. *Nurs Forum* 26(4): 19–24, 1991.

20. Conn V, Taylor SG, Kelley S: Medication regimen complexity and adherence among older adults. *Image J Nurs Sch* 23(4):231–235, 1991.

21. French DG. Avoiding adverse drug reactions in the elderly patient: Issues and strategies. *Nurse Prac* 21(9):90, 1996.

22. Michaud PL: Independent older persons managing medications at home: A grounded theory. Unpublished doctoral dissertation, Boston College, May 1996.

23. Napier K: Unproven medical treatments lure elderly. *FDA Consumer*, March 1994, p 33.

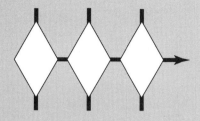

Part 2

DRUG THERAPY ISSUES AND APPLICATIONS

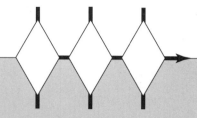

Chapter 8
IMMUNIZATIONS IN ADULTS

Patricia A. Stevenson

OVERVIEW

The Public Health Service receives recommendations from the Advisory Committee on Immunization Practices (ACIP), which meets periodically. No vaccine has 100 percent effectiveness or is completely safe. There are benefits and risks associated with all immunizations. As recommendations are revised, they are published in the Centers for Disease Control (CDC) *Morbidity and Mortality Weekly Report (MMWR),* which is available on the Internet (http://www.cdc.gov/cdc.html).

In the United States, vaccinations against diphtheria, tetanus, pertussis, measles, mumps, rubella, poliomyelitis, and *Haemophilus influenzae* type b meningitis are routinely administered, usually as part of childhood immunizations. (See Table 8-1A. Additional schedules are available for infants and children less than 7 years of age who start the series late and patients 7 years and older who were not vaccinated during early infancy.) The newest addition to the childhood vaccines is the hepatitis B vaccine series, initiated at birth. Recommendations for adults are in Table 8-1B.

TABLE 8-1A

Infant/Childhood Immunization in the United States [Ref.: MMWR 44(No. RR-5), 1995]

Vaccine	Birth	1 Mo.	2 Mos.	4 Mos.	6 Mos.	12 Mos.	15 Mos.	18 Mos.	4-6 Yrs.	11-12 Yrs.	14-16 Yrs.
Hepatitis B[†]	Hep B-1		Hep B-2			Hep B-3				Hep B[§]	
Diphtheria and tetanus toxoids and pertussis vaccine[¶]			DTP	DTP	DTP	DTP (DTaP at ≥15 mo.)			DTP or DTaP		Td
Haemophilus influenzae type b[**]			Hib	Hib	Hib	Hib	Hib				
Poliovirus[††]			OPV	OPV		OPV			OPV		
Measles-mumps-rubella[§§]						MMR	MMR		MMR or MMR		
Varicella-zoster virus[¶¶]							VAR		VAR[***]		

▭ Range of Acceptable Ages for Vaccination ▬ "Catch-Up" Vaccination[§***]

[†] If mother HBsAg neg., recommended 1st dose is 2.5 μg of Recombivax HB (Smith Kline Beecham). If mother HBsAg pos., give infant 0.5 mL HBIG within 12 hrs of birth and either 5 μg of Recombivax HB or 10 μg Engerix-B at separate site.

[¶] Acellular pertussis vaccine is now approved for children 6 weeks to 6 years old.

[**] 3 licensed H. influenzae protein conjugate vaccines. A 4th, available in 1997, combines hemophilus B with hepatitis B.

[††] Inactivated polio vaccine acceptable alternative for pts with congenital or acquired immunodeficiency.

[§§] Second dose anytime > 1 mo. after 1st dose.

[¶¶] Anytime after age 12 mos. If no reliable history of chickenpox, vaccinate at age 11–12 yrs.

TABLE 8-1B

Adult Immunization in the United States[1] (Travelers; see Med Letter 38:17, 1996)

Age Group (years)	Td[2]	Measles	Mumps	Rubella	Influenza	Pneumococcal	Hepatitis B[4]
18–24	x	x	x	x			Individuals at ↑ risk regardless of age.
25–64	x	x[3]	x	x			
≥65	x				x	x	

[1] From *Guide for Adult Immunization*, 3d Ed., Am Coll Physicians, 1994. Also see AnIM 12:35, 1996, and IDCP

[2] TD = tetanus + diphtheria toxoids, adsorbed for adult use (contains 5 Fl units tetanus + 2 Fl units diphtheria vs childhood vaccine, which contains 5 Fl u tetanus + 12.5 Fl u diphtheria)

[3] Indicated for persons born in 1957 or later. 9% hospital workers born before 1957 are not immune, serotest and immunize especially during outbreaks.

[4] Screen all pregnant women for HBsAg (give HBIG and vaccine to infants born to HBsAg-positive mothers). Those at ↑ exposure risk: homosexual males, injecting drug users, multiple partner heterosexual exposure, other sexually transmitted diseases, household and sexual contacts of HBV carriers, health care and public safety workers with exposure to blood, residents and staff of institutions for retarded, hemodialysis patients, recipients of Factor VII or IX concentrates, morticians.

Administration Schedule for Above Plus Other Selected Vaccines*

Hepatitis A (Havrix, Vaqta): 1.0 mL IM and repeat in 6–12 mos. Antibodies detectable after 15 days; use immune serum globulin. 0.02 mL/kg IM for immediate protection. Indication: for travelers to endemic areas. (*Med Letter 37:51, 1995; IDCP 5:122, 1996*)

Hepatitis B (Engerix B, Recombivax HB): 3 doses; initial, 1 month later, 6 months after 1st. Give IM in deltoid (not in buttocks), use 1½-inch needle; give SC only in pts at risk of bleeding (hemophiliacs). (Seroprotection associated with titers ≥ 10 mIU/mL.)

Influenza (killed virus): One dose (0.5 mL) IM Annual reimmunization with current vaccine recommended.

Measles (Attenuvax) (live virus vaccine): Unless contraindicated,§ one dose (0.5 mL) sc preferably in outer aspect upper arm. Booster not required.

Measles + Rubella + Mumps (MMR) (live virus): Unless contraindicated§ (do not give to pregnant women), one dose (0.5 mL) sc as with measles. Booster not required.

Pneumococcal (Pneumovax 23, Pnu-Immune 23) (pure antigens, 23): One dose (0.5 ml) sc. Booster not required except possibly individuals at high risk (nephrotic syndromes, renal failure, transplant recipients, splenectomy, ?HIV who received vaccine > 6 years before).

Td (toxoids, not live): Primary: Two doses IM at least 4 wks apart, 3d dose 6–12 months after 2d. Booster: every 10 years

Typhoid (Typhim Vi): A single IM dose of 25 μg yields 95% seroconversion. Minimal side effects. For travelers & lab workers.

Varicella (Varivax): 0.5 ml subcutan, and repeat 4–8 wks later. For susceptible adolescents/adults who are: (1) health care worker, (2) susceptible household contact of immunocompromised person, (3) work in schools/day care centers, (4) college students/military, (5) non-pregnant women of child-bearing age.

*Review package insert for specific product being administered.

173

GENERAL CONSIDERATIONS

The widespread implementation of childhood vaccination programs has substantially reduced the occurrence of many vaccine-preventable diseases. However, successful immunization programs alone do not eliminate specific disease problems.

Immunizations have long been an integral part of the primary health care of infants and young children and have significantly decreased the morbidity of certain infectious diseases among children, particularly illnesses with serious sequelae. However, nursing has a significant responsibility to improve the incidence of childhood immunizations. The high number of underimmunized children in the United States demonstrates the need for closer surveillance and protection of the population. Nurses must be knowledgeable about the individual vaccines and their efficacy, schedules, side effects, and contraindications.

A substantial proportion of the remaining mortality and morbidity from vaccine-preventable diseases presently occurs among adolescents and adults. Patients who escape natural infection and were not vaccinated as young children against diphtheria, tetanus, measles, mumps, rubella, and polio may be at risk for any of the diseases and their complications. Some factors which influence compliance with vaccine programs include lack of awareness related to safe vaccines, unfounded concerns regarding vaccine side effects, and missed opportunities by health care providers to vaccinate during a follow-up visit to the office, clinic, or hospital.[1]

Vaccines are designed to stimulate an active immunologic response in order to provide a long-term protection against infectious disease. They include killed viruses, toxoids, or live attenuated viruses. Exposure to the vaccines causes an initial response by the body's lymphocytes to form antibodies, primarily IgM initially and later IgG. When a person is exposed to a second vaccine or to the disease, the host sets up a second response. The major antibody that then responds is IgG, providing a higher and more lasting level of protection.[2]

Vaccines may require boosters to give prolonged protection against infectious disease. An example of this is the tetanus-diphtheria booster, which is required every 10 years to give continuing protection.

Vaccines developed for childhood immunizations should have a high degree of efficacy. For example, the oral attenuated polio virus vaccine has an efficacy of 95 percent, which means that 95 percent of the study group seroconverted after immunizations.[3] When products are being considered for distribution to the population, side effects, efficacy, and contraindications are always considered. An example of this is seen with the use of inactivated polio vaccine (IPV) as compared with oral polio vaccine (OPV). The killed virus (IPV) is not used as commonly as OPV because it does not provide immunity that is as durable as with OPV and it was found to not protect the intestine as adequately.

The types of vaccine preparations are as follows:

Toxoid: Preparation formed by the alteration of the substance formed by certain microorganisms during growth and metabolism.
Killed virus: Vaccine that includes dead viruses capable of initiating an immune response because of continuation of certain organism characteristics, i.e., the cell wall. Usually these will require a booster.

Attenuated virus: Preparation composed of live organisms that have been altered so that they are not virulent but are capable of inducing long-lasting immunity. They are either recombinant, conjugated, or both.

Recombinant forms: Organisms that have been genetically altered for use in vaccines.

Conjugated forms: Altered organisms joined with another substance to increase immunogenicity.

NURSING CONSIDERATIONS

Some vaccines require repeat dosing for adequate protection. If the provider administers multiple doses that are less than the recommended dose size or at less than the recommended interval, the antibody response may be lessened. This is not recommended. These doses are not to be counted as part of a patient's vaccination series. Some vaccines may even require a booster dose to maintain protection.

Most vaccines can be given safely on the same day at separate sites. However when the vaccine commonly is associated with a local or systemic reaction, such as cholera, typhoid, and plague, it may cause a reaction to be *accentuated* if given simultaneously. In this case it is safer to have the patient schedule the vaccines for separate days.

According to the Centers for Disease Control, when administered at the same time and at different sites, diphtheria, tetanus, pertussis (DTP), OPV, and measles, mumps, rubella (MMR) produce the same seroconversion rates and rates of side effects as when administered separately. Acceptable response has also been seen with the simultaneous administration of DTP, OPV, MMR and either *Haemophilus influenzae* type b (Hib) or hepatitis B vaccine (HPV).

NURSING'S RESPONSIBILITY FOR IMMUNIZATIONS

There are national and international health care systems in place that support efforts to provide proper immunizations. The goal in theory is to eradicate infectious disease through appropriate immunization. An example of this is smallpox vaccination, which is no longer required in the United States because the incidence of complications from the vaccine is now greater than the risk of acquiring the disease. This decreased incidence of disease is directly attributable to the protection provided by years of smallpox vaccination.

Both education and immunization work together in the treatment of high-risk groups, such as with hepatitis B transmission. It is important to target high-risk groups that may have contact with infected blood, stool, or saliva. This is vital to control the spread of the disease and its associated mortality and morbidity. Immunizations have a significant correlation with reducing the cost of health care, particularly in relation to the number of hospitalizations. Illnesses related to infectious diseases cause lost work hours for parents, lost school days for children, closed facilities if outbreaks occur, and additional money to investigate an outbreak and further immunize the exposed public.[4]

Nurses should emphasize with families the importance of maintaining immunizations on schedule. They should inform parents that children may need more than one injection per visit and that children may still maintain their vaccine schedule despite a recent antibiotic regime, exposure to a recent infectious illness, or breastfeeding practices. Patients will also need additional instructions when immunizations are interrupted by vacations or international travel.

Side effects when administering vaccines are always a possibility. Nurses must be prepared to administer epinephrine 1:1000 (0.01 mL/kg) subcutaneously to treat anaphylaxis. Any additional doses of the vaccine that caused a reaction are contraindicated, and the patient record is marked accordingly.

Providers need to educate patients about the appropriate schedule for administration of vaccines, the possible side effects, specific contraindications, the degree of efficacy, and the need for additional boosters. The Department of Public Health in the closest town or city will answer any questions regarding dose, side effects, and availability of vaccines.

IMMUNE GLOBULIN

Immune globulin (IG) contains antibodies that can prevent or diminish the effect of some infectious diseases. It is acquired naturally through transplacental transfer of maternal immunity in full-term infants. Depending on the immunity experiences of the mother, the child will be selectively protected against those infectious diseases to which the mother is immune. Plasma is pooled from many individuals and available for intramuscular injection; human immune serum globulin (HISG) has been used to prevent poliomyelitis, measles, and infectious hepatitis in exposed persons. Specialized HISG selected for high titers of a specific antibody (convalescent serum) is used prophylactically in the prevention of hepatitis B, varicella zoster, rabies, and tetanus. Human immune globulin for intravenous use (IVIG) has been developed for cytomegalovirus. Specific IVIG for other diseases are in development. These offer the advantage of maximum and specific dosing and offer great hope for the future.

Prophylactic benefit is greatest when given before or soon after exposure. It is not recommended for patients already demonstrating clinical manifestations of illness or for those individuals exposed more than two weeks before. It can be given as a mode of replacement therapy for persons with hypogammaglobulinemia.

IG is urged for both preexposure and postexposure in hepatitis A prophylaxis. One dose of 0.02 mL/kg administered within 2 weeks of exposure may be effective in household and sexual contacts of persons with hepatitis A. Preexposure prophylaxis is discussed in the "Immunizations for Travelers," page 190.

IG is recommended in the prevention or modification of measles (rubeola). It should be administered to any susceptible person exposed less than 6 days previously. A susceptible person is defined as a person not previously vaccinated and who has not had the measles. IG is particularly indicated for at-risk household contacts of measles patients.

Varicella-zoster immune globulin (VZIG) and IG are used for passive immunization after exposure to the varicella-zoster virus. With immunocompromised patients, it is best done using VZIG. If VZIG is unavailable, IG may modify the varicella if given promptly.

The routine use of IG for postexposure prophylaxis of rubella in patients in early pregnancy is not recommended. However, if termination of the pregnancy is not an option for a susceptible woman exposed to rubella infection, IG may be considered. It is important to note that the absence of rubella following administration of IG to the mother does *not* guarantee that infection has been prevented or that the infant will not experience congenital rubella. This is information that nurse practitioners need to incorporate into their prenatal teaching and counseling.

Prophylactic treatment to prevent hepatitis B is best accomplished with the use of hepatitis B immune globulin (HBIG) in combination with hepatitis B vaccine.

Reactions

Systemic reactions to immune globulin administration are rare, but epinephrine should be available for treatment of acute allergic response. No lab tests are required prior to administration for traveling patients. However, because hepatitis A cannot be reliably diagnosed on clinical presentation alone, serologic confirmation of hepatitis A virus (HAV) infection in index patients by IgM anti-HAV testing is recommended before postexposure treatment of contacts. Screening of the contacts for immunity is not recommended because screening is more costly than IG and will delay its administration. When a patient is admitted to the hospital with hepatitis A, the staff need not be given IG; instead good hand-washing and hygienic precautions should be carefully enforced. Should an epidemiological investigation show that an institutional outbreak has occurred, then IG may be recommended.[5]

TETANUS-DIPHTHERIA-PERTUSSIS VACCINE

According to CDC estimates, a large percentage of adults (22 to 26 percent of patients 18 to 35 and 41 to 84 percent of patients over 60) may have insufficient immunization to diphtheria.[6] However, in 1994, only one case of diphtheria occurred in the United States. Diphtheria is an endemic disease in many developing countries. Tetanus is ubiquitous worldwide. Pertussis is common in developing countries as well as in other countries where routine immunization against pertussis is not widely practiced. Pertussis is highly communicable, is often associated with complications, and has a relatively high case-fatality ratio in infants. Because the risk of contracting pertussis in other countries and of diphtheria in developing countries is higher than the United States, it is advised that children leaving the United States should be immunized before departure.

Tetanus-diphtheria (Td) is a toxoid vaccine with 98 percent efficacy. Pertussis is a live attenuated vaccine with 75 to 85 percent efficacy. Optimum protection against diphtheria, pertussis, and tetanus in the first year of life is achieved with the following schedule:

DTP series:
Dose 1: age 2 months (or DTaP)
Dose 2: age 4 months (or DTaP)

Dose 3: age 6 months (or DTaP)
Dose 4: age 12 to 18 months (or DTaP at age 15+ months)
Dose 5: age 4 to 6 years (or DTaP)
Td booster: age 12 (and every 10 years)

Infants traveling to endemic areas should have preferably received three doses. Parents who are traveling with young infants need to be informed that an unimmunized child is at far greater risk of contracting pertussis than a child who has been adequately protected.

A tetanus-diphtheria booster algorithm can be seen in Table 8-2.[7]

Indications for Vaccination during Pregnancy

If a pregnant patient lacks a primary vaccination series or a Td booster within the past 10 years, it is recommended that she receive a vaccination and a booster after the first trimester.[8]

TABLE 8-2

Antitetanus Prophylaxis, Wound Classification, Immunization

Wound Classification			**Immunization Schedule**				
Clinical Features	**Tetanus Prone**	**Non–Tetanus Prone**	**History of Tetanus Immunization**	**Tetanus-Prone Wound**		**Non–Tetanus Prone Wound**	
				Td[1,2]	TIG	Td	TIG
Age of wound	> 6 hours	≤ 6 hours	Unknown or < 3 doses	Yes	Yes	Yes	No
Configuration	Stellate, avulsion	Linear					
Depth	> 1 cm	< 1 cm	3 or more doses	No[3]	No	No[4]	No
Mechanism of injury	Missile, crush, burn,	Sharp surface (glass, knife)					
Devitalized tissue	Present	Absent					
Contaminants (dirt, saliva, etc.)	Present	Absent					

[1] Td = Tetanus & diphtheria toxoids adsorbed (adult)
  TIG = Tetanus immune globulin (human)
[2] Yes if wound > 24 hours old.
  For children < 7 years. DPT (DT if pertussis vaccine contraindicated);
  For persons ≥ 7 years. Td preferred to tetanus toxoid alone.
[3] Yes if > 5 years since last booster
[4] Yes if > 10 years since last booster
SOURCE: From ACS Bull, 69:22.23, 1984, No. 10.   SOURCE: From MMWR 39:37, 1990 (Jan. 26).

Hypersensitivity to Vaccine Components

Vaccine components can cause allergic reactions in some recipients. These reactions can be local or systemic and could possibly include mild to severe anaphylactic-like responses. Vaccine components that are responsible include vaccine antigens, animal proteins, antibiotics, preservatives, or stabilizers.

Bacterial vaccines, such as contained in DTP, are frequently associated with local or systemic adverse effects. On rare occasions, urticarial or anaphylactic reactions have been reported. It is extremely difficult to link a sensitivity reaction to a specific vaccine component. Since the incidence and severity of pertussis decreases with age, and because the vaccine may cause side effects and adverse reactions, pertussis vaccine is not recommended after age 7. Skin testing can be performed to determine sensitivity. Acellular pertussis vaccine causes fewer reactions and is now approved and recommended for infants over 6 weeks.

Adverse Reaction to Td or DTP

Local reactions and erythema or induration with or without tenderness are common after administration of Td or DTP. Mild systemic reactions occur frequently. These include fever, drowsiness, restlessness, and anorexia. Moderate to severe systemic responses would include high fever (temperature at 105°F), persistent or inconsolable crying lasting more than three hours, collapse, or febrile convulsions. These reactions occur infrequently but appear to occur without sequelae. The rate of local reactions, fever, and other common systemic symptoms following receipt of DTaP are lower than those following whole-cell DTP vaccinations.[9]

No causal relationship has been found between DTP and sudden infant death syndrome and no increased risk for Guillain-Barré syndrome (GBS) is observed with DTP vaccine use. A family history of convulsions or other central nervous system disorders is not a contraindication for vaccination.[10]

Special Considerations

The following special considerations apply to immune-compromised populations.

1. Immune-compromised patients: Because of their immunodeficiency, many HIV-infected patients are at increased risk for complications of vaccine-preventable diseases. Thus, the risk-benefit ratio *favors* administration of vaccines to HIV-infected patients. Children with HIV should receive, on schedule, all of the routinely recommended inactivated childhood vaccines (DTP, hepatitis B) whether or not they are symptomatic.
2. Homeless persons: Administer the vaccine; there are no special considerations.

3. Immune-compromised due to large doses of steroids or malignancy: Administer when indicated.
4. Immunosuppression associated with bone marrow transplantation: Administer one year *after* transplant or check titers. Ideally, administration should occur prior to organ donation.

MEASLES, MUMPS, RUBELLA VACCINE

There is only one measles vaccine currently licensed for use in the United States. However, in the past other measles vaccines have been used. The measles, mumps, rubella (MMR) vaccine, produced in the United States, is prepared by chick embryo cell culture. Measles antibodies develop in 95 percent of patients vaccinated with the live attenuated vaccine at age 15 months and older.

Dose Schedule

Usually, two doses of live measles vaccine are recommended, one at 15 months and the second before entering kindergarten or middle school. This may vary according to individual state laws. Live measles vaccine given prior to the first birthday should not be considered as part of the usual series. When measles vaccine is administered, it should be given as a combined measles-rubella or MMR vaccine. The combined vaccine is as effective as each antigen given separately.

Simultaneous vaccination with other live and inactivated vaccines has shown no known decrease in antibody response nor any increase in the risk of side effects. If live vaccines such as measles are not given together, they must be separated by at least 30 days. Advise patients that measles vaccine should be given at least six weeks after immune globulin to ensure adequate antibody response. If a patient received measles vaccine outside of the guidelines, it is recommended to administer a repeat measles vaccine or test the patient for measles antibodies.[9]

Contraindications include infants under 12 months of age; individuals on cortisone, chemotherapy, or radiation therapy; pregnant women, patients having received IgG or blood transfusions within the last 6 months; and those with a known allergy to egg products or neomycin.

Nursing Considerations

With HIV-infected patients, administer if indicated, even though it is a live virus vaccine. Draw serum titers before administration. If a symptomatic HIV patient is exposed to measles, administer immune globulin.

Allowing the second dose of MMR to be given at age 12 emphasizes the importance of routine visits for preadolescents. For those not previously fully immunized this presents an opportunity to review immunizations and administer vaccines not yet added to a patient's schedule.

High-Risk Groups

Certain groups of adults have been identified as at increased risk for measles:
1. Health care workers having direct contact with infected patients.
2. Students attending colleges or post–high school institutions.
3. International travelers.

For each of these adults, it is important to have documented immunity to measles. According to the CDC, documented evidence of measles immunity is defined as:

1. Immunization dates showing two doses of live measles vaccine after age 12 months, spaced at least 30 days apart.
2. Written documentation of physician-diagnosed measles disease.
3. Laboratory evidence of immunity.
4. Birth before 1957.

Criteria may vary from state to state. If there is any doubt as to an individual's measles immune status, it is best to administer at least a single dose of the vaccine. There is *no* risk in receiving the additional dose if already immune. Pregnant women should not receive either the MR or the MMR vaccine. Women who have been immunized within the last 3 months should avoid pregnancy. Since children given MMR vaccine do not transmit the viruses, these vaccines *can* be given to children of pregnant women.

Patients with severe febrile illness should not be given the measles vaccine until recovery. However, minor illnesses, such as upper respiratory illness with or without low-grade fever, are not a reason to postpone the vaccination schedule. Extreme caution must be used with any patient demonstrating a history of anaphylaxis after egg ingestion. Protocols have been developed for vaccinating these patients.[11] There is no evidence that a person is at increased risk if he or she has egg allergies that are nonanaphylactic in nature or if he or she has an allergy to chicken or feathers.[9]

Measles vaccine contains minute amounts of neomycin. Measles vaccine is contraindicated for patients known to have an anaphylactic allergy to neomycin. The vaccine can cause a delayed immune response manifested as a contact dermatitis such as an erythematous pruritic nodule or papule at the injection site for 18 to 96 hours. However, mild contact dermatitis reaction to neomycin is *not* a contraindication for measles vaccine.

Routine skin testing for tuberculosis (Mantoux test) can be done the same day as administration of the measles vaccine. However, if done following measles administration, the testing must be delayed for six weeks.

Immune-Deficient Patients

Patients with the following diseases should not receive the MMR or measles vaccine: leukemia, lymphoma, and malignancies. Patients receiving steroid therapy, alkylating agents, antimetabolites, or radiation should not receive these vaccines. Administration of MMR should be considered for *all* susceptible symptomatic HIV-infected patients.

Side Effects

Mild fever and transient rash occurring 7 to 12 days after vaccination and lasting several days can be associated with primary vaccination. Approximately 5 to 15 percent of patients may develop fever higher than 103°F. Rare instances of encephalitis and encephalopathy have been reported (less than one case per million doses). There is no evidence of greater risk for patients either previously vaccinated or those who had natural measles disease.

Patients who had received killed measles vaccine may be more likely to develop local or systemic reactions following revaccination with live measles vaccine. Despite this, these patients should be revaccinated to avoid the severe atypical form of disease that often occurs after their exposure to measles.[9]

POLIO VACCINE

Trivalent oral polio vaccine (OPV) is the vaccine of choice for all infants, children, and adolescents up to age 18. Killed inactivated polio vaccine (IPV) is the only poliovirus vaccine recommended for immunocompromised children and their household contacts. It is an acceptable alternative for healthy children and adults.

The following schedules are all acceptable by the Advisory Committee on Immunization Practices (ACIP), the American Academy of Pediatrics (AAP), and the American Academy of Family Physicians (AAFP), and parents and providers may choose from among them:

1. IPV at 2 and 4 months; OPV at 12 to 18 months and 4 to 6 years.
2. IPV at 2, 4, 12 to 18 months, and 4 to 6 years.
3. OPV at 2, 4, 6 to 18 months, and 4 to 6 years.

For overall public health benefit, the ACIP recommends a sequential schedule of two doses of IPV followed by two doses of OPV for routine vaccination.[11]

Recent changes have developed in 1997 in regard to the recommendation for the polio vaccination schedule. The new changes have been recommended because of the lack of indigenous polio in the United States and the reduced risk of importation of wild polio virus.

Paralytic polio attributed to indigenously acquired wild polio has not occurred in the United States since 1979. Aggressive immunization practices worldwide have eliminated polio from the western hemisphere. Since 1980, the only indigenous cases of polio in the United States have been cases of vaccine-associated paralytic polio (VAPP), following administration of oral polio vaccine (OPV), with approximately 8 to 10 cases reported annually. The ACIP, the AAP, and the AAFP now recommend an increased use of IPV and decreased use of OPV over the next 5 years. All three schedules of polio vaccination meet acceptable standards of care. Parents should be informed of the benefits and risks of each schedule and should choose among them. In addition, a vaccine information statement (VIS) that describes the three schedules is available from local vaccine distributors or regional immunization offices.

High-Risk Groups

Patients traveling to countries where poliomyelitis is epidemic or endemic are considered to be at increased risk for disease and should be fully immunized. Unvaccinated or partially vaccinated travelers should complete the primary series with the vaccine that is appropriate to their age and previous immunization status. People who have completed the primary series should receive an additional dose of OPV once before traveling to areas with an increased risk of exposure to wild polio virus.

Side Effects

On rare occasions, paralysis has been associated with the administration of OPV to healthy patients and their contacts. Although the risk is extremely small, people should always be informed of the risk. No serious side effects have been documented with the use of IPV.

Since IPV contains trace amounts of streptomycin and neomycin, patients with a known history of anaphylaxis following receipt of these antibiotics should not receive IPV. Patients with a history of nonanaphylactic reactions to neomycin or streptomycin are at *no* increased risk and can be vaccinated. Available data do not support any increased risk of GBS.

Pregnancy

In general, pregnant women should not be vaccinated with polio vaccine. However, if immediate protection against poliomyelitis exposure is needed, OPV (not IPV) is recommended.

Altered Immunity

Patients with an altered immune state due to disease or immunosuppressive therapy are at increased risk for paralysis with OPV. These patients (including symptomatic and asymptomatic HIV-infected patients) and their household members and close contacts should receive IPV, not OPV.

Storage

Polio vaccine is stable only if stored in the refrigerator between 2 and 8°C (35 to 46°F). The vaccine must *not* be frozen.

HEPATITIS B VACCINE

Hepatitis B is a highly contagious, potentially deadly virus. There are as many as 300,000 new cases of hepatitis B every year, many of whom become chronic carriers. It is estimated that 91 percent of patients with hepatitis B infections have acquired the virus during adolescence or early childhood. The previous strategy of preventing hepatitis B emphasized immunization of selected high-risk adults. This failed to show an impact on the prevention of hepatitis B disease. Because of this, a strong plan for disease prevention is now in place targeting newborns and high-risk adolescents with universal immunizations. Infant hepatitis B vaccination has expanded rapidly since national recommendations were made in 1993; however, universal coverage has not yet been achieved.[12]

Dose Schedule

There are two dose schedules for infants born to mothers *not* infected with hepatitis B virus. With the first schedule, the newborn is given the first dose of hepatitis B vaccine (either 2.5 µg of Recombivax HB or 10 µg of Engerix-B) soon after birth, before the hospital discharge. The second dose is given at 1 to 2 months of age. The last dose is given between 6 to 18 months of age. The second schedule shows the first dose being given at 1 to 2 months of age, the second dose at 4 months, and the final dose at 6 to 8 months of age.

Perinatal Information

All pregnant women should be tested for hepatitis B surface antigen. If an infant is born to a mother known to have the hepatitis B virus, it should be treated with hepatitis B immune globulin plus hepatitis B vaccine within 12 hours of birth. The second and third doses of vaccine are given at 1 and 6 months of age. Hepatitis B vaccine may be given simultaneously with other childhood vaccines.

To measure effectiveness, infants should be tested at 3 to 9 months after the completion of the vaccine series, using the hepatitis B surface antigen and the antibody screen. If it is not known that the mother is infected until more than a month after delivery, the infant should be tested first for the hepatitis B surface antigen.

Infants born to HBsAg-positive mothers should receive 0.5 mL hepatitis B immune globulin (HBIG) within 12 hours of birth and either 5 µg of Recombivax HB or 10 µg of Engerix-B at a separate site. The second dose is recommended at 1 to 2 months of age and the third dose at age 6 months. Blood tests should be done at time of birth to determine the mother's HBsAg status; if it is positive, the infant should receive HBIG as soon as possible (no later than 1 week of age). The dosage and timing of subsequent vaccine doses should be based upon the mother's HBsAg status.[13]

Special Considerations

Hepatitis B and *Haemophilus influenzae* type b (Hib) vaccines were approved by the AAP as a combination immunization (COMVAX) for administration at 2, 4, and 12 to 15 months of age. This regimen, as well as other Hib-containing vaccines, should not be administered to infants younger than 6 weeks of age. Further, the AAP states that hepatitis B immunization can now be given at any age in children not previously vaccinated during infancy.

Adverse Reactions

Pain at the injection site, elevated temperatures greater than 37.7°C (98.6°F), anaphylaxis, and hypersensitivity are the main side effects reported with this vaccine. It is contraindicated for any patient that has a known prior history of anaphylactic response. Available data do not indicate any relationship to Guillain-Barré syndrome.[10]

High-Risk Patients

The American College Health Association (ACHA) recommends that all colleges and universities:

- Require hepatitis B vaccine for health care students
- Strongly urge vaccination for all college students
- Give special attention to high-risk students

High-risk students are those who:

1. Are sexually active with more than one sexual partner in six months
2. Engage in unprotected sex
3. Have had another sexually transmitted disease
4. Share needles for injecting drugs
5. Receive blood products on a chronic basis
6. Are students from areas where hepatitis B is endemic (Alaska, Africa, Asia, Brazil, Pacific Islands, northern Canadian provinces, southern Greenland)
7. Are African-Americans raised in urban areas with high hepatitis B prevalence, traveling to endemic areas for six months, and expecting to work in medical settings

In addition, in accordance with CDC guidelines, ACHA recommends screening prior to vaccination for high-risk groups that may already be hepatitis B carriers. This would include the following:[14]

- Students with multiple sex partners (more than one in the last 6 months)
- Male homosexuals
- Students whose parents or grandparents were born in Asia, Africa, Alaska, the Pacific Islands, Brazil, the northern Canadian provinces, or southern Greenland
- IV drug users

HEPATITIS A VACCINE

Hepatitis A vaccine is an inactivated whole virus vaccine derived from hepatitis A virus and grown in cell culture in human MRC-5 diploid fibroblasts. One milliliter of the vaccine contains approximately 50 U of hepatitis A virus antigen, which is purified and formulated without a preservative. The pediatric dose is 0.5 mL IM; the adult dose is 1 mL IM in the deltoid muscle.

Clinical Pharmacology

Hepatitis A virus is one of several viruses that cause a systemic infection with pathology in the liver. The incubation period ranges from 20 to 50 days. Hepatitis A is transmitted most often by the fecal-oral route. A common source of outbreak is contamination of food and water supplies, particularly shellfish, and uncooked foods prepared by an infected handler prior to ingestion (e.g., salads, sandwiches, meat).

Bloodborne transmission is mostly uncommon but is possible via blood transfusions, contaminated blood products, or IV drug use. The United States has seen approximately 143,000 infections per year. Clinical signs of hepatitis A are similar to those associated with other types of viral hepatitis and include anorexia, nausea, fever, chills, jaundice, dark urine, light-colored stools, abdominal pains, malaise, and fatigue.

Dose Schedule

Hepatitis A vaccine, introduced in 1995, is given as one primary dose and one booster dose for all ages 2 years and older by intramuscular injection only. A very high degree of protection has been demonstrated after a single dose of vaccine in children and adolescents. The protective efficacy and safety of the vaccine were evaluated in the Monroe Efficacy Study ($p < 0.001$). This study was a randomized, double-blind, placebo-controlled study involving 1037 children and adolescents 2 through 16 years of age in a U.S. community with recurrent outbreaks of hepatitis A.[15] One hundred percent protection against hepatitis A disease was demonstrated in this efficacy trial. A 95 percent seroconversion in healthy adults 18 years of age and older was noted 4 weeks following a single dose of 50 U/1.0 mL. A 97 percent seroconversion rate was noted in healthy children and adolescents ages 2 to 17 within 4 weeks of a single dose of 25 U/0.5 mL IM.

Patients 2 to 17 years of age should receive 0.5 mL IM and a booster of 0.5 mL IM 6 to 18 months later. Adults 18 years of age and older should receive a single 1.0 mL dose IM of vaccine and a booster dose of 1.0 mL IM 6 months later. It can be administered concomitantly with immune globulin, using separate sites and syringes. The deltoid muscle is the preferred site.

Indications and Use

Hepatitis A vaccine is indicated for preexposure prophylaxis against disease caused by the hepatitis A virus. This vaccine is recommended for all people traveling to countries with high or intermediate risk of infection. These areas include but are not limited to Africa, Asia, the Mediterranean, Central and South America, Mexico, Europe, and the Caribbean. Immunization should be given at least 2 weeks prior to expected exposure. High-risk individuals include travelers, military personnel, persons with multiple sex partners, recipients of therapeutic blood products, and people exposed to a patient with hepatitis A virus.

If hepatitis A vaccine is used in individuals with malignancies or patients receiving immunosuppressive therapy, the expected immune response may not be obtained. Caution is to be used with breastfeeding mothers and pregnant women. It is not known whether the vaccine can cause fetal harm. It has been shown to be well tolerated and highly immunogenic to patients 2 to 17 years of age. However, safety and efficacy in infants under 2 years has not been established.

Adverse Reactions

Side effects which have been reported include: localized pain at the injection site, fever, abdominal pain, headache, myalgia, nausea, vomiting, and diarrhea.

HAEMOPHILUS INFLUENZAE TYPE b CONJUGATE VACCINE

Haemophilus influenzae type b is an endemic disease worldwide. This virus causes meningitis and several other severe bacterial illnesses that affect primarily children under age 5. These include pneumonia, septic arthritis, epiglottitis, and sepsis. In the past it was the most common cause of bacterial meningitis in the United States. The use of *Haemophilus influenzae* type b conjugate vaccine (HbCV) dramatically reduced the incidence of this disease. Risk of acquiring the disease may be higher during travel to developing countries outside of the United States.

H. influenzae organisms are gram-negative coccobacilli with six distinct antigenically capsular types (types A to F). Invasive disease is almost always carried by type b. The mode of transmission is droplet inhalation and direct contact. The incubation period is widely variable but usually is 2 to 4 days.

In the United States, two types of HbCV were licensed in 1990 for use in infants starting at age 2 months. These include *Haemophilus* b conjugate vaccine, HbOC, and PRP-OMP. A third type of vaccine (PRP-D) is licensed only for use in children age 15 months and older. The same conjugate vaccine should be used for all doses in the primary series and ideally for the booster dose as well. A schedule for these vaccines is shown in Table 8-3.

Travel

Infants and children should be fully immunized prior to travel. If previously unvaccinated, children less than 15 months of age should be given two vaccine doses prior to travel. Doses should be given at least one month apart. Children between 15 months and 2 years of age require a single dose of vaccine.

TABLE 8-3

Vaccine Schedule for HbCV Vaccines

Vaccine	2 months	4 months	6 months	12 months	15 months
HbOC	Dose 1	Dose 2	Dose 3		Booster
PRP-OMP	Dose 1	Dose 2		Booster	
PRP-D					Single dose

SOURCE: Centers for Disease Control.[11]

Adverse Reactions

HbCV is considered relatively free of side effects. Redness and swelling at the injection site, as well as fevers (103°F or higher), have been reported. These reactions begin 24 h after vaccination and generally subside rapidly. Severe hypersensitivity reactions are rare.

PNEUMOCOCCAL VACCINE

Pneumococcal vaccine contains inactivated antigen that has an overall efficacy of 61 to 81 percent in preventing virulent *Streptococcus* pneumonia. Efficacy depends on the patient's age and underlying illness. Efficacy declines with age and after 65 years of age is 44 to 61 percent.

The following groups are targeted for the one-time injection:

Adults over 65 years of age (consider after age 50 years)
High-risk adults and children:
    asplenics
    those with heart and lung diseases [congestive heart failure (CHF), chronic
        obstructive pulmonary disease (COPD), asthma]
    immune-compromised persons (sickle cell disease, AIDS)
    household contacts of high-risk individuals.

Only those at highest risk receive a second or booster dose from 4 to 6 years after the first immunization. Mild pain or redness at the injection site occurs in 50 percent of those immunized, although severe reactions are rare.

INFLUENZA VACCINE

Influenza is a major cause of morbidity and mortality among persons 65 and older, causing an estimated 20,000 deaths per year. It is estimated that fewer than 50 percent of senior citizens receive the protection of influenza vaccine despite its availability within the community.

Influenza vaccine is an inactivated type A and type B. It is inactivated, safe, and seldom produces side effects. It is highly recommended for at-risk patients, particularly the elderly and patients with severe underlying disease or chronic respiratory conditions. Vaccination should be avoided during the first trimester of pregnancy or if the person has an allergy to eggs. A nasal spray vaccine is under investigation.

TUBERCULIN TESTING

Pathogenesis

Tuberculosis (TB) is an airborne communicable disease caused by *Mycobacterium tuberculosis,* or the tubercle bacillus. The disease is spread primarily by tiny airborne particles expelled by a person who has infectious TB. The following persons are most likely to be exposed to or infected with *M. tuberculosis:*

- Close contacts of person with infectious TB
- Foreign-born persons from endemic areas such as Asia, Africa, and Latin America
- Medically underserved, low-income populations including high-risk racial groups such as Asians, Pacific Islanders, African-Americans, Hispanics, and Native Americans
- The elderly

Infection begins with the multiplication of tubercle bacilli in alveolar macrophages, some of which spread through the bloodstream. These patients are considered infected but not infectious. They are asymptomatic and do not have tuberculosis but will have a positive tuberculin skin test. Approximately 10 percent of infected patients will develop TB at some time in their lives. The risk is significantly higher for HIV patients. Although the majority of TB cases are pulmonary, TB can occur in almost any anatomical site. The groups that should be screened with the tuberculin skin test include:

- Persons with or at risk for HIV infection
- Close contacts of patients with infectious TB
- Persons with certain chronic conditions (i.e., diabetes, prolonged corticosteroid therapy, cancer, leukemia, Hodgkin's disease, intestinal bypass, end-stage renal disease, gastrectomy)
- IV drug users
- Residents of long-term care facilities, correctional institutions, and nursing homes
- Medically underserved, low-income populations, including homeless persons, and high-risk racial and ethnic groups

Administration

Mantoux skin testing is the standard method of identifying patients infected with *M. tuberculosis.* The Mantoux test is performed by giving an intradermal injection containing 5 tuberculin units (TU) into the volar or dorsal surface of the forearm. By using a tuberculin syringe with the bevel up, a discrete elevation (wheal) of the skin is produced that is 6 to 10 mm in diameter. The reaction to the Mantoux test should be read 48 to 72 hours after the injection. If a patient fails to return, a positive reaction may still be measurable up to one week after testing. The results are recorded in millimeters of induration.

Classifying the Tuberculin Reaction

An induration of 5 mm or greater is positive in:

- Persons known to have or suspected of having HIV infection
- Close contacts of a person with infectious TB
- Persons whose chest x-rays show suggestion of prior TB
- IV drug users (HIV status unknown)

An induration of greater than 10 mm is positive in:

- Persons with certain medical conditions
- IV drug users (HIV negative)
- Persons from endemic areas
- Medically underserved, low-income populations
- High-risk ethnic and racial groups
- Residents of long-term care facilities
- Children under 4 years of age
- Migrant workers and homeless persons

An induration of 15 mm or more is positive in all persons with no known risk factors for TB.

A chest x-ray is recommended following a positive TB skin test. This will be used to rule out the possibility of pulmonary TB in an otherwise asymptomatic person. Prophylactic use of isoniazid (INH) is recommended for 6 months, 300 mg PO daily.

IMMUNIZATIONS FOR TRAVELERS

Immune Globulin

Immune globulin (IG) prophylaxis against the hepatitis A virus is recommended for travelers to developing countries, especially those who will be living in or visiting rural areas, eating or drinking in poor sanitation, or having close contact with local inhabitants, particularly children. U.S. citizens who reside in developing countries should receive IG regularly.

The recommended dose for travelers is 0.02 mL/kg. For prolonged travel or residence greater than 3 months, 0.06 mL/kg should be given every 5 months. Dose volume is adjusted according to body weight and length of stay. The vaccine schedule is shown in Table 8-4.

TABLE 8-4

Vaccine Schedule for Immune Globulin for Travelers

Length of Stay	Weight, lb	Weight, kg	IM dose, mL
< 3 months	< 50	< 23	0.5
	50–100	23–45	1.0
	> 100	> 45	2.0
> 3 months	< 22	< 10	0.5
	< 50	< 23	1.0
	50–100	23–45	2.5
	> 100	> 45	5.0

SOURCE: Centers for Disease Control.[9]

Side Effects

Immune globulin prepared in the United States has few side effects, primarily soreness at the injection site. It has never been shown to transmit infectious agents such as hepatitis B virus, hepatitis C virus, or HIV. Pregnancy is not a contraindication to receiving immune globulin.

Precautions

MMR vaccination should be administered at least 14 days prior to or deferred at least 3 months after administration of IG because passively acquired antibodies may interfere with the response to the vaccine.

Typhoid Vaccine

Typhoid vaccine is not routinely required for international travel but is recommended for travelers to areas where there is risk of exposure to *Salmonella typhi,* the organism which causes typhoid fever. *Salmonella typhi* is transmitted by contaminated food and water and is prevalent in many countries of Africa, Asia, and Central and South America.

The oral typhoid vaccine licensed for use in the United States is a live attenuated bacterial vaccine of the Ty21a *S. typhi* strain. The parenteral vaccine is an inactivated vaccine. Both the oral and parenteral preparations have been shown to protect 70 to 90 percent of recipients, depending on the severity of exposure. However, even after vaccination, travelers should use particular caution with food and water selection and use good hand-washing technique.

Dosage Schedule

For the oral typhoid primary series, take 1 tablet with a cool liquid one hour before a meal, every other day for four doses. Keep the tablets refrigerated. This also applies to the booster, which is required every 5 years if exposure continues.

The parenteral typhoid primary series consists of two doses more than 4 weeks apart—0.25 mL for persons under 10 years of age and 0.5 mL for those over 10 years by the subcutaneous route. The booster is on the same schedule. By the intradermal route, the dose is 0.1 mL for all ages, with a repeat dose every 3 years for repeated exposures.

Contraindications

Typhoid vaccine is contraindicated in pregnant women and HIV patients.

Reactions

Oral typhoid produces few adverse reactions. Abdominal discomfort, nausea, vomiting, and rash have been reported as possible rare reactions. Parenteral typhoid vaccine often results in discomfort at the injection site. This local reaction can occur along with fever, malaise, and headache.

Cholera Vaccine

Cholera is an acute intestinal infection caused by the *Vibrio cholerae* O group 1. The infection is often mild and self-limited or subclinical. Patients with severe cases respond well to simple IV fluids and electrolyte replacement. Cholera is acquired by ingesting contaminated water or food; person-to-person transmission is rare.

The risk of cholera to U.S. travelers is so low that it is questionable whether vaccination is of any benefit. Currently no country or territory requires vaccination as a condition for entry. However, if local authorities require documentation of cholera vaccination, a single dose of vaccine will be sufficient.

To prevent the disease, travelers should be advised to avoid eating uncooked food, especially fish and shellfish, as well as to peel fruits themselves. Carbonated water and soft drinks are usually safe. Available vaccines only provide 50 percent effectiveness in reducing illness for 3 to 6 months after vaccination, with the maximum protection in the first 2 months.

Reactions

Pain, erythema, and induration at the injection site for one to two days has been noted. This local reaction may be associated with fever, malaise, and headache. Severe reactions are rare.

Contraindications

Cholera vaccine is contraindicated during pregnancy.

Table 8-5 illustrates the dosage schedule for cholera vaccine.

Malaria Treatment

Malaria in humans is caused by one of four protozoan species of the genus *Plasmodium: P. falciparum, P. vivax, P. ovale,* and *P. malariae.* All are transmitted by the bite of an infected female *Anopheles* mosquito. Transmission may also occur by blood

TABLE 8-5

Dosage Schedule for Cholera Vaccine

Doses	Intradermal Route	SC/IM Route		
	Age 5 or older	6 months– 4 years	5–10 years	>10 years
Primary series 1 and 2 (Give doses 1 week to 1 month apart)	0.2 mL	0.2 mL	0.3 mL	0.5 mL
Booster (Give one dose every 6 months)	0.2 mL	0.2 mL	0.3 mL	0.5 mL

transfusion or congenitally from mother to fetus. Symptoms of malaria are fever, chills, headache, malaise, and myalgias. Malaria can be associated with anemia and jaundice and can cause kidney failure, coma, and death.

The World Health Organization gathers information on malaria risk in specific countries around the world. Malaria transmission occurs in large areas of Central and South America, Hispaniola, sub-Saharan Africa, India, Southeast Asia, the Middle East, and Oceania. The risk to travelers of acquiring malaria varies markedly from area to area depending on local weather conditions, mosquito vector density, and prevalence of infection.

Table 8-6 gives drugs and dosage used in the prevention of malaria.

The drug used in the presumptive treatment of malaria is pyrimethamine-sulfadoxine (Fansidar), three tablets orally in one single dose.

Contraindications

Mefloquine and doxycycline are contraindicated with pregnancy and for use with children. Use of chloroquine in pregnancy is advised only if the benefits outweigh the risks of disease.

Drug Resistance

Resistance of *P. falciparum* to the following agents has been confirmed

1. to chloroquine everywhere except the Dominican Republic, Haiti, Central America, Egypt, and the Middle East.
2. to both chloroquine and Fansidar in Thailand, Myanmar, Cambodia, the Amazon basin, and sub-Saharan Africa.
3. to mefloquine in Thailand.

TABLE 8-6

Drugs Used in Prophylaxis of Malaria

Drug	Adult Dose	Comments
Mefloquine (Larium)	228 mg PO once per week	Begin 2 weeks before travel and continue 4 weeks after return.
Doxycycline	100 mg PO daily	Begin 2 days before departure and continue 4 weeks after return.
Chloroquine (Aralen)	500 mg PO once per week	Begin 2 weeks before departure and continue until 8 weeks after return. Take same time of day.

Travel Advice

Travelers staying in air-conditioned hotels may be at lower risk than backpackers, adventure travelers, Peace Corps volunteers, or missionaries. Patients should be advised to take maximum protective measures primarily between dusk and dawn, because of the nocturnal feeding habits of the *Anopheles* mosquito.

Travelers should also be informed that regardless of preventive methods taken, malaria may still be contracted. Symptoms of malaria can occur as early as 8 days after exposure to several months after chemoprophylaxis has been terminated. Travelers should seek medical evaluation as soon as possible.

Meningococcal Vaccine

Neisseria meningitidis causes endemic and epidemic diseases, particularly meningitis and meningococcemia. It is the second most common cause of bacterial meningitis in the United States, causing an estimated 3000 to 4000 cases per year. Within the United States, serogroup B, for which a vaccine is not currently available, accounts for 50 to 55 percent of all cases. Serogroup C accounts for 20 to 25 percent, serogroup W-135 for 15 percent, serogroup Y for 10 percent, and serogroup A for 1 to 2 percent. The most common cause of meningococcal epidemics *outside* of the United States is serogroup A, but serogroups B and C can also cause epidemic disease.

Vaccination against meningococcal disease is not a requirement for entry into any country but is required for pilgrims to Mecca, Saudi Arabia, for the annual hadj. Vaccine is indicated for travelers to countries having epidemics of meningococcal disease. The sub-Saharan African countries have epidemics frequently during the dry season,

December through June. One formulation of meningococcal polysaccharide vaccine is currently available in the United States.

Dosage

The dosage is a single injection of 0.5 mL subcutaneously. Its efficacy rate is 85 to 95 percent against serogroup A, with comparable efficacy against serogroup C. Contraindications include pregnant women and any patient with an acute illness. Adverse reactions include localized erythema and transient fever lasting 1 to 2 days.

Yellow Fever Vaccine

Yellow fever, a viral disease transmitted by mosquito, occurs in parts of Africa and South America. This illness is characterized by severe hepatitis and hemorrhagic fever. Although yellow fever is a rare illness among travelers, it is important because of its high mortality rate. Travelers to high-risk areas should be vaccinated and educated in precautions against exposure to mosquitoes.

For purposes of international travel, yellow fever vaccine must be administered at an approved Yellow Fever Vaccination Center. Travelers should receive an International Certificate of Vaccination completed, signed, and validated with the center's stamp when the vaccine is given.

Dosage for yellow fever vaccine is 0.5 mL subcutaneously for all patients older than 9 months of age. Contraindications include pregnant women, infants less than 6 months of age, and patients demonstrating an allergy to chicken embryos or eggs. The decision to immunize an immunocompromised patient with yellow fever vaccine should be based upon a physician's evaluation of the patient's state of immunosuppression weighed against the risk of exposure to the virus. The freeze-dried vaccine must be maintained continuously at a temperature between 0 to 5°C (32 to 41°F).

Adverse reactions include fever or malaise (10 percent of patients) usually occurring 7 to 14 days after administration.

REFERENCES

1. Centers for Disease Control: *Health information for international travel.* 1995; 77–94, 100, 103–106, 111–118, 120–126, 129–134, 137–140.
2. Ballanti J: Basic principles underlying vaccination procedures. *Pediatr Clin North Am* 37:516–517, 1990.
3. Fulginiti VA: Current topics in immunizations. *Pediatrics* 4:2, 1985.
4. Bellig L. Immunization and the prevention of childhood diseases. *J Obstet Gynecol Neonatal Nurs* 24(7):669–677, 1995.
5. Centers for Disease Control: Recommendations for use of hepatitis A vaccine and immune globulin. *MMWR* 45:20–25, 1996.
6. Centers for Disease Control: Update on adult immunization. Recommendations of the immunization practices advisory committee (ACIP). *MMWR.* 1991; 40(RR-12): 1–88.
7. Sanford JD: *Guide to Antimicrobial Therapy.* Dallas: Antimicrobial Therapy, p 179.

8. Massachusetts Department of Public Health. *Guidelines for the control of vaccine-preventable diseases.* 1993; 3–35.

9. Centers for Disease Control: *Health information for international travel.* 1993; 65–122, 126, 130–136.

10. Buck ML: Vaccine update: New policies and products. *Pediatric Pharmacotherapy 1997* 3(7):03–07 (http://www.medscape.com/UVA/PedPharm/1997/v03.007/pp0307.buck.html).

11. Centers for Disease Control: Poliomyelitis prevention in the United States: Introduction of a sequential vaccination schedule of inactivated poliovirus vaccine followed by oral poliovirus vaccine. Recommendations of the Advisory Committee on Immunization Practices (ACIP) document. *MMWR,* 1997.

12. Woodruff BA: Progress toward integrating hepatitis B vaccine into routine infant immunization schedules in the United States, 1991 through 1994. *Pediatrics, 1996* 97(6): 798–803, 1996.

13. Centers for Disease Control: *Universal infant hepatitis B immunization.* Document #361351. November 27, 1995; 1–2.

14. American College Health Association: Task Force on Vaccine Preventable Diseases. Institutional statement on hepatitis B vaccination. 1996, 1–2.

15. Centers for Disease Control: CDC travel information: Hepatitis A vaccine and immune globulin (IC) disease and vaccine information. http://www.cdc.gov/travel/hepa—ig.htm:1996

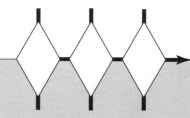

Chapter 9

USE OF HORMONES IN CONTRACEPTION AND REPLACEMENT THERAPY

Margaret A. Murphy

OVERVIEW OF THE DRUG THERAPY AND PATHOPHYSIOLOGY

The female sex hormones estrogen and progesterone are necessary for conception, maintenance of pregnancy, and secondary sexual characteristics. Release of these hormones is controlled by a feedback system involving the ovaries, the gonadatrophin-releasing hormone (Gn-RH) produced by the hypothalamus, and the luteinizing hormone (LH) and follicle-stimulating hormone (FSH) produced by the anterior pituitary gland. The ovaries are stimulated to produce estrogen and progesterone in a cyclic pattern that promotes nutritive changes in the uterus, ovulation and implantation, or shedding of the hypertrophied endometrium if fertilization does not take place. Combination oral contraceptives containing fixed dosages of estrogen and progesterone prevent ovulation by inhibiting Gn-RH affecting both pituitary and hypothalamic centers. The progestational agent suppresses LH secretion, preventing ovulation. Low basal plasma levels of estrogen inhibit FSH secretion, preventing emergence of a dominant follicle. Midcycle surges of endogenous estrogen, FSH, and LH do not occur and ovulation is not supported in 95 to 98 percent of women. Figure 9-1 illustrates specifically the regulation of the female sex hormones. Figure 9-2 shows basic hormonal relationships in humans.

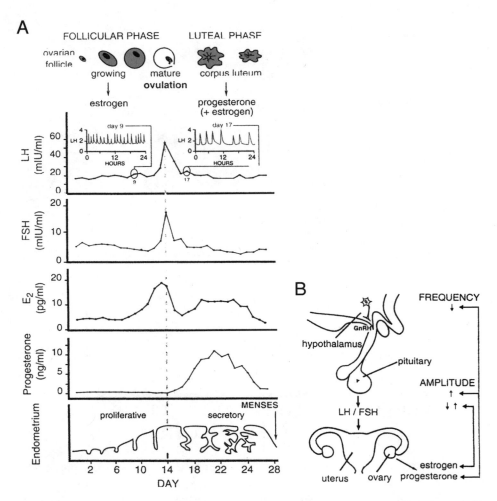

Figure 9-1. Hormonal relationships of the human menstrual cycle. **A.** Average daily values of LH, FSH, estradiol (E$_2$), and progesterone in plasma samples from women exhibiting normal 28-day menstrual cycles. Changes in the ovarian follicle (*top*) and endometrium (*bottom*) also are illustrated schematically.

Frequent plasma sampling reveals pulsatile patterns of gonadotropin release. Characteristic profiles are illustrated schematically for the follicular phase (day 9, inset on left) and luteal phase (day 17, inset on right). Both the frequency (number of pulses per hour) and amplitude (extent of change of hormone release) of pulses vary throughout the cycle. **B.** Major regulatory effects of ovarian steroids on hypothalamic-pituitary function. Estrogen decreases the amount of follicle stimulating hormone (FSH) and luteinizing hormone (LH) released (*i.e.,* gonadotropin pulse amplitude) during most of the cycle and triggers a surge of LH release only at midcycle. Progesterone decreases the frequency of Gn-RH release from the hypothalamus, and thus decreases the frequency of plasma gonadotropin pulses. Progesterone also increases the amount of LH released (*i.e.,* the pulse amplitude) during the luteal phase of the cycle. *(From Hardman et al.[1])*

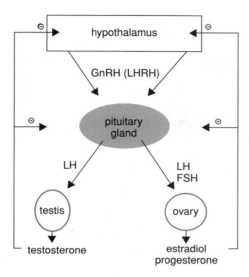

Figure 9-2. Regulation of sex hormones.

This is a very simplified scheme to remind you of the regulation of the sex steroids. There is additional positive and negative feedback to the pituitary. Gn-RH is gonadotropin-releasing hormone, which is sometimes called LH-RH (luteinizing hormone-releasing hormone). *(From Stringer.[2])*

Natural Estrogens

The major estrogens produced by women are estradiol, estrone, and estriol (see Fig. 9-3). Androgens can be converted into estrogens by fat tissue, hair follicles, the liver, and skeletal muscles. Postmenopausal women produce estrogens in the adrenal glands.[3]

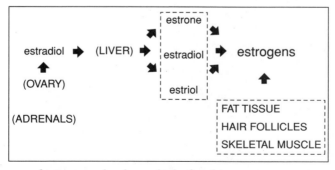

Figure 9-3. Sources of estrogen and androgen in the female.

The ovaries produce estradiol that is processed in the liver to produce the three main estrogens in the human female. The adrenal glands produce estrogen in the postmenopausal woman. Fat tissue, hair follicles, and skeletal muscle convert androgens to estrogens.

Synthetic Estrogens

Ethinyl estradiol (EE) and to a lesser extent mestranol (ME) are the synthetic estrogens found in contraceptive pills. Mestranol undergoes rapid demethylation in the liver to EE, which is its active form. Both are highly effective as contraceptives.[4] Substitution of the ethynyl group protects estradiol from hepatic metabolism and makes it effective when taken orally. Nonsteroidal compounds with estrogenic activity have been synthesized and some are used clinically. These synthetic estrogen analogues are well absorbed by the gastrointestinal tract and through the skin and mucous membranes. They are fat soluble, stored in adipose tissue, and slowly released. One such synthetic estrogen, diethylstilbestrol (DES), is no longer used except in breast cancer chemotherapy due to reproductive tract adenocarcinoma observed in female offspring of mothers taking it early in pregnancy. Hormone-specific RNA synthesis occurs with the commonly used synthetic estrogens and has a wide effect on target organs.

The two most common uses of estrogens are for oral contraception to suppress ovulation and in hormone replacement therapy (HRT) to maintain secondary sex characteristics after menopause, while decreasing vasomotor symptoms and vaginal dryness and increasing bone density. Both uses have other health benefits across a woman's life cycle (see Fig. 9-4). Hormone replacement therapy in the United States primarily utilizes conjugated estrogens. The use of estradiol is more common in Europe and other countries. Plant estrogen products are now available and their use is growing. Estropipate tablets utilize plant-derived estrogens and are preferred by some women. The advantages of "designer HRT" may include wider use for health promotion among perimenopausal and postmenopausal women.

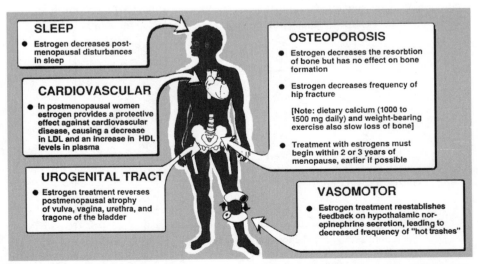

Figure 9-4. Benefits associated with postmenopausal estrogen replacement. *(From Harvey RA, Champe PC: Hormones, in Lippincott's Illustrated Reviews: Pharmacology. 1992, p 245. Used with permission.)*

Synthetic Progesterones

Synthetic progesterones, in addition to short-circuiting the LH surge and preventing ovulation, induce a leuteal phase and withdrawal bleeding. Progesterone use in HRT is necessary in a woman with a uterus to prevent increased risk for endometrial cancer associated with the use of estrogen alone. Since progesterone is not absorbed by the gastrointestinal tract, the use of progestins (synthetic progesterones) is necessary to enable women to take the drug by mouth. Many progestins with varying chemical compounds and different degrees of potency are in use today. All four generations of progestins induce secretory changes in the endometrium after priming with estrogen. The third- and fourth-generation progestins provide as high a degree of endometrial activity as other progestins but without the androgen effect responsible for an adverse effect on serum lipids. The progestin effect is more powerful than that of estrogen and provides adequate contraceptive action. In addition to suppressing the LH surge and preventing ovulation, progestins decrease ovum transport by altering tubal secretions and peristalsis. An increased risk for ectopic pregnancy may result in women on progesterone-only pills. Thick cervical mucus creates an unfriendly environment for sperm and decreases the ability of the sperm to penetrate the ovum.

Synthetic progesterones (progestins) are classified according to their derivation from progesterone (C21) or testosterone (C19) (see Table 9-1). Progestational activity is most

---

TABLE 9-1

Evolution of Synthetic Progestins

First & Second Generation
Estrane progestins (C19-nor compounds)
   Norethynodrel (NOR) no androgenic effect, but most estrogenic effect (in
      Enovid-E, Enovid 5 mg)
   Norethindrone intermediate in estrogenic and androgenic effect but strong
      antiestrogenic effect (Ortho-Novum, Norinyl, Loestrin, Nor-O.D.,
      Micronor, Ovcon, Tri-Norinyl, Nelova, Brevicon, Modicon)
   Ethynodrel decreased androgenic activity (Demulin)
Third & Fourth Generation
Gonane progestins
   Di-norgestrel greater progestational and androgenic effect, but no estrogenic
      activity (Ovral, Lo/Ovral, Nordette)
   Levonorgestrel (LNG) greater progestational and androgenic effect, but no
      estrogenic activity (Triphasils, Tri-Levlen, Nordette, Levlen)
   Desogestrel less androgenic effect (Desogen and Ortho-Cept)
   Gestodene less androgenic effect (not available yet in U.S.)
   Norgestimate reduced androgen binding (Ortho-Tri-Cyclen and Ortho-Cyclen)
   Pregnane (C21 compounds) strongest progestational effect, no androgen or
      estrogen activity but may be metabolized to androgens and estrogens
      (chlormadinone acetate, megestrol acetate, medroxyprogesterone acetate
      (MPA))

widely indicated by the Clauberg test, which measures the dose of the progestin needed for complete transformation of the endometrium into full secretion in immature estrogen-primed rabbits. The test is poorly standardized, and the results in immature rabbits do not translate well to humans. The Kaufman test (human equivalent of Clauberg) and the Goldblatt (menstrual delay) test hopefully give more clinically useful measures of the potency of progesterone. Unfortunately, results are dependent on the test system, and agreement across systems is poor. Experts agree that C21 progestins are poor ovulation inhibitors compared to C19 progestins. Tests of potency are also affected by concurrent estrogen presence, increasing the potency of progestins in nonuniform ways. The progestins can augment or inhibit estrogenic activity in combination oral contraceptive pills.

The only clinically significant differences in the progesterones are the androgenic effect of many of them. This effect, more closely associated with the first and second generation testosterone-derived nor-19 compounds, is associated with increased hyperlipidemia and significant carbohydrate metabolism effects and therefore weight gain, acne, and cardiovascular disease. The third-generation nor-19 derivatives of norethisterone (gestodene and desogestrel) have been chemically altered to achieve a more favorable selectivity ratio (progestin/androgen ratio) and theoretically offer a diminished androgenic effect with diminished associated atheroma risks.[5]

Oral Contraceptives

The first combination oral contraceptive pill was approved by the FDA in 1960. The combination contained 200 mg of norethynodrel (NOR) and 3000 μg of the estrogen mestranol in one cycle.[6] These are incredibly high doses compared to the low-estrogen or even progestin-only pills used today. Oral contraceptives remain the most highly used and most effective means of delaying or avoiding pregnancy.[7,8] The composition of various oral contraceptives is shown in Table 9-2. Estimate of effectiveness of all methods of contraception is shown in Table 9-3.

The oral contraceptives currently available consist of combined estrogens and progestin pills or pills with progestin only (see Table 9-4). The goal is to provide the lowest dose of each hormone that will ensure the lowest possible pregnancy rate. Combination agents (those containing estrogen and progestin) act by preventing ovulation. The progestin also inhibits implantation and capacitation of sperm. Progestin-only minipills are almost as effective in preventing ovulation and may be taken by women who cannot take estrogen (nursing mothers, women with chronic diseases, and smokers over 35 years of age). More breakthrough bleeding (BTB) may be experienced with progestin-only pills, and alopecia can be a problem.

Postcoital contraception can be achieved in most patients with estrogens alone or in combinations of estrogen and progestin if given within 24 hours of unprotected intercourse. These contraceptives may be effective up to 72 hours afterwards. High doses are used, resulting in nausea and vomiting in about 40 percent of patients. Following FDA-mandated package instructions will yield 75 percent efficacy in preventing pregnancy, which could prevent up to 2 to 3 million unplanned pregnancies per year, 1 million of which now end in abortion. The pills prevent a fertilized egg from implanting into the uterus. If the woman is already pregnant, the pills will have no effect.[10]

TABLE 9-2

Composition of Various Oral Contraceptives

Classification of oral contraceptives based upon the composition of estrogen/ progestin combination products and progestin-only products.

TYPE Estrogen/ progestin	Preparation	Manufacturer or Distributor	Estrogen (mcg)	Progestin (mg)	Color of active tablets
Combination	Loestrin 1/20	Parke-Davis	20	1*	white
Monophasic	Loestrin Fe 1/20	Parke-Davis	20	1*	white
Ethinyl estradiol/	Loestrin 1.5/30	Parke-Davis	30	1.5*	green
norethindrone	Loestrin Fe 1.5/30	Parke-Davis	30	1.5*	green
	Brevicon	Searle	35	0.5	blue
	Modicon	Ortho	35	0.5	white
	Norinyl 1+35	Searle	35	1	yellow-green
	Ortho-Novum 1/35	Ortho	35	1	peach
	Ovcon-35	Mead Johnson	35	0.4	peach
	Ovcon-50	Mead Johnson	50	1	yellow
Ethinyl estradiol/	Alesse	Wyeth-Ayerst	20	0.10	pink
levonorgestrel	Levlen	Berlex	30	0.15	light orange
	Nordette	Wyeth-Ayerst	30	0.15	light orange
Ethinyl estradiol/	Lo/Ovral	Wyeth-Ayerst	30	0.3	white
norgestrel	Ovral	Wyeth-Ayerst	50	0.5	white
Ethinyl estradiol/	Demulen 1/35	Searle	35	1	white
ethynodiol	Demulen 1/50	Searle	50	1	white
diacetate					
Mestranol/	Norinyl 1+50	Searle	50	1	white
norethindrone	Ortho-Novum 1/50	Ortho	50	1	yellow
Ethinyl estradiol/	Desogen	Organon	30	0.15	white
desogestrel	Ortho-Cept	Ortho	30	0.15	orange
Ethinyl estradiol/	Ortho-Cyclen	Ortho	35	0.25	blue
norgestimate					
Combination	Ortho-Novum 10/11	Ortho	35	0.5	10 white tabs
Biphasic			35	1	11 peach tabs
Ethinyl estradiol/	Jenest-28	Organon	35	0.5	7 white tabs
norethindrone			35	1	14 peach tabs
Combination	Ortho-Novum 7/7/7	Ortho	35	0.5	7 white tabs
Triphasic			35	0.75	7 light peach tabs
Ethinyl estradiol/			35	1	7 peach tabs
norethindrone	Tri-Norinyl	Searle	35	0.5	7 blue tabs
			35	1	9 yellow-green tabs
			35	0.5	5 blue tabs
Ethinyl estradiol/	Ortho-Tri-Cyclen	Ortho	35	0.18	7 white tabs
norgestimate			35	0.215	7 light blue tabs
			35	0.25	7 blue tabs
Ethinyl estradiol/	Tri-Levlen	Berlex	30	0.05	6 brown tabs
levonorgestrel			40	0.075	5 white tabs
			30	0.125	10 light yellow tabs

*as norethindrone acetate

(continued)

TABLE 9-2

Composition of Various Oral Contraceptives (continued)

Classification of oral contraceptives based upon the composition of estrogen/progestin combination products and progestin-only products.

TYPE Estrogen/ progestin	Preparation	Manufacturer or Distributor	Estrogen (mcg)	Progestin (mg)	Color of active tablets
	Triphasil	Wyeth-Ayerst	30	0.05	6 brown tabs
			40	0.075	5 white tabs
			30	0.125	10 light yellow tabs
Combination	Estrostep 21	Parke-Davis	20	1	5 white triangle tabs
Estrophasic			30	1	7 white square tabs
Ethinyl estradiol/			35	1	9 white round tabs
norethindrone	Estrostep Fe	Parke-Davis	20	1	5 white triangle tabs
acetate			30	1	7 white square tabs
			35	1	9 white round tabs
Progestin-Only	Micronor	Ortho	none	0.35	lime green
Norethindrone	Nor-QD	Searle	none	0.35	yellow
Norgestrel	Ovrette	Wyeth-Ayerst	none	0.075	yellow

SOURCE: Murphy J (ed): *Nurse Practitioners' Prescribing Guide.* New York: Prescribing Reference, Fall, 1997, p 194.[9]

TABLE 9-3

Percent of Women Experiencing an Accidental Pregnancy in First Year of Use of Contraceptives

	% Pregnant in First Year	
Method	**Typical Use[a]**	**Perfect Use (Estimated)[b]**
Male sterilization	0.15	0.10
Female sterilization	0.40	0.40
Implant (Norplant)	0.09	0.09
Injectable progestogen (Depo-Provera)	0.30	0.30
Intrauterine device (IUD)		
Progestasert	2.00	1.50
Copper T 380A	0.80	0.60
LNg 20	0.10	0.10
Pill		
Progestin only		0.50
Combined		0.10

(continued)

TABLE 9-3

Percent of Women Experiencing an Accidental Pregnancy in First Year of Use of Contraceptives (continued)

Method	% Pregnant in First Year	
	Typical Use[a]	Perfect Use (Estimated)[b]
Condom		
Male (without spermicide)	12.00	3.00
Female (Reality)	21.00	5.00
Diaphragm with spermicide	18.00	6.00
Cervical cap with spermicide	18.00 (nulliparous)	9.00 (nulliparous)
	36.00 (parous)	26.00 (parous)
Vaginal sponge	18.00 (nulliparous)	9.00 (nulliparous)
	36.00 (parous)	20.00 (parous)
Withdrawal	19.00	4.00
Periodic abstinence	20.00	
Calendar		9.00
Ovulation method		3.00
Sympto-thermal		2.00
Post-ovulation		1.00
Spermicide[c] (alone)	21.00	6.00
None	85.00	85.00

[a]Among typical couples who initiate use of a method (not necessarily for the first time), the percentage who experience an accidental pregnancy during the first year if they do not stop use for any other reason.
[b]Among couples who initiate use of a method (not necessarily for the first time) and who use it perfectly (both consistently and correctly), the percentage who experience an accidental pregnancy during the first year if they do not stop use for any other reason.
[c]Foams, creams, gels, vaginal suppositories, and vaginal film.
SOURCE: Adapted with permission from Hatcher RA, Trussell J, Stewart F, et al: *Contraceptive Technology*, 16th ed. New York: Irvington, 1994–1996, pp 69, 113, 243–248.[8]

TABLE 9-4

Combination Oral Contraceptives

	Name	Estrogen	Progestin
First generation	Enovid 10	150 µg	10 mg
Second generation	Oracon, C-Quens	>50 µg (14–15 days)	2 mg (5–6 days)
Third generation	LDCOC	35–50 µg	1.5 mg or less
Fourth generation	bi- and triphasic	35 µg	0.5–1 mg
New	VLDCOC	20 µg	0.10 mg

LDCOC = low dose combination oral contraceptives; VLDCOC = very low dose oral contraceptives.

Mifepristone (RU-486) with an affinity five times that of progesterone is a synthetic antiprogesterone that binds to progesterone receptors and to a lesser extent, glucocorticoid receptors. It is thought to increase endometrial prostaglandin secretions which stimulate uterine contraction and softening of the cervix.[11] As a potent antiprogesterone it is effective for pregnancy termination. Its use as an abortifacient has been accompanied by controversy in the United States. A single 600-mg oral dose followed within 72 hours by a prostaglandin analogue, misoprostol (Cytotec) 400 mg, resulted in termination of pregnancy in 98.7 percent of patients from 7 to 14 days after treatment. Other potential uses include chemotherapy of progestin-dependent tumors and meningiomas and as a treatment for secreting adrenal tumors.[12]

Depo-Medroxyprogesterone (DMPA) is an injectable progestin-only contraceptive that prevents ovulation by inhibiting production of human gonadotropin, the LH surge and ovulation, and prevents fertilization by interfering with capacitation of sperm and hostile cervical mucus. The contraceptive effect is reversible within 1 to 2 years for most women. Injections are required every 3 months and start to work immediately when given within 5 days of the start of the menstrual cycle. Accidental pregnancies that occur when DMPA is given outside this time frame are associated with higher neonatal infant mortality rates. Therefore, patients presenting for a subsequent injection more than 91 days later should be screened for pregnancy twice, 2 weeks apart with serum beta-human chorionic gonadotropin (hCG). The drug has had extensive use in third world countries and has been found safe and effective. It is an option for those unable or unwilling to take a pill every day. It shares risks and benefits with progestin-only pills and additionally has been found to reduce seizure activity and sickle cell crises. Most users will eventually be amenorrheic. It is not reversible until after the 3 months of activity has expired.[13]

Norplant progestin implants (levonorgestrel) are effective contraceptives for a 5-year period. They are the most effective method even including sterilization. They are implanted subdermally in the upper arm and release from 85 (initially) to 30 µg mg/day into the blood stream. Prolonged or irregular bleeding and amenorrhea are common during the first year, but menses resumes in most women by year two. There are occurrences of infection associated with insertion and removal. Difficulty in removing the silastic capsules has been experienced and should only be attempted by those with special training. Fertility has been known to return as early as 4 weeks after removal.

Bibliography for Basic Information on the Pharmacology of Drugs

Dickey RP: *Managing Contraceptive Pill Patients,* 8th ed. Durant, OK:EMIS, 1996.

Hardman JG, Limbird LE, Molinoff PB, et al: *Goodman & Gilman's The Pharmacological Basis of Therapeutics,* 9th ed. New York: McGraw-Hill, 1996, pp 1411–1440.

Hatcher RA, Trussell J, Stewart F, et al: *Contraceptive Technology, 1994–1996.* New York: Irvington, 1994.

Hawkins JW, Roberto-Nichols DM, Stanley-Haney JL: *Protocols for Nurse Practitioners in Gynecologic Settings,* 5th ed. New York: Tiresias, 1995.

Katzung B: *Drug Therapy,* 2d ed. Norwalk, CT: Appleton & Lange, 1991.

Murphy J (ed): *Nurse Practitioners' Prescribing Guide.* New York: Prescribing Reference, 1997.

Ruggiero R: Contraceptives, in Young LL, et al (eds): *Applied Therapeutics: The Clinical Use of Drugs,* 6th ed. Vancouver, WA: Applied Therapeutics, 1996, pp 67-1 to 67-21.

Yuzpe AA: Contraception, in Gray J (ed): *Therapeutic Choices.* Ottawa, Canada: Canadian Pharmaceutical Association, 1995, p 442–449.

ISSUES IN DRUG THERAPY

Prescribing Considerations

There are numerous issues involved in the choice to use natural or so-called artificial methods of contraception (see Fig. 9-5). The ideal situation is one in which the decision

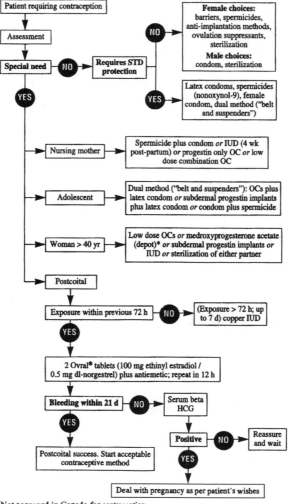

Figure 9-5. Contraceptive choices. *(From Yuzpe AA: Contraception, in Gray J (ed): Therapeutic Choices. Ottawa, Canada: Canadian Pharmaceutical Association, 1995, p 443.)*[14]

is made jointly with two responsible and committed sexual partners. Statistics on unintended pregnancies tell us that this is not always the case. The patient assessment process preceding contraceptive decision making provides an opportunity to offer teaching and counseling on sexually transmitted diseases. The time taken can save lives and fertility as well as offer choices for the kind of contraception that will fit the patient and her family values and beliefs. Adequate patient teaching may avoid situations in which 40 to 60 percent of women discontinue use because of BTB or other discomfort or inconvenience.

Abstinence, barrier methods, and natural family planning are all options that should be discussed with patients. These are outside the scope of this book and will not be discussed here.

The provider takes the lead from the patient in terms of what the priorities are: effectiveness and tolerance of initial side effects including BTB, nausea, vomiting, weight gain, and breast tenderness. The provider attends to patient reliability; age; possibility of pregnancy; presence of disease or risk factors for a hormone-dependent tumor, hypertension, diabetes mellitus, hyperlipedemia, and thrombophlebitis; and risks associated with concurrent drug use. Factors of efficacy, safety, and acceptability must be carefully weighed. The reliability of the patient in adhering to prescribing instructions and the socioeconomic consideration of factors that may interfere with adherence are all important.

Prescribing Variables

Patient Variables

Differences in physiological responses to estrogens and progestins make it very difficult to prescribe with accuracy for individual women. Little is known about the biological availability of the oral progestins since blood levels after a standard dose vary up to tenfold.[5] Thus standard doses are too high for some women and too low for others. This accounts for the wide variety of side effects associated with oral contraceptive (OC) pill regimens. Dickey in 1977 presented the first logical plan for selecting an initial OC based on patient clinical profiles and knowledge of the estrogenic and progestational clinical effects of the drugs.[15] Measures of endometrial activity may be more reliable since they take into consideration all these effects.

Clinical information must be elicited from the patient regarding onset and character of menses and perceived hormone sensitivity. Side effects may be reduced if a patient's menstrual pattern and history of hormone-related symptoms are taken into consideration before initial choices are made and subsequently when side effects develop.[15]

Noncontraceptive Benefits   Oral contraceptives offer women an extremely effective method of birth control, as well as a number of other benefits.[16]

Ovarian Cancer   Ovarian cancer is the most commonly fatal cancer of the female reproductive system in the United States. A 40 percent reduction in risk for ovarian cancer is associated with OC use. Nulliparous women enjoy the greatest protection. The protective effect occurs even with short-term use, increases with duration of use, and may continue up to 15 years in former users. Estrogen and progesterone block ovulation, decreasing the incidence of benign ovarian cysts as well.

Endometrial Cancer Endometrial cancer is the third leading cause of cancer deaths in women in the United States. Those who use oral contraceptives have a risk 40 percent lower than the general population. The protective effect is greater with increased duration of use and nulliparity. The benefits are noted after 1 year of use and continue at least 10 years after cessation of use.

Benign Breast Disease Most data support a decreased incidence of benign breast disease with OC use. Up to 50 to 75 percent, or 20,000, surgical cases are prevented annually. Increased duration of use and low progestin potency appear to provide the greatest protection.

Pelvic Inflammatory Disease and Salpingitis There is evidence that the incidence of pelvic inflammatory disease (PID) in women on OCs is up to 50 percent less than in nonusers. The protective effect is noted after the first year of use and disappears after the pill is discontinued. It is estimated that hospitalizations for PID are reduced by 70 percent among OC users. Theories relate to a decrease in menstrual blood, reducing the availability of this rich medium for incubation and growth of bacteria, and the hostile cervical mucus in women taking progestational agents, deterring potential pathogens (as well as sperm) from entering the uterine cavity. This may not be true for chlamydia, which is an intracellular organism. Higher rates of chlamydial cervicitis may be related to cervical ectropion often seen in women taking OCs.[17]

Other Benefits Reduced menstrual flow and associated iron deficiency anemia, and lower incidence of acne, premenstrual syndrome, and dysmenorrhea have all been noticed among users of OCs.[18]

Contraindications for Use Pathophysiologic conditions or risk factors for such conditions can serve as absolute or relative contraindications for OC use. Use of OCs is not without risk, and the risk is increased in the presence of other health conditions. The list below of pathologic contraindications is adapted from Hatcher, Trussell, and Stewart.[8] OCs should not be started or continued in the presence of any absolute contraindication. Strong relative contraindications may also be significant enough to discontinue or switch oral contraceptives. Everyone taking oral contraceptives should be familiar and have at the ready another method of birth control. For women with certain relative risk factors, such as diabetes and sickle cell anemia, physician consultation should be considered.[8]

Refrain from providing oral contraceptives for women with the following diagnoses:

1. Current or past thromboembolic disorder
2. Current or past cerebrovascular disease
3. Current or past coronary artery disease
4. Known or suspected or past carcinoma of breast cancer
5. Known or suspected current or past estrogen dependent neoplasia
6. Current pregnancy, known or suspected
7. Current or past benign hepatic adenoma or liver cancer
8. Current markedly impaired liver function

Exercise caution if combined oral contraceptives are used or considered in the following situations and carefully monitor for adverse effects:

9. Over 35 years old and currently a heavy smoker (> 15 cigarettes a day)
10. Classic migraines or undiagnosed headache
11. Hypertension with resting diastolic blood pressure of 90 or greater, or a resting systolic blood pressure of 140 or greater, on three or more separate visits, or an accurate measurement of 110 diastolic or more on a single occasion
12. Diabetes mellitus or positive glucose tolerance test
13. Surgery planned within the next 4 weeks or major surgery requiring immobilization
14. Undiagnosed abnormal vaginal or uterine bleeding
15. Sickle cell (SS) anemia or sickle cell–hemoglobin C(SC) disease
16. Lactation
17. Gestational diabetes
18. Active gallbladder disease
19. Congenital hyperbilirubinemia (Gilbert's disease)
20. Over 50 years of age
21. Completion of term pregnancy within past 10 to 14 days
22. Current or past cardiac or renal disease
23. Conditions likely to make the woman unreliable in following pill instructions (mental retardation, major psychiatric problems, alcoholism or other drug abuse, or history of repeated incorrect use of oral contraceptives or other medication)
24. Family history of hyperlipidemia
25. Family history of death of a parent or sibling due to myocardial infarction before age 50

Breast Cancer   It remains unknown, after many studies whether exogenous estrogen influences breast cancer risk. Several studies have indicated an increase in relative risk for women taking exogenous estrogen. Duration of treatment and high doses associated in the past with both OC and HRT use may influence the results of studies. Women with first-degree risk (mother or sister with breast cancer) may wish to take no chances on increasing breast cancer risk. However, others may reason that low doses of estrogen for up to 10 years may do no harm. There is research to support both positions.

Long-term prospective studies are warranted to clarify any association, delineate the risk groups, and demonstrate the findings of lifetime follow-up. Unfortunately, several such studies have failed to resolve the question absolutely. Women who start OCs before age 20 or have 5 years of use before the first full-term pregnancy show a 1.5 fold increase in relative risk for breast cancer before age 45. It is wise to consider using a low-estrogen pill in the premenopausal period. The National Women's Health Network[19] recommends that young women should consider pill use for a maximum of 7 years and that all women, particularly long-term pill users, should follow preventive and early detection measures for breast cancer.

Birth Defects   Many studies have failed to find any association between the use of OCs during pregnancy and birth defects. Nevertheless, estrogen is contraindicated during pregnancy. Women who become amenorrheic (missed 2 periods) while on the pills, should use a backup method until pregnancy is ruled out. If the women have missed pills, they should seek advice at the time of the first missed period.[20]

Dickey[15] offers the following options if pregnancy is ruled out:

1. Continue with OCs with no monthly bleeding
2. Switch to an OC with a lower progestin dose; the endometrium will thicken and monthly periods will resume
3. Switch to a pill with higher estrogen component (up to 50μ of EE); the endometrium will thicken and monthly periods will resume
4. Take extra estrogen tablets (premarin 0.125μ for 10 days) that can be repeated for 2 cycles.

Risks to Adolescents   One million U.S. teens become pregnant every year. In 1990 48 percent of females and 61 percent of male high school students reported having sexual intercourse. No deaths related to serious cardiovascular complications have been reported for women under 18; however, the practitioner should be aware of some special considerations when prescribing OCs to teenage women in order to promote more efficient and safe fertility control. Teenagers using OCs are almost twice as likely to become pregnant than adults using OCs. Postpill amenorrhea and infertility resulting from the effects of OCs on the hypothalamic-pituitary-ovarian axis, though rare, is a potential problem for adolescent pill users. Hatcher et al.[8] recommend waiting until the teenager has had 6 to 12 regular periods before providing her with OCs. They urge practitioners to be sensitive to the individual who is already sexually active with irregular and/or few menses. The risks of postpill amenorrhea and potential infertility associated with premature use of OCs must be weighed against the risks associated with adolescent pregnancy. Women with a history of irregular menses, which includes many adolescents, are likely to return to a similar pattern and take longer to conceive after discontinuing use of the pill.

To prevent unplanned pregnancy, the practitioner should initiate low dose combination oral contraceptives (LDCOC) and provide anticipatory guidance with a discussion about relative risks of side effects versus pregnancy. The adolescent must be encouraged to take OCs correctly, to call in case of side effects, and not stop OCs without using another method.

Psychological factors should be reviewed with patients. A history of impulsive behavior or depression may make a long-acting choice more effective for these patients. DMPa or Norplant are good choices for those who find it difficult to adhere to daily schedules. Very low dose combination oral contraceptives (VLDCOC) should not be used in adolescents because of the high rate of missed pills. The average adolescent misses an estimated 2.7 pills per month.

Drug Variables

Antacids and antibiotics may inhibit absorption.[9] Oral contraceptives are antagonized by hepatic enzyme-inducing drugs (e.g., carbamazepine, phenytoin, phenobarbital, rifampin, gliseofulvin, tetracyclin). Those on antibiotics are well advised to use a backup method.[15]

Laboratory tests may be affected by OCs. The following FDA package insert labeling indicates major laboratory testing affected by oral contraceptives.[15] For an exhaustive listing, the reader is referred to Dickey.[15]

Drug Selection and Dosing

Drug selection is based on endometrial activity as well as estrogen activity, progestin activity, androgenic activity, and antiestrogenic activity (see Table 9-5). Unfortunately, there is no standardized in vivo testing that is useful because of the wide range of human responses to hormones. Dickey[15] and Hatcher, Trussell, Stewart, et al.[7] offer specific choices for starting and switching OCs based on patient profiles and patient responses to those choices. In general, the goal is to start everyone on low dose combination oral contraceptive pills. Based on patient responses, a more potent progestin may be prescribed.[15] Perimenopausal women are often started on or switched to an OC containing 20 μg of estradiol.

Initiating oral contraceptives is associated with symptoms of early pregnancy, nausea, breast tenderness, weight gain, increased vaginal infections, mild headaches, bloating, chloasma, BTB, and amenorrhea.

EXHIBIT 9.1

Laboratory Tests Affected by OCs

Certain endocrine and liver function tests and blood components may be affected by oral contraceptives:

- Increased prothrombin and factors VII, VIII, IX, and X; decreased antithrombin 3; and increased norepinephrine-induced platelet aggregability

- Increased thyroid-binding globulin (TBG) leading to increased circulating total thyroid hormone, as measured by protein-bound iodine (PBI), T_4 by column or by radioimmunoassay. Free T_3 resin uptake is decreased, reflecting the elevated TBG. Free T_4 concentration is altered

- Other binding proteins may be elevated in serum

- Sex steroid binding globulins are increased and result in elevated levels of total circulating sex steroids and corticoids; however, free or biologically-active levels remain unchanged

- Triglycerides may be increased

- Glucose tolerance may be decreased

- Serum folate levels may be depressed by oral contraceptive therapy. This may be of clinical significance if a woman becomes pregnant shortly after discontinuing oral contraceptives

TABLE 9-5

Estimated Relative Oral Contraceptive Estrogen/Progestin Activity

↑ Progestins ↓		Low Estrogens		Intermediate
	High			Ovral
		Demulen 1/35	Lo/Ovral	Demulen 1/50
	Intermediate	Desogen	Nordette	
		Levlen	Ortho-Cyclen	
		Monophasic	Nelova 0.5/35 E	*Monophasic*
		Brevicon	Nelova 1/35 E	Ovcon-35
		Genora 0.5/35	Nelova 1/50 M	Ovcon-50
		Genora 1/35	Norethin 1/35 E	
		Genora 1/50	Norethin 1/50 M	
	Low	Loestrin 21 1/20	Norinyl 1/35	
		Loestrin Fe 1/20	Norinyl 1/50	
		Loestrin 21 1.5/30	Ortho-Novum 1/35	
		Loestrin Fe 1.5/30	Ortho-Novum 1/50	
		Modicon		
		Biphasic		
		Nelova 10/11	Ortho-Novum 10/11	
		Triphasic		
		Ortho-Novum 7/7/7	Tri-Norinyl	
		Tri-Levlen	Triphasil	
		Low		Intermediate
		← Estrogens →		

SOURCE: Cada D (ed): *Drug Facts and Comparisons*. St Louis: Facts and Comparisons, 1997, p 435.[21]

CONTEXTUAL ISSUES

Increased competition among drug manufacturers and financial pressures associated with managed care have resulted in some hospitals and managed care organizations agreeing to carry only certain brands of each class of drugs. In general, there are probably many more choices of OCs than needed to suit most patients. Patients do resent being switched for monetary reasons and may choose to let their concern be known to the managed care company. Cost has been an issue for a long time (see Table 9-6), but generic estrogens reduce the cost somewhat.

TABLE 9-6

Costing out Some Contraceptives

Contraceptive Method	Total Cost at 4 yr	Average Annual Cost Over 4 yr
Condom	$200	$50
Diaphragm	$516	$129
DMPA (Depo-Provera)	$480	$120
Intrauterine device		
Copper T 380A (ParaGard)	$140	$35
Progesterone T (Progestasert)	$344	$86
Levonorgestrel implants (Norplant)	$360–$600	$90–$150
Oral contraceptive	$676	$169
Vaginal contraceptive sponge (Today)	$660	$165

SOURCE: Mastroianni L Jr, Robinson JC: Contraception in the 1990s. *Patient Care* 28(1):109, 1994.[22]

Women should not have to choose between protection from unplanned pregnancy and food or household needs. Debates go on regarding the advantages and preferences for natural versus synthetic hormones. Questions remain regarding standardization of generic and natural drug components, especially plant-derived hormones.

Monitoring and Evaluation Requirements

Complete health assessment is ideal before starting OCs. A history, a physical examination including pap smear within the last year, and a functional health pattern assessment each contribute unique information to assist in choices to be made. A consent form is signed, and lipid and liver profiles and fasting blood sugar (FBS) are drawn if indicated by age, family, and personal history. Patient teaching may be more important than the choice of a particular pill. Fortunately, the FDA has directed drug companies to use standard directions for use with oral contraceptive labeling. The standardized OC pill use instructions are as follows:[23]

1. Start oral contraceptive on day 1 (first day of menses) or on Sunday of week menses start.
2. Oral contraceptive must always be taken at the same time of day (within an hour either way).
3. Backup contraception is necessary for 7 days with Sunday start, *except* in those cases where pill is *first day* of menstrual cycle start, in which case no backup is required.

4. Missed pills
    a. One pill missed: woman to take pill when she remembers, and then take scheduled pill at regular time.
    b. Two pills missed in first 2 weeks: take two pills at regular time for 2 days. Use backup contraception for 7 days.
    c. Two or more pills missed in third week, or three or more pills missed any time (and woman starts on Sundays), she should keep taking a pill each day until Sunday, then start a new packet that Sunday. Instruct woman to use a backup method for 7 days. If woman does not start on Sundays, she should throw out pill pack and start a new pack that day. A backup method of birth control should be used for the first 7 days of this new pill pack.
    d. If one or more pills are missed and no backup contraception is used and no withdrawal bleeding occurs, woman should be instructed to call to discuss a pregnancy test.

Monitoring of the patient's degree of comfort or discomfort is part of a planned follow-up visit that will occur according to one of the following schedules:[20]

3 months, 6 months, annually
3 months, q 6 months
q 6 months

The procedure for pill check (3 to 6 months) is as follows:[23]

1. All women will have routine screening of
    a. Blood pressure, weight
    b. Urine, for protein and glucose
    c. Last menstrual period
2. Review side effects and danger signals
3. Allow time for client to ask questions
4. If problems are elicited or suspected, consultation with other nurse practitioners and/or physician as necessary
5. Teach about prescription: one and only one pharmacy (individual state pharmacy regulations)
6. Six-month check: bimanual examination and breast examination

It should be remembered that the risk of pregnancy must always be balanced against the risks associated with OCs. Healthy nonsmoking women over 40 with negative family histories may be better served by assuming a small increased cardiovascular risk rather than an increased risk of pregnancy and its attendant problems. The degree of acceptable risk varies among women and for individual women at different times in the life cycle. The practitioner may decide to withhold a method based on her judgment of the limits of safety. In these instances, the provider assists the patient in accepting this by offering an alternative method of family planning that will not compromise her health status. Choices available currently are much wider than in the past although few methods offer equivalent protection from unplanned pregnancy.

Stopping OCs prior to the tenth day of the cycle may result in a skipped or very heavy period; therefore, when prudent OCs should be stopped after the tenth day. The FDA package insert calls for stopping OCs after two missed periods. A more conservative approach (one missed period or 45 days since the last period) should be used with those who have missed OC doses and those on progesterone-only pills.

Amenorrhea is frequently due to estrogen deficit. This can be recognized by atrophic changes with BTB during pill days, which frequently occur during the first three cycles of pill taking. Doses may be adjusted after a pregnancy test and normal pelvic exam. Due to the risk of deep vein thrombosis, combination OCs should be stopped 4 weeks presurgery through 2 weeks postsurgery and not initiated until 4 weeks postpartum. Other methods should be used during periods of prolonged immobilization. Nursing mothers may use the progestin-only minipills although their effect on the milk supply must be monitored. Menses will normally resume between 5 weeks and 3 months of stopping the pill.

HORMONE REPLACEMENT THERAPY

Hormone replacement therapy (HRT) refers to provision of estrogen and progestin to a woman with a uterus. Estrogen replacement therapy (ERT) refers to estrogen replacement only for women who have had a hysterectomy. Use of estrogen for HRT and ERT is at much lower doses than for OCs. Conjugated estrogens at 0.625 to 1.25 µg/day constitute the usual dose of estrogen in the United States. The dose for women over 60 may be reduced to 0.3 µg/day. A dose of 0.625 µg of conjugated estrogen is equal to 5 to 10 mg of EE. Side effects are similar to those from OCs but much less intense with the lower dosage used for perimenopausal and postmenopausal women.

Reasons for using HRT in this midlife transition include symptom management and health promotion. Symptoms accompany the gradual depletion of estrogen production associated with natural cessation of menses as well as the sudden cessation induced by hysterectomy, oophorectomy, chemotherapy, or radiation. One-third to one-fourth of American women are said to experience such a sudden decline in estrogen levels.[24] Menopause, a natural, permanent cessation of menstruation, occurs between 48 and 55 years. Premature menopause occurs before age 40. Unopposed estrogen increases risk of endometrial cancer, and progestin is given concurrently with estrogen to prevent this increased risk. Medroprogesterone acetate (MPA), a C-21 progestin compound, is given for a minimum of 13 daily doses each month with estrogen. Continuous daily dosing of MPA 2.5 mg/day prevents the cyclic bleeding that occurs when progestin is delivered cyclically at 10 mg/day from day 12 or 16 until the last day of the cycle.

Changes Attributed to Estrogen Level Decline

Vasomotor flushing is experienced by 75 to 80 percent of menopausal women. This may occur anywhere from 4 to 6 years before the last period and continue for several years thereafter. This is severe enough in 25 percent of women to require drug therapy.

Therapy with estrogens is highly specific and very effective after 2 to 4 weeks of treatment.[25] Progestins are also effective as is clonidine (0.1 to 0.2 mg bid).

Urogenital atrophy presents as pain when intercourse is attempted. In response to decreased estrogen levels, the thickness of vaginal epithelium is decreased with an accompanying change in pH. Vaginal dryness is a major concern. Symptoms of dysuria, frequency, and urgency may occur. Administration of estrogen by any route discussed above is effective in relieving symptoms. Additionally, an estradiol vaginal ring offers local relief for 90 days with one insertion (Estring). Progestins must also be administered to counteract the risk associated with unopposed estrogen in women with a uterus.

Bone loss Following natural menopause, estrogen-dependent bone loss is rapid, averaging one to two percent per year. Bone loss averages 3.9 percent for the first six years after hysterectomy; then one percent thereafter. During 10 years of estrogen deprivation, a woman may lose one-third of her total bone mass.[26] ERT slows the rate of bone loss to 0.05 percent each year.[27] Substantial impairments are associated with vertebral fractures that are a result of bone loss.[28] As many as 20 percent of patients sustaining a hip fracture die within one year of the fracture, and the majority require daily assistance following this injury. The costs associated with osteoporosis exceed $10 billion annually.

Issues in Drug Therapy

Prescribing Considerations

Some degree of symptoms are experienced by up to 80 percent of women during menopause. Vasomotor instability, insomnia, and genitourinary atrophy may be accompanied by dizziness, headache, palpitations, and diaphoresis.[25] Hormone deficiency is said to contribute to psychological as well as physical symptomatology. In postmenopausal women, a positive correlation has been found between plasma estrogen and tryptophan levels.[27] These findings are suggestive of a relationship between estrogens and depression; however, there is no clinical evidence to date that estrogen deficiency causes depression.

Risk factor modifications shown to be effective against osteoporosis include smoking cessation, increased aerobic and weightbearing exercise, and adequate dietary intake or supplements of 1500 mg or more of calcium per day and, for those over 65 years of age, 800 units of vitamin D.[29]

Behavioral interventions related to risk reduction for myocardial infarction include:

> Control of hypercholesterolemia
> Weight reduction
> Low-dose aspirin
> Control of hypertension

Smoking cessation, exercise, and weight reduction may be as effective as HRT in preventing coronary artery disease. Col and colleagues estimate that the only women who would not benefit from HRT are those at highest risk of breast cancer and those with no risk factors for cardiovascular disease.[30] He estimates that less than 1 percent of healthy women are in this category.

Prescribing Variables

Patient Variables   Loss of the protective estrogen effect is associated with increased deaths from diseases of the circulatory system. The cardioprotective effect is the single most important health benefit associated with HRT. Epidemiologic studies have shown that women who take estrogen after menopause have a lower rate of heart disease than untreated women. Heart disease is four times as likely to cause death in women than is breast cancer.

A recent study published in *The New England Journal of Medicine* notes that mortality among women who have used HRT within the past 6 months is lower than among those who have not.[31] This is particularly true for heart disease. A 53 percent decrease in mortality is noted in women on HRT. The benefit continues for 5 years after stopping HRT. The survival benefit for heart disease after 10 years or more of use is diminished. It is also diminished for those with a beginning low relative cardiovascular risk. The Postmenopausal Estrogen/Progestin Interventions Trial noted that in 850 healthy women, estrogen alone or in combination with progestins increased high-density lipoproteins (HDLs) when compared with a placebo group.[32] Low-density lipoproteins (LDLs) were reduced, and systolic blood pressure and serum insulin levels were not affected.

Benefits of Hormone Replacement Therapy   There are well-documented benefits to HRT, especially in preventing hot flashes and urogenital atrophy (UGA). Estrogens probably do have a cardioprotective effect, but neither the degree of the protection nor the mechanism is understood. Although there is no question that estrogens protect against the osteoporosis-related fractures of relatively young postmenopausal estrogen users, it is not so certain that this benefit is retained in the older patient (greater than age 75 to 80 years) in which these fractures most often occur. The risk of unopposed estrogen-related endometrial cancer is eliminated by adding a progestin in those women with a uterus. Prescription of combination pills ensures that the progestin will be taken with the estrogen.

Risks Associated with Hormone Replacement Therapy   The postmenopausal woman who takes a combination of estrogen and progesterone has a lower risk of uterine cancer than the woman who takes no hormone at all. It is now considered malpractice to use an estrogen without a progestin for the woman who has a uterus.

It is not known with certainty whether estrogens increase the risk for breast cancer. In 1989, a Swedish study reported that the relative risk of developing breast cancer increased to 1.7 in those women who took estrogen for a total of 9 years. (The estrogen employed was not available in the United States and was used in doses that are not comparable to those used in the United States.) There are reports that estrogen replacement therapy of greater than 10 years duration is associated with a threefold increase in the risk of developing breast cancer and that the use of a dose of greater than 2.5 mg of estrogen increases the relative risk to 1.7. The estrogen-related increase in breast cancer risk is thought to relate to the longer duration of exposure to estrogen.

Estrogens do not appear to increase the risk for breast cancer for the first 5 to 7 years, after age 50. Thus, a woman who has undergone a surgical menopause can be treated until age 50 years with no increased risk. Starting at age 50 years, there may be an increased risk of breast cancer after 7 to 10 years of estrogen replacement therapy in some women.[33]

In the most recent study the risk of breast cancer was elevated by 43 percent after 10 years of HRT.[31] Women with a family history of breast cancer may be at an increased risk introduced by HRT, but other studies report no increase in risk. It is of interest that to date there is no study that demonstrates that HRT places women already treated for breast cancer at increased risk of recurrence. In a recent investigation of 145 breast cancer survivors who took conjugated estrogen, only 13 had recurrences of breast cancer during a 31-month follow-up. This was no different from the recurrence rate in those who did not take estrogen.[34] Studies with longer follow-ups and studies corrected for the effects of exercise and diet are needed, as well as randomized, longitudinal samples.

Breast cancer survivors must be fully informed of the issues and agree that the desire to take estrogen takes precedence over the potential that an already increased risk will be magnified.

Almost 50 percent of women have fibroids by age 50 years. The doses of estrogen employed for postmenopausal replacement therapy are relatively low, and they are not anticipated to stimulate fibroid growth. Should the fibroid be in a submucous location, however, withdrawal bleeding may be copious. If there is a strong desire to continue estrogen therapy, referral for fibromyomectomy should be advised.

Delivery Systems   Careful consideration of a woman's current health, possible adverse effects, and medical and family history continues to establish the database for HRT prescription. Common HRT regimens include estrogen, progestins, and androgens in various combinations (see Table 9-7). All of the orally administered estrogens undergo extensive first-pass metabolism in the liver. When administered transdermally, parenterally, or vaginally, estrogens do not undergo first-pass metabolism. Use of transdermal estrogens with liver disease or prior phlebitis is controversial. Although the transdermal delivery system does not appear to alter the coagulation profile, the use of any form of ERT in the patient with a history of phlebitis or venous thrombotic disease is relatively contraindicated.

Vaginal estrogens are absorbed systematically. If estrogens are absolutely contraindicated, then it will not be possible to prescribe topical estrogen therapy. Absorption is variable and although not fully studied, it is suspected that initially, when vaginal mucosa is thin, there will be rapid absorption of topical estrogen. As vaginal tissue recovers, there may be a lessening of systemic absorption. If vaginal estrogens are to be used with regularity (for example, three times per week) and the uterus is present, a progestin should be given for a 13-day period at least once every 2 to 3 months in order to reduce endometrial hyperplasia and the risk of endometrial cancer.

Contraindications and Side Effects   Contraindications include active thrombophlebitis, breast cancer or estrogen-dependent tumor, pregnancy, active liver disease, undiagnosed or abnormal vaginal bleeding, undiagnosed headache, or cholelithiasis. The most common side effects of HRT include vaginal bleeding, breast tenderness, bloating, and headache. The symptoms are usually mild and may be alleviated by switching to a different preparation or adjusting the dose. About half the women on continuous combined estrogen/progestin therapy will have irregular vaginal bleeding

TABLE 9-7

Commonly Used HRT Regimens

Hormone Regimen	Recommended Dosage Range and Average dose/day	Average AWP Pricing for 30 days	Patient Considerations
Oral Formulations			
Conjugated estrogens (CE) (Premarin)	0.3 mg to 1.25 mg (Range) 0.625 mg qd	<$10.96	Risk of endometrial hyperplasia if woman has intact uterus (all dosage forms).
Esterified estrogens (Estratab) (Menest)	0.3 mg to 1.25 mg (Range) 0.625 mg qd	$ 4.45	Continuous daily use preferred in those women with surgical menopause who have symptoms on E-free days (headaches, hot flashes).
Estradiol, micronized (Estrace)	0.5 mg to 2 mg (Range) 0.5 mg qd	$ 5.70	
Estropipate (Ogen, Ortho-est)	0.625 mg to 5 mg (Range) 0.75 mg qd	$ 8.61	Side effects include breast tenderness or sensitivity, nausea, change in weight, loss of appetite, withdrawal bleeding (cyclic use).
Transdermal Patches			
Estradiol-transdermal system (Estraderm)	0.05–0.1 mg/day twice weekly (.05 mg qd)	<$13.79	Transdermal system may be preferred in women with history of venous thromboembolism or stable liver disease.
(Vivelle)	0.0375–0.1 mg/day applied twice weekly (0.5 mg qd)	<$15.17	
(Climara)	0.05–0.1 mg/day applied weekly (.05 mg qd)	$14.81	

Oral Formulations Progestin Products

Taken with one of the estrogen products listed under "Estrogen"

Monitor for any irregular bleeding.

P-related side effects include mood changes, acne, abdominal bloating, weight gain, tiredness.

| Medroxyprogesterone (MPA): (Provera, Cycrin, Amen, Curretab, Generic) | 5-10 mg/day in a cyclic regimen or 2.5 to 5 mg/day continuously | $14.03 | All progestins may lower HDL levels. The 19-nortestosterone derivatives (e.g., norethindrone) particularly lower HDL by 15% to 20%. |

Combination Products (E–P)

| CE 0.625 mg/tab and MPA 5 mg/tab on days 15–28 (Premphase) | One tab daily | <$18.33 |
| CE 0.625 mg/tab and MPA 2.5 mg/tab (Prempro) | One tab daily | <$21.60 |

Table was adapted from *F&C*,[21] *Applied Therapeutics*, 6th edition,[6] and Hardman JG et al.[1]

<Drug is less expensive than price listed due to volume discounts.

E = Estrogen, P = Progesterone, CE = Conjugated Estrogen,

MPA = Medroxyprogesterone, AWP = average wholesale price.

for several months before menses ceases entirely. Vaginal bleeding may occur with either too much or too little estrogen. Some women will not take hormone therapy as directed. Self-adjustment of dosage can cause untoward effects. It is also an indication that the patient is having side effects. Many of these women subsequently discontinue the progestin or both hormones. Attention should be directed at solving dosing problems and preventing discontinuation. New natural and designer estrogens may tailor therapy to each woman's needs and result in improved compliance.

Contextual Issues   The primary care provider must recognize that many biases can be introduced when case-controlled studies are employed to make clinically important decisions. Prescribers create biases that are difficult to control. Patients tend to self-select. General population surveys show that women who take HRT are leaner and more health conscious than those who do not. Additionally, studies are often performed in academic centers, where the patient population is frequently more educated and more affluent than it is representative. Studies do not give us definitive answers on the issues of cardiac benefit and prevention of bone loss versus risk of breast cancer. Very little has been said regarding the two- to threefold increase in gallbladder disease following oral HRT. Risks and benefits must be weighed for each woman as an individual. Unfortunately, no matter what the benefit, U.S. women do not initiate or continue HRT in great numbers. Population-based prevalence rates range from 8 percent in Massachusetts to 30 percent on the West Coast.[35] This is in spite of the fact that many more women die from heart disease than from breast cancer. Women may have other reasons for not initiating or continuing HRT. Studies currently underway may shed some light on the reasons women give for not taking or continuing HRT.

REFERENCES

1. Hardman JG, Limbird LE, Molinoff PB, et al: *Goodman & Gilman's The Pharmacological Basis of Therapeutics,* 9th ed. New York: McGraw-Hill, 1996, p 1416. Used with permission.
2. Stringer J: *Basic Concepts in Pharmacology.* New York: McGraw-Hill, 1996, p 245. Used with permission.
3. Harvey RA, Champe PC: Hormones, in *Lippincott's Illustrated Reviews: Pharmacology.* Philadelphia: Lippincott, 1992, pp 243, 245.
4. Sweeney G: *Clinical Pharmacology: A Conceptual Approach.* New York: Churchill-Livingstone, 1990, p A18.
5. Barentsen R, Van De Weijer PHM: Progestins: Pharmacological characteristics and clinically relevant differences. *Eur Menopause J* 3(4):266–271, 1996.
6. Ruggiero R: Contraception, in Young LL, Koda-Kimble MA (eds): *Applied Therapeutics: The Clinical Use of Drugs,* 6th ed. Vancouver, WA: Applied Therapeutics, 1995, pp 43–44.
7. U.S. Public Health Service: Put prevention into practice: Unintended pregnancy. *J Am Acad Nurse Pract* 9(4):193, 1997.
8. Hatcher RA, Trussell J, Stewart F, et al: *Contraceptive Technology,* 16th ed. New York: Irvington, 1994–1996, pp 69, 113, 243–248.
9. Murphy J (ed): *Nurse Practitioners' Prescribing Guide.* New York: Prescribing Reference, 1997, p 192.

10. Painter K: Morning after pill receives FDA backing. *USA Today* Feb. 25, sec A, p 1, col 6, 1997.
11. DiPierri D: RU-486, Mifepristone: A review of a controversial drug. *Nurse Practit* 19(6):59–61, 1994.
12. Aguillaume CJ, Tyrer LB: Current status and future role of RU-486 in the US, *Contemp Nurse Practit* 1(4):32, 1997.
13. Mastroianni L Jr, Robinson JC: Hassle-free methods of contraception, *Patient Care* 29(5):46–58, 1995.
14. Yuzpe AA: Contraception, in Gray J (ed): *Therapeutic Choices.* Ottawa, Canada: Canadian Pharmaceutical Association, 1995, p 443.
15. Dickey RP: *Managing Contraceptive Pill Patients,* 8th ed. Durant, OK: EMIS, 1996, pp 6–7, 64–65, 82, 146–147, 154–155, 228.
16. Mastroianni L Jr: Noncontraceptive benefits of oral contraceptives. *Postgrad Med* 93(1):193, 1993.
17. Ness RB, Keder LB, Soper DE, et al: Oral contraception and the recognition of endometritis. *Am J Obstet Gynecol* 176(3): 580, 1997.
18. Goldzieher JW: Are low dose contraceptives safer and better? *Am J Obstet Gynecol* 171:587–590, 1994.
19. National Women's Health Network: *Recommended Guidelines on Birth Control Pills.* Washington, DC: National Womens' Health Network, Feb. 23, 1989.
20. Federal Drug Administration package insert labeling.
21. Cada D (ed): *Drug Facts and Comparisons.* St Louis: Facts and Comparisons, 1997, p 435.
22. Mastroianni L Jr; Robinson JC: Contraception in the 1990s. *Patient Care* 28(1):109, 1994.
23. Hawkins JW, Roberto-Nichols DM, Stanley-Haney JL: *Protocols for Nurse Practitioners in Gynecologic Settings,* 5th ed. New York: Tiresias, 1995, pp 16–17, 21.
24. Brown J: Women's health: A look at mid-life transitions and hormone replacement therapy. *Drug Utiliz Pract* 4(4):1, 1997.
25. Belchetz PE: Hormonal treatment of postmenopausal women. *New Engl J Med* 330: 1062–1071, 1994.
26. Hammond CB: Climacteric, in Scott JR, DiSaia PJ, Hammond CB, Spellacy WN: *Danforth's Obstetrics and Gynecology,* 7th ed. Philadelphia: Lippincott, 1994.
27. Ettinger B, Grady D: The waning effects of postmenopausal estrogen therapy on osteoporosis. *N Engl J Med* 329:1192–1193, 1993.
28. Evan MP, Feming KC, Evans JM: Hormone replacement therapy: Management of common problems. *Mayo Clin Proc* 70:800–805, 1995.
29. Speroff L: The case for postmenopausal hormone therapy. *Hosp Pract* 31(2):75–89, 1996.
30. Col N, Eckman MH, Karas RH, et al: Patient-specific decisions about hormone replacement therapy in women. *J Am Med Assoc* 277:1140–1147, 1997.
31. Grodstein F, Stampfer MJ, Colditz GA, et al: Postmenopausal hormone therapy and mortality. *New Engl J Med* 336(25):1769–1775, 1997.
32. The Writing Group for the PEPI Trial: Effects of estrogen and estrogen/progestin regimens on heart risk factors in post-menopausal women. *J Am Med Assoc* 273:199–208, 1995.
33. Schiff I: Estrogen replacement therapy, *Prim Care News* 3(3):4, 1993.
34. Saltus R: Findings encouraging on estrogen therapy. *Boston Globe,* March 25, 1997, sec A, p 1, col 1.
35. Harris RB, Laws A, Reddy VM, et al: Are women using post-menopausal estrogens? A community survey. *Am J Public Health* 80:1266, 1990.

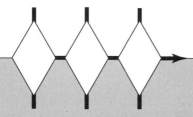

Chapter 10

DRUG THERAPY IN SIMPLE EPISODIC CONDITIONS

Constance F. O'Connor

OVERVIEW OF THE DRUG THERAPY FOR UNCOMPLICATED HEALTH PROBLEMS IN WELL PEOPLE

Drug therapy for episodic illness in the healthy adult is primarily directed at providing relief of symptoms and treatment of the specific health problem. A careful drug history should be taken to avoid unexpected drug interactions, allergic reactions, or any other adverse effects. Before prescribing a specific drug regime to treat an illness, the nurse practitioner needs to have a thorough understanding of the pathophysiology of the disease in order to make effective pharmacotherapy decisions.

Resources

Di Piro T, Talbert L, Yee GC, et al (eds): *Pharmacotherapy: A Pathophysiologic Approach.* Stamford, CT: Appleton & Lange, 1997.

Hardman JG, Limbird LE, Molinoff PB, et al: *Goodman & Gilman's The Pharmacological Basis of Therapeutics,* 9th ed. New York: McGraw-Hill, 1996.

Nurse Practitioner's Drug Handbook. Springhouse, PA: Springhouse, 1997.

Nurse practitioners treat a variety of uncomplicated episodic illnesses in the clinical setting. For the advanced practice nurse, the right to prescribe medication differs from state to state. The role of the nurse practitioner in prescribing the most effective medication for episodic health problems is the key for patient wellness and satisfaction. This chapter will present an overview of drug therapy for common, uncomplicated illnesses frequently encountered in the clinical area.

Head, Neck, and Chest

Headache is a common complaint that requires a thorough patient history taken to assist in determining the headache characteristics. When investigating the headache condition, the nurse practitioner should ensure that the history includes the following information:[1]

1. Duration of headache: How long has the patient been experiencing the headache?
2. Frequency and duration of the headache
3. Site of pain
4. Intensity and quality of pain
5. Time of onset of the headache
6. Associated symptoms: neurological symptoms (visual changes, dizziness, weakness), nausea, vomiting, photophobia
7. Aggravating and relieving factors of the headache

If a careful systematic history and physical examination reveal no abnormalities, treatment for a suspected tension or migraine headache can be initiated. The first-line approach to treatment is for the patient to avoid the trigger factors that may precipitate the headache. Common factors may include stress; certain foods, such as cheese, chocolate, monosodium glutamate, alcohol, and citrus fruits; sleep deprivation or prolonged sleep, delayed or missed meals, dehydration, and caffeine withdrawal.

The pharmacotherapy of choice for headaches is an analgesic such as aspirin or acetaminophen and nonsteroidal anti-inflammatory drugs (NSAIDs). When the drug therapy with simple analgesics is not effective in headache management, antimigrainous agents should be instituted (see Table 10-1).

The majority of patients with headache are experiencing a benign condition such as a migraine or a tension-type headache.[1] A referral to a specialist is necessary when the patient has been compliant in taking the medication as prescribed, but the headache has not improved.

A condition that is frequently seen in ambulatory medicine is conjunctivitis, referred to as "pink eye" or *red eye*. Inflammation and infection of the conjunctiva is the most common disease, and it accounts for more than 90 percent of red eye.[2] When taking a patient history for red eye, the clinician should ask the following questions:

1. Have you ever had this condition before?
2. Do your eyes stick together in the morning? (Eyes that stick together in the morning indicate bacterial conjunctivitis 99 percent of the time.)
3. Is there any pain?
4. Is there a family history of serious eye disease?
5. Has there been any trauma to the eye?
6. Does bright light bother your eyes?
7. Do you wear contact lenses?
8. Do you have any allergies?
9. Can you see as usual?

After a systematic eye examination is performed and conjunctivitis is suspected, follow the red eye chart (see Table 10-2) for specific causes and treatment. If the patient does

(text continues on page 232)

TABLE 10-1

Drug Treatment for Headaches

Drug	Indication, Route, and Dosage	Adverse Reactions	Interactions	Contraindications and Precautions	Patient Education
Acetaminophen	Mild pain Adults: 325–650 mg PO or rectally q 4 h PM; do not exceed 4 g/day	Hematologic: hemolytic anemia, neutropenia, leukopenia, pancytopenia, thrombocytopenia Hepatic: jaundice, severe liver damage with toxic doses Dermatologic: rash, urticaria Other: hypoglycemia	Ethanol: ↑ risk of hepatic damage Caffeine: ↑ analgesic effect Anticoagulants and thrombolytic drugs: may ↑ hypoprothrombinemic effects Phenothiazines: may result in hypothermia with large doses of acetaminophen	Known hypersensitivity to acetaminophen Administer cautiously to patients with anemia or hepatic or renal disease Persistent pain or fever may indicate serious illness	Instruct patient drug is for short-term use and if symptoms persist to see PCP for further evaluation
Ibuprofen	Mild to moderate pain Adults: 400 mg PO 4–6 hours PM	CNS: headache, dizziness, drowsiness, lightheadedness, weakness, vertigo, aseptic meningitis CV: peripheral edema, water retention, CHF, hypertension, tachycardia, palpitations	Furosemide: ↓ diuretic effect Lithium: ↑ plasma levels of lithium Thiazide diuretics: ↓ diuretic effect	Hypersensitivity to aspirin, iodides, or any NSAID; not recommended during pregnancy	Inform patient to take with food or milk to reduce GI upset Report any evidence of side effects to PCP immediately

(continued)

TABLE 10-1

Drug Treatment for Headaches (continued)

Drug	Indication, Route, and Dosage	Adverse Reactions	Interactions	Contraindications and Precautions	Patient Education
		Dermatologic: pruritus, rash, urticaria, Steven-Johnson syndrome	Beta blockers: Antihypertensive effect ↓		
		GI: nausea, vomiting, GI bleeding, anorexia, constipation, occult blood loss	Methotrexate: ↑ plasma levels		
		GU: acute renal failure, cystitis, hematuria, azotemia	Warfarin: ↑ risk of GI bleeding		
		Hematologic: Prolonged bleeding time, anemia			
		Hepatic: elevated enzymes			
		Respiratory: bronchospasm			

| Aspirin (acetylsalicylic acid) | Mild to moderate pain
Adults: 325 to 650 mg PO or rectally q 4 h PM | EENT: tinnitus and hearing loss

GI: nausea, GI distress, occult bleeding, dyspepsia, GI bleeding

Hematologic: leukopenia, thrombocytopenia, prolonged bleeding time

Hepatic: abnormal liver function studies, hepatitis

Dermatologic: rash, bruising

Other: hypersensitivity reactions manifested by anaphylaxis or asthma | Alcohol: ↑ chance of GI ulceration and bleeding

Antacids: urinary alkalinizers and corticosteroids, ↓ aspirin levels

Anticoagulants and thrombolytic drugs: ↑ risk of bleeding

NSAIDs: ↓ serum levels of NSAIDs and ↑ ulcerogenic effects

Beta blockers: ↓ antihypertensive effect

Methotrexate: ↑ toxicity

Oral hypoglycemics: ↑ hypoglycemic effect

Probenecid sulfinpyrazone: ↓ uricosuric effect

Valproic Acid: ↑ serum concentrations | Children and teenagers who have flu symptoms or chicken pox should avoid ASA because it has been associated with Reye's syndrome

Hypersensitivity to salicylates

Patients with asthma, nasal polyps, hay fever, and chronic urticaria have a ↑ incidence of hypersensitivity

Contraindicated for patients with GI history

Pregnancy, lactation

Vitamin K deficiency, severe anemia, renal or liver disease, or in conjunction with anticoagulant therapy | Advise patient to take with food or milk to reduce GI side effects

Instruct patients taking prescription drugs to check with the pharmacist or PCP before taking drugs |

TABLE 10-2

Red Eye Chart

Problem	Signs/Symptoms	Additional Points	Treatment	Medication	Patient Education
Bacterial conjunctivitis	Itching Tearing Moderate amount of discharge Moderate conjunctival hyperemia No pain, vision disturbance No preauricular adenopathy Cornea clear	Bilateral or unilateral involvement Mucopurulent (yellow-green) discharge Red, shiny appearance to lower lids More common in winter and spring	General measures Cold compresses to periocular area Artificial tears frequently Warn the patient of the contagiousness of disease Inform others to avoid close contact with infected persons Use separate towels, frequently wash hands, avoid hand-shaking Always wipe eye from inside to outside to prevent self-inoculation of other eye	Sulfacetamide Sodium ophthalmic drops Adults and children: instill 1–2 drops of 10% solution into lower conjunctival sac q 1–4 h; doses may be tapered by increasing time interval between doses as condition responds	Warn patient the drops may burn slightly Ophthalmic products may cause light sensitivity; wear sunglasses Instruct patients on installation of drops, not to touch the tip of dropper to eye or surrounding tissue
Viral conjunctivitis	Burning Itching	Watery, mucoid discharge	Symptomatic treatment		Use separate towels and wash cloths

Signs/Symptoms	Findings	Management	Medication	Patient Education
Conjunctival infection Tearing Recent contact with another person with "red eye" Recent URI Unilateral initial presentation followed by bilateral infection	Moderate amount of debris Follicular pattern on lower eyelid Usual causes are human adenovirus 8 to 19 Transmission is from direct contact or from contaminated objects	Cold compresses Gently cleanse with water to remove debris (remember to wipe from inside of eye to outside) Artificial tears to decrease irritation Warn the patient of contagiousness of disease Frequently wash hands, use separate towels, avoid hand-shaking	Erythromycin ophthalmic ointment 0.5% Adults and children: 1 cm in length applied to affected eye TID or q 4 h for severe infections	Alert patient to signs of sensitivity and report immediately Remove any purulent eye drainage as this interferes with sulfacetamide Instruct patient on application of ophthalmic ointment; cleanse the eye of excess exudate before applying Warn patient not to touch the eye or surrounding area with tube Instruct patient to report any adverse reactions immediately Stress importance of medication compliance Warn patient that ointment can cause temporary blurred vision after application
Iritis Redness in the area surrounding the cornea called "ciliary flush" Photophobia caused by movement of iris	Causes are trauma, recent ocular surgery, ankylosing spondylitis, Reiter's syndrome, arthritis, psoriasis	Referral to an ophthalmologist		

SOURCE: Fenstermacher and Hudson.[3]

not respond to the prescribed treatment within 2 days, a referral to an ophthalmologist is necessary.

Ears, Nose, and Throat

Disorders of the upper respiratory tract that include the ears, nose, and throat are commonly treated in the ambulatory setting.

Ceruminosis, a common problem, usually presents with the patient complaining of decreased hearing. Ceruminolytic agents that are equally effective for impacted wax are hydrogen peroxide and carbamide peroxide in glycerol (Debrox). The patient should be instructed to instill the ear drops the evening before the ear irrigation to ease the procedure. The dosage for carbamide peroxide for adults and children is 5 to 10 drops into the ear canal bid for up to 4 days. The solution should remain in the ear canal for 15 to 30 min and be removed with warm water. There are no adverse reactions or drug interactions reported. The patient should return if redness, pain, or swelling continues.

External otitis, better known as *swimmer's ear*, often presents with ear pain, a decrease in hearing, pruritus, a sensation of obstruction in the ear, and discharge. A history of recent water exposure or trauma from cotton swabs, scratching, or other foreign objects is frequently given. Treatment is initiated after careful and thorough removal of exudate from the external ear canal to allow the topical medication to penetrate the inflamed tissue. Cortisporin otic solution, 4 drops in the affected ear qid for 10 to 14 days is the treatment of choice. Cortisporin otic suspension may be used if the ear canal is swollen, because this is less viscous and may allow better distribution of the medication. The suspension may be prescribed to avoid pain if there is a concern about a perforation of the tympanic membrane. The drops should be instilled with the patient lying flat with the affected ear up for 5 min. Counsel patient on care of ears, keeping water out of ear canals for 2 weeks, and avoiding putting foreign objects in the ear canals to scratch or clean them.

Another frequently encountered condition of the ear is *serous otitis media*. The patient may complain of a hearing loss, fullness in the ear, or a popping sensation with nose blowing, swallowing, or yawning. Often a patient gives a history of having a recent upper respiratory infection. If the symptoms are mild, no therapy is indicated, because the condition will usually spontaneously resolve itself in 2 to 3 weeks. However, if the patient is symptomatic a course of topical nasal decongestants or a trial of oral decongestants may be beneficial (see Table 10-3 for decongestant therapy).

Acute otitis media is an inflammation of the middle ear usually precipitated by an upper respiratory tract infection. The patient complains of an earache, decreased hearing, and often fever. Perforation of the tympanic membrane is present when there is a purulent discharge in the external ear canal. The management of acute otitis media is antibiotic therapy. Amoxicillin 500 mg PO tid for 10 days is the first line of therapy. Adverse reactions to the medication may include nausea, vomiting, and diarrhea. Hypersensitivity to the drug may present with a maculopapular rash and urticaria. Amoxicillin is contraindicated with patients with a history of an allergy to penicillins or to cephalosporins. Patients with mononucleosis should not take amoxicillin because a rash may develop during treatment. The antibiotic course should be finished in

(text continues on page 236)

TABLE 10-3

Decongestant Therapy

Drug	Indication, Route, and Dosage	Adverse Reactions	Interactions	Contraindications and Precautions	Patient Education
Oxymetazoline hydrochloride (Afrin) Available in solution or spray	Treatment of upper respiratory infection and congestion around eustachian tube in middle ear infections Adults and children over 6 years: 2–3 sprays or 2–3 drops of 0.05% solution in each nostril every 10–12 h	Topical use: stinging, sneezing, burning, local irritation, mucosal dryness, and rebound congestion	May increase the pressor effect of tricyclic antidepressants from significant systemic absorption of the decongestant	Do not give to breastfeeding mothers Contraindicated in patients with narrow-angle glaucoma or hypersensitivity to any of the components of the drug Monitor carefully in patients with cardiovascular disease, diabetes mellitus, or prostatic hypertrophy, because systemic absorption can occur	Advise patient not to exceed recommended dosage and that the drug is for short-term use and to notify provider if symptoms persist Instruct patient how to administer Warn patient that excessive use can cause hypotension, dizziness, weakness, and bradycardia
Phenylephrine HCl (Neo-Synephrine)	Nasal, sinus, or eustachian tube congestion	Can cause temporary stinging or burning on instillation, rebound congestion and blurred vision	None significant	Contraindicated in patients with hypersensitivity to the drug	Instruct patient to clear nasal passage before using medications

(continued)

233

TABLE 10-3

Decongestant Therapy (continued)

Drug	Indication, Route, and Dosage	Adverse Reactions	Interactions	Contraindications and Precautions	Patient Education
	Adults and children over 12 years old: Apply 2–3 drops or 1–2 sprays of 0.25, 0.5, or 1% solution in each nostril q 3–4 h as needed			Use caution in patients with hypertension, hyperthyroidism, diabetes mellitus, or cardiac disease	Teach patient instillation of solution; instruct to hold head upright, then sniff spray quickly into each nostril After use, rinse tip of bottle with hot water and dry with clean tissue Caution patient not to exceed recommended dosage and to notify provider if no relief in 3 days or if side effects are experienced
Pseudoephedrine HCl	Relief of nasal or eustachian tube congestion	CNS: nervousness, excitability, dizziness, tremor, insomnia, depression, restlessness	Antihypertensive: may increase hypotensive effect, closely monitor blood pressure	Contraindicated in patients with severe hypertension or coronary artery disease, breastfeeding patients,	Remind patients not to take medication within 2 h of bedtime to minimize insomnia effects

Adults: PO 60 mg q 4–6 h or 120 mg sustained-release q 12 h, not to exceed 240 mg/day	CV: tachycardia, arrythmias, bradycardia, cardiovascular collapse, palpitations GI: nausea, vomiting, dry mouth, anorexia GU: dysuria Dermatologic: pallor	MAO inhibitors: potential of causing severe hypertension and in patients receiving MAO inhibitors Extended-release preparations are contraindicated in children under 12 years old Use cautiously in patients with hypertension, cardiac disease, diabetes mellitus, glaucoma, hyperthyroidism, and prostatic hyperplasia	Dry mouth may occur; suggest taking sips of water, ice chips, or chew gum Tell patient to swallow sustained-release preparations whole and not to chew or crush medications Advise not to take other OTC medicines containing sympathomimetics, which can cause hazardous reactions Instruct patient to report any side effects or lack of improvement to provider

entirety even if the patient feels well. Erythromycin 250 mg PO qid for 10 days should be prescribed if the patient is allergic to penicillin derivatives. Possible adverse reactions of the medication are abdominal discomfort, nausea, vomiting, diarrhea, hepatitic dysfunction, rash, urticaria and hearing loss (with high doses). Drug interactions to be considered when prescribing erythromycin are increased anticoagulant effects, increased theophylline plasma levels, and increased risk of nephrotoxicity with cyclosporine. Erythromycin preparations should never be used concurrently with terfenadine or astemizole because it increases levels of these antihistamines and potentially could cause serious cardiovascular effects. The patient should be instructed to take the medication with a glass of water and 2 h after a meal to avoid GI side effects. Instruct the patient to finish all medication and report immediately any adverse reactions.

The *common cold* or upper respiratory tract infection (URI) is an acute infection lasting several days; adults average 2 to 4 colds a year. Symptoms of a URI are malaise, headache, nasal congestion, scratchy throat, sneezing, watery rhinorrhea, and nonproductive cough. There is no specific treatment for the common cold, but supportive measures such as decongestant therapy (see Table 10-3) and analgesics are used as necessary for fever and myalgias.

Sinusitis is an inflammation of the mucous membrane lining of the paranasal sinuses causing obstruction of normal sinus drainage. In uncomplicated, nonbacterial sinusitis symptoms may be clear nasal discharge, headache, malaise, a feeling of fullness or pressure over the involved sinus, and postnasal drip. Symptoms should last no longer than 10 days; otherwise the patient should notify the provider. Treatment consists of aggressive use of decongestant therapy, especially the use of topical decongestants to decrease edema and discomfort. Analgesic therapy with aspirin or acetaminophen may be given as needed (see Table 10-1).

When the sinus drainage tract becomes obstructed secondary to mucosal edema, the retention of secretions in the sinus cavity leads to the bacterial stage of sinusitis. Patients may present with mucopurulent discharge, pain, or tenderness over the affected sinus area, facial pain, toothache, and pressure behind the eyes. The first line of treatment in acute bacterial sinusitis is vigorous use of decongestant therapy. Oxymetazoline (Afrin) should be used for no longer than 5 days to avoid the rebound effect. Amoxicillin 500 mg PO tid for 2 weeks is the first choice for antibiotic therapy. However, if the sinus condition does not respond or if the patient becomes reinfected during the amoxicillin therapy, an alternative or second-line antibiotic is Augmentin 500 mg bid for 14 days. Augmentin is expensive, and it is contraindicated in patients with known hypersensitivity to the penicillins or cephalosporins. As with amoxicillin, the administration of Augmentin may reduce the efficacy of oral contraceptives. The adverse reactions may include nausea, vomiting, diarrhea, acute interstitial nephritis, rash, and urticaria. Patients should be instructed to take the medication on an empty stomach for maximal effectiveness and to take the medication in its entirety.

Pharyngitis is the final condition of the upper respiratory tract to be discussed. Pharyngitis is an inflammation of the pharynx, the tonsils, or both. Clinical features may include fever, cervical adenopathy, sore throat, headache, and malaise. There is still a debate among providers whether to treat the condition before a positive throat culture is identified or to treat it empirically based on symptoms. Viral pharyngitis is managed with symptomatic relief. Acetaminophen can be given for throat pain, fever, and myalgias. Penicillin is the first choice of antibiotics for beta hemolytic streptococcal pharyngitis. Penicillin VK 250 mg PO qid for 10 days is the recommended dosage. However, if the patient is allergic to Penicillin VK, erythromycin 250 mg PO qid for 10 days is the substitute choice. Penicillin VK may reduce the effectiveness of oral contraceptives, and beta blockers may increase risk of anaphylactic reactions with penicillin. Penicillin VK is to be used cautiously with renal impaired patients. Adverse reactions to Penicillin VK can be nausea, vomiting, diarrhea, neuropathy, hemolytic anemia, eosinophilia, leukopenia, thrombocytopenia, pruritus, and rash.

Acute bronchitis is a lower respiratory tract infection that involves inflammation of the tracheobronchial tree. The condition is often preceded by a URI, and presenting symptoms may be a nonproductive cough that usually develops into a mucopurulent productive cough accompanied by a low-grade fever, headache, and malaise. Often the patient complains of substernal chest discomfort worsened with coughing. Treatment is aimed at the symptoms. Guaifenesin, an expectorant, aids in decreasing the viscosity of the sputum and helps with expectoration of the secretions. There are no significant interactions; however, it is contraindicated with any allergy to this medicine and its efficacy is debated. A persistent cough may be treated with dextromethorphan 10 to 20 mg PO q 4 h or 30 mg q 6 to 8 h. Side effects of this medicine include dizziness, nausea, and vomiting. Instruct patient to notify the provider if cough worsens or there is no improvement. Acetaminophen or ibuprofen may be used for myalgias and/or fever. An inhaled bronchodilator such as albuterol or metaproterenol, 2 puffs every 4 h as needed, should be given if wheezing or chest tightness is present.[4] The patient should be instructed on the use of inhalers and that side effects include bad taste or change in taste, rash, and diarrhea. Antibiotics may be indicated with a persistent cough productive of mucopurulent secretions and a fever that may be indicative of a secondary bacterial infection. Careful antibiotic therapy may be used; tetracycline 500 mg PO qid for 10 days or erythromycin 500 mg PO qid for 10 days. Physical examination is necessary to rule out community-acquired pneumonia (CAP) or other conditions.

Musculoskeletal Pain

Musculoskeletal pain is frequently seen in the clinical setting. A history of pain noted after recent trauma or straining the involved area such as the neck, shoulder, knee, or lower back is often elicited. The patient should be asked about recent changes in physical activity that may have contributed to the condition. The conservative treatment of musculoskeletal pain is to advise the patient to ice the involved area initially and then use alternate ice with heat (heating pad, hot water bottle, hot tub bath). The affected area should be rested and analgesics given for discomfort. Ibuprofen (see Table 10-1) 800 mg PO tid should be prescribed or if NSAIDs are contraindicated give acetaminophen (325 mg) 2 tablets PO every 4 to 6 h as needed. If musculoskeletal pain continues or worsens after treatment, an orthopedic referral is needed.

Gastrointestinal Disorders

Nausea is a complaint that refers to a sick, queasy feeling a patient experiences that may or may not be accompanied by vomiting. Vomiting is the expulsion of gastric materials brought on by gastric, abdominal, and thoracic contractions. Acute symptoms without abdominal pain are usually caused by gastroenteritis, food poisoning, or medications. A thorough history and physical examination are essential in finding and treating the underlying cause of vomiting. Usually, the causes of acute nausea or vomiting are mild and require no specific treatment. The patient needs to be instructed on a clear liquid diet along with dry foods; hydration is important to avoid any metabolic complications. Antiemetic medications are given to prevent or control vomiting. In the ambulatory clinic setting, the antiemetic medication most frequently prescribed is prochlorperazine (Compazine). Compazine can be given PO 5 to 10 mg tid or qid, PR 25 mg suppository bid or 5 to 10 mg IM every 3 to 4 h as needed for severe nausea and vomiting. Adverse reactions may be sedation, dizziness, extrapyramidal reactions, pseudoparkinsonism, orthostatic hypotension, tachycardia, ECG changes, dry mouth, constipation, blurred vision, urine retention, dark urine, inhibited ejaculation, agranulocytosis, cholestatic jaundice, menstrual irregularities, exfoliative dermatitis, allergic reactions, and mild photosensitivity. Antacids inhibit absorption of phenothiazines. Anticholinergic drugs including antidepressants and antiparkinsonian agents will have an increased anticholinergic activity as well as aggravated parkinsonian symptoms. Barbiturates may decrease the effectiveness of the medication. The patient should be advised on side effects and to notify the provider immediately if they become evident. Antacids may also control simple nausea and vomiting by neutralizing gastric acid. Over-the-counter antacid products containing magnesium hydroxide, aluminum hydroxide, and/or calcium carbonate may provide relief. There is a potential for side effects from these products in the antacids, such as magnesium causing diarrhea and constipation from the aluminum. In general, when antacids are used intermittently for the relief of acute episodic nausea and vomiting, they do not cause serious side effects.

Constipation is a common complaint that is often defined as hardness of stool with straining during defecation. Constipation is not an illness but a symptom of an underlying problem. Common causes of constipation are poor dietary and behavioral habits such as low-fiber diet, poor bowel habits, and lack of exercise, structural abnormalities, medications, and systemic disease. All patients should have a careful history taken and have a physical examination including stool testing for occult blood to assist in determining the cause of constipation. The standard treatment for this problem is patient education on proper dietary fluid and fiber intake. Studies show that diet is a crucial factor in bowel functioning and that greater amounts of crude dietary fiber are associated with lesser prevalence of constipation as well as other gastrointestinal disorders. Fibers can be given through a high-fiber diet or fiber supplements such as bran powder. If these measures along with a regular exercise program do not solve the patient's constipation problem, laxatives may be introduced, starting with the milder products. Psyllium hydrophilic mucilloid (Metamucil) 2 teaspoons PO in 8 oz of liquid up to tid or 1 packet dissolved in water 1 to 3 times a day may be given. Contraindications to psyllium are severe abdominal pain or intestinal obstruction or ulceration. Patients who need to restrict their sodium intake should be instructed to avoid psyllium products containing sugar or salt. Osmotic laxatives may be used to soften stools and may be given in combination with fiber supplements. These agents have a prompt onset of action in 1 to 3 h and may be used safely long term. Magnesium hydroxide (Milk of Magnesia) with dosages of 15 to 40 mL once daily with water, preferably at bedtime, may be used and takes about 8 h to be effective. Adverse reactions include hypermagnesemia in patients with renal failure and hypocalcemia from phosphate overdoses. Emollients or stool softeners are another choice of treatment. Docusate sodium (Colace) promotes defecation by softening the stool, and onset of action is 24 to 72 h. Dosage is 100 mg capsules given 1 to 3 times per day with water. Adverse reactions are mild abdominal cramping. This medication may provide a bitter taste. Enemas provide an immediate relief from acute constipation and may be necessary in severe cases.

Acute *diarrhea* is a condition that is usually an annoying, self-limiting illness that produces frequent, loose, watery stools. With this disorder, the patient complains of a sudden onset of loose stools, flatulence, malaise, and mild abdominal cramping. In 90 percent of patients with acute diarrhea, the illness is benign and responds within 5 days to simple rehydration therapy or antidiarrheal agents. However, it is important to keep in mind that a percentage of patients will have a significant illness for which specific therapy is needed. If diarrhea continues for more than 72 h or if there is blood in the stool, a further evaluation is indicated.[5] Treatment for acute diarrhea is for the patient to rest the bowel and rehydrate. High-fiber foods, milk products, fats, and caffeine should be avoided. Frequent small amounts of fruit drinks, tea, flat carbonated beverages, and bland soft foods such as soup, dry toast, and crackers are advised. Rehydration in severe diarrhea is essential and fluids containing glucose, Na+, K+, CL−, and bicarbonate or citrate (e.g., Gatorade, Pedialyte) should be given frequently. Antidiarrheal agents can be given to help relieve diarrhea symptoms; however, they are contraindicated in patients with high fever, bloody diarrhea, or systemic toxicity. The patient should be instructed to discontinue the antidiarrheal medication if diarrhea is not getting better or is worsening despite the therapy. Lopermide hydrochloride (Imodium) is the preferred drug given in a dosage of 4 mg PO, then 2 mg after each loose stool with a maximum dosage of 16 mg daily. It is contraindicated in patients with a known hypersensitivity to the drug, ulcerative colitis, or where constipation should be avoided. Adverse reactions reported are drowsiness, fatigue, dizziness, dry mouth, abdominal cramping or distention, nausea, vomiting, and constipation. Instruct patients to use caution while driving because loperamide can cause drowsiness.

Bismuth subsalicylate (Pepto-Bismol) is an antidiarrheal medication that is effective in treatment and prevention of traveler's diarrhea. The dosage for acute diarrhea is 30 mL or 2 tablets PO every ½ to 1 h, up to a maximum of 8 doses in 24 h for no longer than 2 days. The dosage for the prevention and treatment of traveler's diarrhea prophylactically is 60 mL qid during the first 2 weeks of travel. It is contraindicated in patients with a known hypersensitivity to salicylates. Bismuth subsalicylate may interfere with tetracycline absorption, and it may increase the risk of aspirin toxicity. Adverse reactions include temporary tongue and stool darkening and salicylism with high doses. Advise patients who are taking medication for diabetes, gout, and anticoagulant therapy to seek medical advice. If diarrhea persists with treatment, patients should inform their provider for further evaluation.

Urinary Tract Infection

Another common disorder seen in ambulatory medicine is *urinary tract infection* (UTI). It is frequently seen in women, and the history may include increased sexual activity (or newly sexually active), use of a spermicide or a diaphragm, and failure to void after intercourse. The patient may typically complain of frequency and urgency of urination, dysuria, and occasionally hematuria. The urine dipstick is a rapid diagnostic test that is often used in the ambulatory clinic setting to assist in the diagnosis. When there are positive findings for the nitrate test and leukocyte oxidase, a UTI is present 90 percent of the time. Treatment for the uncomplicated UTI is usually antibiotic therapy for 3 days. The cure rates are the same for the traditional 7- to 10-day course as with the 3-day treatment. Antibiotic therapy for uncomplicated UTIs is given in Table 10-4. Preventive measures include:

1. Avoid a full bladder
2. Void after sexual intercourse
3. Wear cotton-lined underwear and avoid tight-fitting clothing
4. Increase fluid intake to assist in eradicating an infection that has just become symptomatic

Skin

One of the common skin disorders that is frequently seen in ambulatory medicine is *acne vulgaris*. Its onset often occurs at puberty and is more common in males. The skin lesions may be blackheads, whiteheads, comedones, pustules or cysts on the face, neck, chest, shoulders, and back. Symptoms that the patient may complain of are painful lesions or itching. In order to treat acne, the type and the severity of the lesion need to be evaluated. There are different modes of treatment for comedones, papules, and pustules and cystic lesions as well as different levels of severity of the condition. The primary treatment for inflammatory acne is antibiotics. They may be used topically or orally. Mild acne requires a topical antibiotic with the first choice being erythromycin with benzoyl peroxide topical gel (Benzamycin). The patient should be instructed to keep the medication refrigerated to prevent inactivity. The medication can be applied bid; however, if benzoyl peroxide causes irritation and dryness, frequency should be reduced to daily use. Patients should be instructed to apply the medication to dry skin 30 min after washing to avoid irritation. The drug therapy of choice for moderate acne is tetracycline 500 mg PO bid or erythromycin 333 mg PO tid. Tetracycline is contraindicated in pregnancy and young children because it interferes with enamel formation and dental pigmentation. It therefore should be given only with great caution in females of childbearing age. The common side effects are gastrointestinal, such as nausea, vomiting, diarrhea, anorexia, flatulence, and epigastric distress. Instruct patients not to use outdated medicine because a Fanconi-like syndrome may occur with nausea, vomiting, acidosis, proteinuria, glycosuria, polydipsia, polyuria, or hypokalemia. Patients should take the medication on a full stomach to enhance absorption. However, it should not be taken with foods

(text continues on page 243)

TABLE 10-4

Antibiotic Therapy for Uncomplicated UTI

Drug	Indication, Route, and Dosage	Interactions	Contraindications and Precautions	Adverse Reactions	Patient Education
First choice: trimethoprim-sulfamethoxazole (Bactrim, Septra) Inexpensive: $18.00 for 6 tablets	Urinary tract infection Dosage: 160/800 mg 1 tablet (double strength) PO q 12 h for 3 days	Oral anticoagulants may ↑ anticoagulant effect Oral diabetic agents may ↑ hypoglycemic effect Oral contraceptives: decreased effectiveness and increased risk of breakthrough bleeding Phenytoin: may inhibit metabolism Zidovudine: may ↑ serum levels due to decreased renal clearance	Contraindicated in patients with known hypersensitivity to sulfonamides or any drug containing sulfur, in patients with renal or hepatic impairment, or during pregnancy or lactation Adverse reactions occur more frequently in AIDS patients, especially hypersensitivity reactions of rash and fever	CNS: headache, mental depression, seizures, hallucinations Dermatologic: erythema multiforme (Stevens-Johnson syndrome), generalized skin rash, epidermal necrolysis, exfoliative dermatitis, photosensitivity, urticaria, pruritus GU: toxic nephrosis with oliguria and anuria, crystalluria, hematuria Hematologic: agranulocytosis, aplastic anemia, megaloblastic anemia, thrombocytopenia, leukopenia, hemolytic anemia Hepatitic: jaundice	Encourage adequate fluid intake Report any adverse reactions such as drug fever, vasculitis, nausea and vomiting, or CNS disturbances immediately

TABLE 10-4

Antibiotic Therapy for Uncomplicated UTI (continued)

Drug	Indication, Route, and Dosage	Interactions	Contraindications and Precautions	Adverse Reactions	Patient Education
Ciprofloxacin hydrochloride (Cipro) Expensive: $27.00 for 6 tablets	Effective against both gram-positive and gram-negative organisms Urinary tract infection: PO 250 (mild to moderate) to 500 mg (severe infection) every 12 h for 3-day course	Aluminum- and magnesium-containing antacids may interfere with ciprofloxacin absorption Space doses at least 2 h apart Probenecid: may ↑ serum level of Cipro Theophylline: may ↑ plasma theophylline concentrations	CNS: headache, restlessness, dizziness, lightheadedness, insomnia, nightmares, hallucinations, depression, seizures, paresthesia GI: nausea, vomiting, diarrhea, abdominal pain, thrush, dysphagia, GI bleeding, intestinal perforation Dermatologic: rash, pruritus, urticaria, photosensitivity, flushing, hyperpigmentation, erythema, nodosum GU: crystalluria, ↑ serum creatinine, and BUN levels, interstitial nephritis CV: hypertension, angina pectoris, atrial flutter, MI, cerebral thrombosis Other: ↑ liver enzymes, Stevens-Johnson syndrome, unpleasant taste	

containing calcium (e.g., milk, ice cream, yogurt, cheese). For severe cystic acne that needs to be treated with Accutane, a referral to a dermatologist is appropriate.

A skin disorder often seen in the clinical environment is *contact dermatitis*, which may be from an irritant or an allergen. Irritant contact dermatitis usually is caused by excessive exposure to irritants such as soaps, detergents, or organic solvents. Allergic contact dermatitis is caused by a delayed hypersensitivity reaction. Some irritants that may precipitate contact allergic rashes are poison ivy, oak, or sumac, topical medications, hair dyes, adhesive tape, and latex. A detailed history needs to be elicited concerning the exposures to various plants, personal products, soaps, medicines, and occupational exposures, so that an allergen may be identified. Signs and symptoms of the condition are tiny vesicles, papules, or erythematous macules in the areas of contact to the allergens, along with pruritus. Acute weeping dermatitis may be treated with saline compresses and potent topical corticosteroids bid to tid. Fluocinonide gel 0.05% is a recommended topical corticosteroid used 2 to 3 times daily that will help resolve the contact dermatitis and relieve itching. When the condition begins to subside, a midpotency steroid such as triamcinolone 0.1% is the treatment of choice. When the condition is severe with widespread pruritic lesions involving the face, eyes, and genitalia, a regime of oral steroids (prednisone) in tapering dosages is recommended. It is at the discretion of the clinician as to what dosage regimen is prescribed (prednisone 0.7 mg/kg/day tapered over 1 to 2 weeks) and consultation is advised. Short-term high-dosage corticosteroid therapy given for acute conditions rarely causes side effects. Prednisone is contraindicated in patients with systemic fungal infections and in those with hypersensitivity to the drug. It is to be used with caution in patients with GI ulceration, renal disease, hypertension, osteoporosis, diabetes mellitus, thromboembolic disease, seizures, myasthenia gravis, CHF, tuberculosis, hypoalbuminemia, hypothyroidism, cirrhosis of the liver, hyperlipidemia, psychotic episodes, glaucoma, or cataracts. When prednisone is administered in high doses or long term, it suppresses release of adrenocorticotropic hormone (ACTH) from the pituitary gland and the adrenal cortex stops secreting endogenous corticosteroids. Patients should be instructed to take the medication with food to reduce GI irritation and not to discontinue medication abruptly or without the provider's consent. Topical corticosteroids should be discontinued as soon as lesions are healed. Contact dermatitis is self-limited and usually takes 2 to 3 weeks to completely resolve with proper therapy. Patients should be assisted in avoiding exposure to causitive irritants and allergins.

ISSUES IN DRUG THERAPY

Prescribing Considerations

Nurse practitioners need to be knowledgeable about many different variables that affect the choice of therapy. Patient variables may include age, sex, weight, education, medical history, allergies, health and nutritional factors, functional status, effectiveness of past drug therapy, compliance, psychological status, religious or cultural beliefs, and economic factors. Clearly, a number of factors need to be considered when making pharmacotherapy decisions to ensure safe and cost-effective use of medications. Route of administration, dosing, drug selection, drug interactions, and side effects are addressed throughout the chapter in reference to specific episodic illnesses.

Contextual Issues

Patient lifestyle, socioeconomic status, and beliefs are factors that influence decisions in drug therapy selection. The nurse practitioner should inquire about the patient's medical insurance status because this information may be significant for patient compliance. Often poor compliance results from the patient's inability to pay for medication, from the patient's daily routine not fitting the drug regimen, or from the patient's lack of understanding of the importance or need for the drug therapy. Economic considerations become increasingly important in formulating a pharmacotherapy plan. Increased competition among pharmaceutical companies has resulted in hospitals and managed care organizations becoming very selective as to what drugs they use in the agency formulary.

Monitoring/Evaluation Requirements

When evaluating the drug therapy of a patient, the clinician needs to evaluate the therapeutic effectiveness and whether there are adverse effects. Monitoring techniques used to evaluate drug therapy are discussed throughout the chapter in regard to the specific medication.

REFERENCES

1. Edmunds J: *Which Headache? A Guide to the Diagnosis and Management of Headache.* Worthing, UK: Professional Postgraduate Services, Europe Ltd, 1992, pp 8–9.
2. Miller D: The red eye. *Prim Care Newsletter* 8:190–192, 1996.
3. Fenstermacher K, Hudson B: *Practice Guidelines for Family Nurse Practitioners.* Philadelphia: Saunders, 1997, pp 98–100.
4. Tierney M, McPhee SJ, Papadakis MA (eds): *Current Medical Diagnosis and Treatment.* Stamford, CT: Appleton & Lange, 1997, pp 260, 1372.
5. Barker RL, Burton JR, Zieve PD: *Principles of Ambulatory Medicine.* Baltimore: Wilkins & Wilkins, 1995, pp 482, 496.

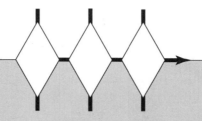

Chapter 11

PAIN MANAGEMENT

Laurel A. Eisenhauer

OVERVIEW

The effective management of pain involves integration of medical, nursing, and pharmacological approaches.

Pain usually occurs as a result of a series of neurological processes beginning with the stimulation/activation of peripheral nerves and transmission through the spinal cord tracts to the cerebrum, where impulses are interpreted and experienced as pain. Drugs and other nonpharmacological pain management work at various points along this pathway. For example, many nonopioid drugs such as aspirin and the nonsteroidal anti-inflammatory drugs act in the periphery to control the production of substances (e.g., prostaglandins) that produce inflammation or irritate nerve endings, while other agents such as the opioids act in the central nervous system (CNS) to block the transmission of pain impulses in the spinal cord or brain and/or their interpretation as pain by the brain.

Drugs used in the treatment of pain in patients in ambulatory settings are primarily the nonsteroidal anti-inflammatory agents (NSAIDs), acetaminophen, and some opioids. Adjuvants such as antidepressants, neuroleptics, anticonvulsants, and centrally acting alpha$_2$ agonists are also used in certain situations. In some cases of neurological pain, low-dose antidepressants have been found to be effective. Management of cancer pain involves these medications plus other medications such as steroids that may help to decrease pain caused by pressure.

Selected Bibliography

The Agency for Health Care Policy and Research (AHCPR) clinical guidelines on pain are excellent resources for the clinician and represent a multidisciplinary review and synthesis of the research on pain management, particularly for acute pain and cancer pain.

Acute Pain Management Guideline Panel. *Acute Pain Management: Operative or Medical Procedures and Trauma. Clinical Practice Guideline*. AHCPR Pub. No. 92-0032. Rockville, MD: Agency for Health Care Policy and Research, Public Health Service, U. S. Department of Health and Human Services, 1992.

Jacox A, Carr DB, Payne R, et al: *Management of Cancer Pain. Clinical Practice Guideline No. 9*. AHCPR Publication No. 94-0592. Rockville, MD: Agency for Health Care Policy and Research, Public Health Service, U. S. Department of Health and Human Services, 1994.

ISSUES IN DRUG THERAPY

Prescribing Considerations

Approaches to pain management depend on the nature, causes, and duration of the pain experience as well as knowledge of the patient and his or her responses. An initial concern is to recognize pain as a symptom that needs to be diagnosed and the underlying pathological mechanism treated whenever possible. Because of the diagnostic value of pain, it may be desirable to delay the use of full analgesia until a diagnosis has been established. A specific example is the case of undiagnosed abdominal pain wherein the characteristics and severity of the pain are particularly important in establishing an accurate diagnosis. Opioids and other CNS depressants should be avoided in head injury or other situations in which assessment of level of consciousness is essential to diagnosis and/or if the drug would contribute to respiratory depression; narcotic analgesics also increase intracranial pressure.

Nonpharmacological techniques should be used in conjunction with drug therapy. The use of diversion, relaxation, visual imagery, applications of heat or cold, and electrical stimulation (TENS) have been found to be effective in preventing or decreasing the need for pain medication and/or enhancing analgesic effects when used in appropriate patients.

When drug therapy is indicated, the type and level of analgesic need to be determined. Usually the least potent analgesic that will give satisfactory relief with minimal side effects is the therapeutic goal. The choice among NSAID, acetaminophen, or opioid analgesics will depend upon the cause and severity of the pain and the characteristics of the patient, which need to be considered in relation to drug effects.

The management of mild to moderate pain usually begins with the use of an NSAID or acetaminophen. The use of NSAIDs and acetaminophen avoids the side effects of respiratory depression, sedation, constipation, and bladder dysfunction that occur with opioids. If opioids are needed, they are usually used in conjunction with these drugs in order to decrease the dose of opioid needed and thereby help to minimize these side effects. Figure 11-1 illustrates the process of medication selection in the treatment of pain.

The choice of approach may depend on whether the pain is acute or chronic in nature. Patients experiencing chronic pain usually do not exhibit the classical external signs of acute pain such as increased blood pressure, pulse, and respiration or grimacing and moaning since they may have adapted these responses to pain to varying degrees. However, this can result in a misinterpretation by clinicians and others of the reality and severity of the pain being experienced. Chronic pain may have developed as a neurological response after prolonged and insufficiently treated acute pain; therefore, the original cause of the pain may no longer be present. The treatment approaches to

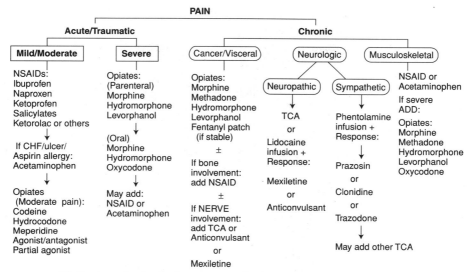

Figure 11-1 Medication selection in the treatment of pain. (*From Reisner-Keller LA: Pain management, in Herfindal ET, Gourley DR (eds): Textbook of Therapeutics: Drug and Disease Management, 6th ed. Baltimore, MD: William & Wilkins, 1996. Used with permission.*)

chronic pain control usually avoid the use of opioids and often involve the use of nonpharmacologic techniques.

A common concern in pain management with opioids is the possible development of tolerance, physical dependence, and psychological dependence (addiction). This concern has unfortunately led to underdosing and undertreatment of pain in some patients by both health care professionals and patients.

Prescribing Variables (Patient-Drug-Context)

Patient Variables

Concurrent conditions and concurrent drug therapy may affect the choice of analgesic. Consider not only the disease state itself but variables (especially liver and renal function) that may affect the absorption, distribution, metabolism, and excretion of analgesics.

Pathology and Characteristics of Pain The pathology causing pain provides guidance to the selection of pain interventions. Aspirin and NSAIDs produce their pain relief through inhibition of prostaglandins in the peripheral nerves and therefore are particularly effective when inflammation is the cause (e.g., arthritis) or contributes to pain (e.g., sports injury). Neuropathic pain may respond to low doses of tricyclic antidepressants.

Allergies   Patients allergic to aspirin may have cross-sensitivity to NSAIDs. In patients with asthma, opioids may precipitate an acute attack through release of histamine.

Peptic Ulcer   Aspirin and NSAIDs can produce GI bleeding that is due not only to a local irritation but to the inhibition of prostaglandins, which results in a break in the gastric mucosa. See below for a more detailed discussion. Acetaminophen does not produce gastric irritation.

Gallbladder Disease   The use of morphine should be avoided because it constricts Oddi's sphincter, and pressure in the common bile duct may increase tenfold within 10 minutes after SC morphine 10 mg. This effect may last for two hours and can be relieved by opioid antagonists or SL nitroglycerin.[1]

Uncontrolled High Blood Pressure   The use of aspirin or NSAIDs could contribute to a stroke in patients with uncontrolled hypertension.

Pregnancy   The use of aspirin in the last trimester may increase the risk of maternal and fetal bleeding during delivery and the risk of a stillbirth. NSAIDs also could cause premature closing of the patent ductus arteriosus.

Renal Dysfunction   In patients with renal disease the use of NSAIDs should be avoided because they can decrease the glomerular filtration rate by 25 to 50 percent; this effect is usually reversible, but it may be as long as a month after discontinuation before a return to baseline function. The effect on renal function occurs because of the inhibition of renal prostaglandin synthesis; sulindac is believed to have less of an effect than other NSAIDs on renal prostaglandin synthesis. Patients with renal failure who take NSAIDs need to be monitored for salt retention, hyponatremia, and hyperkalemia.[2]

Renal excretion of metabolites of opioids may be impaired in renal dysfunction, which can result in prolongation of some side effects produced by these metabolites. In patients with renal dysfunction, CNS adverse reactions may be increased because of the accumulation of the active metabolite normeperidine.

Liver Dysfunction   In patients with liver dysfunction analgesics metabolized or excreted in the liver (especially first-pass effect drugs) should be avoided. If these are used, the dosage needs to be carefully decreased (see Chapter 5). The metabolism of NSAIDs via glucuronidation may be impaired in liver dysfunction, and this may impair the renal excretion of NSAIDs.

Alcoholics or persons ingesting more than two alcoholic beverages a day are at risk for liver toxicity (possibly fatal) if they take acetaminophen. This hepatotoxicity is characterized by high levels of hepatic aminotransferases (e.g., AST of 3000 to 14,920 IU/L and ALT of 290 to 4100 IU/L) and prothrombin times greater than 25 seconds. One recommendation is that persons ingesting more than two alcoholic drinks per day should not take more than 2 g of acetaminophen a day.[3] The use of alcohol with aspirin and NSAIDs can also result in impaired liver function as well as increased gastric irritation. The use of alcohol with opioids can greatly increase the CNS depressant effects and pose danger from respiratory depression.

Respiratory Diseases   Patients with respiratory conditions such as asthma and chronic obstructive pulmonary disease (COPD) may be much more likely to develop respiratory depression from opioids and may need a reduction in dosage and careful titration while oxygen saturation and respiratory rate are monitored.

Other Drug Therapy   Patients on anticoagulants or with bleeding disorders should avoid use of aspirin or NSAIDs because of the effects on platelets and gastric irritation. Aspirin produces an irreversible effect on platelets that affects coagulation for up to 10 days. Salicylate salts such as choline magnesium trisalicylate do not significantly affect platelet function but still may cause gastric irritation and bleeding. NSAIDs produce a reversible effect on platelet aggregation that lasts for 2 to 3 days. Acetaminophen does not affect platelets.

CNS depressants that the patient is receiving need to be considered in the dosing since there may be a synergistic effect. Patients with renal failure on angiotensin-converting enzyme (ACE) inhibitors or potassium-sparing diuretics are at risk for hyperkalemia if they take NSAIDs.

Meperidine should not be used in patients taking monamine oxidase inhibitors (MAOIs) or who have received them within 14 days.

Psychosocial Variables   The expression of pain varies from individual to individual and is often culturally based. The meaning of pain to the individual will affect not only the way pain is expressed but also may influence the actual pain experience. For example, a patient for whom the pain represents a serious worsening of a condition will probably be more anxious, resulting in increased muscle tension, loss of sleep, and increased pain. Anxiety can also be a result of fear that the pain will become uncontrollable or that addiction to pain medications will occur.

Since there is considerable variation in the expression of pain from individual to individual and also in its interpretation by clinicians and others, a careful assessment of the pain is necessary. The only true measure of pain is the subjective experience of the patient. Pain is whatever the patient says it is. The use of visual scales (e.g., visual analogues or pictures of faces) or oral reports of pain intensity (e.g., 1 to 5 or 1 to 10) are useful in assessing the severity of pain as well as the effectiveness of analgesia and other interventions in each individual patient.

Drug Variables

Drug variables include route, monitoring requirements, interactions with other drugs, foods, and laboratory tests.

Nonopioid Analgesics   The two major types of analgesics used in ambulatory care are the nonopioids (e.g., ASA, NSAIDs) and the opioids. Discussions of the class of NSAIDs sometimes include aspirin, while other authors discuss aspirin as a separate class. Both aspirin and NSAIDs share common mechanisms of action and side effects. Aspirin, while one of the most widely used analgesics in the world and one that has been used for many years, has now relatively less use as an analgesic because of the increased number and availability of other anti-inflammatory analgesics and because of aspirin's effects on platelets and its implication in the development of Reye's syndrome when used in children with viral infections.

NSAIDs   Aspirin's effect on platelets is irreversible and the effects last up to 10 days or the lifespan of the platelet. Bleeding time can be prolonged by a factor of 1.5 to 2 when aspirin is given to a normal person. NSAIDs cause a reversible effect on platelets that lasts only while the drug is present.[4]

NSAIDs' advantages when compared to opioids is that they do not produce tolerance or physical or psychological dependence and do not cause any significant respiratory depression or inhibitory bowel or bladder effects. NSAIDs are antipyretic; there is a ceiling effect on their analgesia.

A major disadvantage of NSAIDs are their irritating effects on the GI system (with possible GI bleeding) and their prolongation of bleeding time further increasing the risk of GI bleeding. An estimated 38 to 50 percent of patients taking NSAIDs experience dyspepsia.[5] The GI bleeding caused by NSAIDs can occur without any warning of gastric discomfort or pain. Risk factors for NSAIDs-induced GI bleeding are age (older people over 60 are more likely to develop it), sex (GI bleeding is somewhat more frequent in men), and history of peptic ulcer disease and concurrent use of steroids or anticoagulants.[5] NSAIDs differ in their relative ability to cause GI bleeding; piroxicam (Feldene) has a high risk and low-dose ibuprofen has the smallest risk.[5] NSAIDs also can reduce renal function (see discussion above under patient variables).

In patients at high risk for developing gastric ulceration, misoprostol (Cytotec) has been used. Misoprostol is a synthetic prostaglandin E_1 analogue that can increase the bicarbonate and mucus production decreased by the antiprostaglandin effects of NSAIDs and aspirin. It also causes a moderate decrease in pepsin concentration during basal conditions. It should not be used in patients who are pregnant since it causes uterine contractions; women of child-bearing age need to use an effective contraceptive method while on misoprostol. GI symptoms (e.g., diarrhea, abdominal pains, cramping, nausea, flatulence) also can occur. The diarrhea usually develops after 13 days of therapy and often resolves in about a week. It can be decreased by the administration of misopostol after meals and at bedtime with food.[6]

The NSAIDs share many characteristics but also have some differences that may affect the choice of a particular NSAID for a specific patient. Variation in analgesic effectiveness of a particular NSAID may be idiosyncratic to the patient. NSAIDs are believed to produce analgesia primarily through peripheral effects in inhibiting prostaglandin synthesis; prostaglandins are believed to either produce painful stimuli and/or sensitize the receptors to other chemical mediators such as bradykinin, 5-HT, substance P, and histamine. The analgesic effect of NSAIDs may occur also in the CNS.

Table 11-1 summarizes dosages and other information on nonopioid analgesics.

Acetaminophen   Acetaminophen (e.g., Tylenol) is a metabolite of phenacetin and acetanilid but has less toxicity when used at the recommended dosage levels. It has anti-

TABLE 11-1

Nonopioid Analgesics

Drug	Usual Adult Dose	Comments
Oral		
Acetaminophen	650–975 mg q 4 hr	Acetaminophen lacks the peripheral anti-inflammatory activity of other NSAIDs
Aspirin	650–975 mg q 4 hr	The standard against which other NSAIDs are compared. Inhibits platelet aggregation; may cause postoperative bleeding
Choline magnesium trisalicylate (Trilisate)	1000–1500 mg bid	May have minimal antiplatelet activity; also available as oral liquid
Diflunisal (Dolobid)	1000 mg initial dose followed by 500 mg q 12 hr	
Etodolac (Lodine)	200–400 mg 6–8 hr	
Fenoprofen calcium (Nalfon)	200 mg q 4–6 hr	
Ibuprofen (Motrin, others)	400 mg q 4–6 hr	Available as several brand names and as generic; also available as oral suspension
Ketoprofen (Orudis)	25–75 mg q 6–8 hr	
Magnesium salicylate	650 mg q 4 hr	Many brands and generic forms available
Meclofenamate sodium (Meclomen)	50 mg q 4–6 hr	
Mefenamic acid (Ponstel)	250 mg q 6 hr	
Naproxen (Naprosyn)	500 mg initial dose followed by 250 mg q 6–8 hr	Also available as oral liquid
Naproxen sodium (Anaprox)	500 mg initial dose followed by 275 mg q 6–8 hr	
Salsalate (Disalcid, others)	500 mg q 4 h	May have minimal anti-platelet activity
Sodium salicylate	325–650 mg q 3–4 hr	Available in generic form from several distributors

(continued)

TABLE 11-1

Nonopioid Analgesics (continued)

Drug	Usual Adult Dose	Comments
Parenteral		
Ketorolac	30 or 60 mg IM initial dose followed by 15 or 30 mg q 6 hr. Oral dose following IM dosage: 10 mg q 6–8 hr	Intramuscular dose not to exceed 5 days

SOURCE: Acute Pain Management Guideline Panel.[7]

prostaglandin activity in the CNS equivalent to aspirin but has minimal antiprostaglandin action in the periphery. Therefore, it is not as effective as NSAIDs and aspirin for pain from inflammation. Its advantages are that it does not cause GI irritation or produce effects on platelets or prothrombin response. It does have antipyretic effects. It has been used routinely in all stages of pregnancy and appears to be safe for short-term use.[6]

Its main adverse effect is on the liver. The use of alcohol concurrent with large therapeutic doses or overdosages of acetaminophen increases the hepatotoxicity of acetaminophen. Hepatotoxicity and hepatic failure can occur with therapeutic doses in chronic alcoholics. (See also the above discussion of liver dysfunction.) Hepatotoxicity of acetaminophen may be increased by long-term or high doses of barbiturates, carbamazine, hydantoins, rifampin, and sulfinpyrazone.

Opioid Analgesics The use of opioids may be necessary for adequate control of moderate to severe pain. The use of opioids and acetaminophen is adequate for most patients seen in ambulatory care settings.

Opioids offer analgesia but also present the problems of constipation, respiratory depression, and the development of tolerance and dependence. Some patients may respond to opioids with nausea.

Opioids may also be called narcotics; however, there is some confusion about the meaning of the term since *narcotic* may refer to drugs that have been regulated and classified for legal control purposes as narcotics. Also, some drugs that have not been derived or synthesized from opium have been classified as having similar pharmacologic characteristics.

Opioids are drugs that are derived from opium or have characteristics similar to them. They are classified pharmacologically as agonists, mixed agonist-antagonists, and antagonists. This classification is related to which types of opioid receptors they affect. The opioid agonists have agonist action primarily at the mu and kappa receptors (see Table 11-2). Mixed agonist-antagonist drugs have agonist effects at certain receptors and antagonist effects at others. Antagonists do not have agonist effects at any of the receptors but prevent the effects of an agonist on the receptors; this results in withdrawal symptoms in patients with dependence. A major concern in changing to a different type of opioid drug is to avoid causing withdrawal symptoms in a dependent patient (some degree of physiological dependence can develop after only a few days on opioid drugs) by giving a mixed agonist-antagonist. Use of a mixed agonist-antagonist while a patient is also receiving an agonist also could cause a sudden loss of the analgesic effects of an opioid agonist, which could be quite difficult in certain patients with high levels of pain.

Agonist-antagonists have a "ceiling" effect indicating that there is no increase in analgesia or respiratory depression from giving doses above the threshold or ceiling

TABLE 11-2

Side Effects of Opioids Related to Receptor Type

Receptor Type	Effects	Examples
Mu	Supraspinal analgesia, euphoria, respiratory depression, physical depression, constipation; also responsible for habituating and withdrawal effects	Natural opium alkaloids (e.g., morphine, codeine), semi-synthetic analogues (e.g., hydromorphone, oxymorphone, oxycodone), and synthetic compounds (e.g., meperidine, levorphanol, methadone)
Kappa	Spinal analgesia, miosis, sedation	morphine
Sigma	Dysphoria, psychomimetic effects (e.g., hallucinations), respiratory and vasomotor stimulation	Drugs with antagonist activity (antagonists and agonist-antagonists)
Delta	May have role in euphoria and analgesia at spinal cord level	
Epsilon	Function not definitive	

level. Agonist-antagonists produce varying effects on different types of receptors. For example, pentazocine (Talwin) produces analgesia but does not cause a decrease in the propulsive activity of the intestines; however, it is contraindicated in patients with myocardial infarction because it may cause increased systemic vascular resistance and elevated blood pressure.[8] It also may cause a high incidence of vivid dreams or hallucinations.

Side effects need to be considered when choosing an opioid (see comparisons in Tables 11-2 and 11-3) and while managing pain with an opioid. Tolerance to miosis and constipation does not develop; therefore, a prophylactic bowel regimen should be initiated in patients receiving opioid agonists. The use of an antiemetic along with an opioid analgesic may be advisable in those patients who experience nausea and/or vomiting with opioids. Respiratory depression is a concern but usually would not occur at dosage levels and regimens usually used in patients in ambulatory care settings.

Table 11-4 provides dose equivalents for opioid analgesics and combination opioid/NSAID preparations.

TABLE 11-3

Comparison of Effects of Selected Opioid Agonists

Drug	Analgesic	Antitussive	Constipation	Respiratory Depression	Sedation	Emesis	Physical Dependence
codeine	+	+++	+	+	+	+	+
hydrocodone	+	+++	nd	+	nd	nd	+
hydromorphone (Dilaudid)	++	+++	+	++	+	+	++
meperidine (Demerol)	++	+	+	++	+	nd	++
methadone (Dolophine)	++	++	++	++	+	+	+
morphine	++	+++	++	++	++	++	++
oxycodone (Oxycontin, Roxicodone)	++	+++	++	++	++	++	++
propoxyphene	+	nd	nd	+	+	+	+

nd = no data available.

SOURCE: ©1997 by Facts and Comparisons. Used with permission from *Drug Facts and Comparisons*, 1997 ed. St. Louis, MO: Facts and Comparisons, a Wolters Kluwer Company, 1997, p. 1297.

TABLE 11-4

Dose Equivalents for Opioid Analgesics in Opioid-Naive Adults and Children ≥ 50 kg Body Weight[1]

Drug	Approximate Equianalgesic Dose		Usual Starting Dose for Moderate to Severe Pain	
	Oral	Parenteral	Oral	Parenteral
Opioid Agonist[2]				
Morphine[3]	30 mg q 3–4 h (repeat around-the-clock dosing) 60 mg q 3–4 (single dose or intermittent dosing)	10 mg q 3–4 h	30 mg q 3–4 h	10 mg q 3–4 h
Morphine, controlled-release[3,4] (MS Contin, Oramorph)	90–120 mg q 12 h	N/A	90–120 mg q 12 h	N/A
Hydromorphone[3] (Dilaudid)	7.5 mg q 3–4 h	1.5 mg q 3–4 h	6 mg q 3–4 h	1.5 mg q 3–4 h
Levorphanol (Levo-Dromoran)	4 mg q 6–8 h	2 mg q 6–8 h	4 mg q 6–8 h	2 mg q 6–8 h
Meperidine (Demerol)	300 mg q 2–3 h	100 mg q 3 h	N/R	100 mg q 3 h
Methadone (Dolophine, other)	20 mg q 6–8 h	10 mg q 6–8 h	20 mg q 6–8 h	10 mg q 6–8 h
Oxymorphone[3] (Numorphan)	N/A	1 mg q 3–4 h	N/A	1 mg q 3–4 h

(continued)

255

TABLE 11-4

Dose Equivalents for Opioid Analgesics in Opioid-Naive Adults and Children ≥ 50 kg Body Weight[1] (cont'd.)

Drug	Approximate Equianalgesic Dose		Usual Starting Dose for Moderate to Severe Pain	
	Oral	Parenteral	Oral	Parenteral
Combination Opioid/NSAID Preparations[5]				
Codeine[6] (with aspirin or acetaminophen)	180–200 mg q 3–4 h	130 mg q 3–4 h	60 mg q 3–4 h	60 mg q 2 h (IM/SC)
Hydrocodone (in Lorcet, Lortab, Vicodin, others)	30 mg q 3–4 h	N/A	10 mg q 3–4 h	N/A
Oxycodone (Roxicodone, also in Percocet, Percodan, Tylox, others)	30 mg q 3–4 h	N/A	10 mg q 3–4 h	N/A

[1]Caution: Recommended doses do not apply for adult patients with body weight less than 50 kg. For recommended starting doses for children and adults < 50 kg body weight.

[2]Caution: Recommended doses do not apply to patients with renal or hepatic insufficiency or other conditions affecting drug metabolism and kinetics.

[3]Caution: For morphine, hydromorphone, and oxymorphone, rectal administration is an alternate route for patients unable to take oral medications. Equianalgesic doses may differ from oral and parental doses because of pharmacokinetic differences.

[4]Transdermal fentanyl (Duragesic) is an alternative option. Transdermal fentanyl dosage is not calculated as equianalgesic to a single morphine dose. See the package insert for dosing calculations. Doses above 25 μg/h should not be used in opioid-naive patients.

[5]Caution: Doses of aspirin and acetaminophen in combination opioid/NSAID preparations must also be adjusted to the patient's body weight. Aspirin is contraindicated in children in the presence of fever or other viral disease because of its association with Reye's syndrome.

[6]Caution: Codeine doses above 65 mg often are not appropriate because of diminishing incremental analgesia with increasing doses but continually increasing nausea, constipation, and other side effects.

Note: Published tables vary in the suggested doses that are equianalgesic to morphine. Clinical response is the criterion that must be applied for each patient; titration to clinical responses is necessary. Because there is not complete cross-tolerance among these drugs, it is usually necessary to use a lower than equianalgesic dose when changing drugs and to retitrate to response.

Codes: q = every; N/A = not available; N/R = not recommended; IM = intramuscular; SC = subcutaneous.

SOURCE: Jacox et al.[9]

CONTEXTUAL ISSUES

An important aspect of the nurse practitioner's ability to prescribe drugs for pain is whether or not she or he has the legal authority to prescribe controlled substances. This will depend on the particular state. NPs can obtain a DEA number for prescribing controlled substances if this is allowed by the state in which the NP practices. It also may depend on the particular arrangement the NP has with a supervising physician (if this is a requirement in that state). State laws about controlled substances may also apply.

If the APN is involved in prescribing controlled substances, he or she must be careful to adhere to all the policies and procedures of the DEA and the practice setting. The rationale for the prescription of a controlled substance should be carefully documented in the patient's record (since one of the concerns of the DEA is the prescription of controlled substances without a medical indication). Clinicians need to be cautious and wary of individuals who seek medical attention solely in order to obtain a prescription for narcotics.

The availability of OTC formulations of NSAIDs provides greater patient access to these medications; however, OTC drugs are not reimbursed by third-party payers. Therefore, if a patient has prescription coverage, the prescription formulation and strength (and a prescription) will be necessary for payment by a third-party payer.

Education of the patient (and the caregiver) is important in establishing an optimal approach to the management of pain. Patients need to be encouraged to use analgesics wisely. This includes using the analgesic on a regular basis with acute pain in order to promote adequate analgesia. In other patients it may be necessary to encourage the use of alternate methods of pain control in order to prevent or decrease the need for analgesic medications in order to prevent or decrease side effects. Patients need to warned of any sedation that may impede their functioning and cautioned not to engage in driving, operation of dangerous machinery, or other activities requiring judgment and/or rapid response.

With NSAIDs and aspirin there is concern for the development of gastric irritation and bleeding, which may occur without symptoms, especially in elderly. Effects on platelets are also of concern with prolonged therapy. Since most of the drugs in these groups are available OTC, patients may be taking them on their own either intentionally or inadvertently without realizing the similarity of many brands of the same drugs or the similarity of effects of similar drugs. A careful history of the patient's use of all medications is essential.

REFERENCES

1. Reisine T, Pasternack G: Opioid analgesics and antagonists, in Hardman JG, Limbird LE (eds): *Goodman & Gilman's The Pharmacological Basic of Therapeutics,* 9th ed. New York: McGraw-Hill, 1996.
2. Briefel GR: Chronic renal insufficiency, in Barker L, Burton JR, Zieve PD, (eds): *Principles of Ambulatory Medicine,* 4th ed. Baltimore, MD: Williams & Wilkins, 1955, pp 554–578.

3. Warning label recommended for acetaminophen. Medical Sciences Bulletin, January 1994. (http://pharminfo.com/pubs/msb/acetwarn;html)

4. Noguchi JK, Stephens M: Coagulation disorders, in Herfindal ET, Gourley DR, (eds): *Textbook of Therapeutics. Drug and Disease Management,* 6th ed. Baltimore, MD: Williams & Wilkins, 1996, pp 245–283.

5. Nonprescription NSAIDs: Efficacy and Safety, MSB June 1994. (http.//pharminfo.com/pubs/msb/nsaids.html)

6. *Drug Facts and Comparisons.* St. Louis, MO: Facts and Comparisons, a Wolters Kluwer Company, 1997, pp 1949–1950.

7. Acute Pain Management Guideline Panel. *Acute Pain Management: Operative or Medical Procedures and Trauma. Clinical Practice Guideline*. AHCPR Pub. No. 92-0032. Rockville, MD: Agency for Health Care Policy and Research, Public Health Service, U. S. Department of Health and Human Services, 1992.

8. Reisner-Keller LA: Pain management, in Herfindal ET, Gourley DR (eds): *Textbook of Therapeutics: Drug and Disease Management,* 6th ed. Baltimore: Williams & Wilkins, 1996, pp 1047–1072.

9. Jacox A, Carr DB, Payne R, et al: *Management of Cancer Pain.* Clinical Practice Guideline No. 9. AHCPR Publication No. 94-0592. Rockville, MD: Agency for Health Care Policy and Research, Public Health Service, U. S. Department of Health and Human Services, 1994.

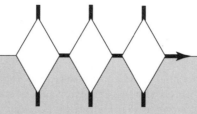

Chapter 12

DRUG THERAPY IN INFECTIOUS DISEASE

Margaret A. Murphy

OVERVIEW OF ANTIBIOTIC THERAPY AND PATHOPHYSIOLOGY

Since the beginning of recorded history man has coexisted with microorganisms. Some are beneficial, and some are killers. Mechanisms of coexistence and infectious disease are complicated and poorly understood. Early disease models include sites of infection, usually a wound or organ, as well as infectious diseases which could be transmitted from an insect, an animal, or a person. Infections were treated as local or systemic.

Local and systemic diseases were considered to be the result of introduction of organisms into the body from the environment. Florence Nightingale wrote of the struggle of the body's immune defenses against organisms. Later the concept was broadened to include an overgrowth of organisms resulting in an imbalance in the bacterial, fungal, and viral body "flora." A variety of animal parasites are included in the category of infectious disease. Experience with immune-compromised individuals has expanded our knowledge of this delicate balance.

Before the 1935 discovery of sulfonamides, treatment for infection was limited to symptom relief. Aspirin relieved fever, and antiseptic powders and ointments created an unfriendly environment for organisms. Homeopathic remedies that supported the patient's own immune defenses were the main tools against infection.

Since the advent of antibiotics and their subsequent worldwide use and overuse during the past 60 years, infectious diseases remain the biggest killer globally. Bacteriostatic and bactericidal agents were followed by development of antifungal and antiviral agents.

Combinations of agents have been found to be useful in protecting against development of resistant organisms in some diseases (TB and AIDS). Drug resistance, the major problem associated with antiinfectives, is thought to be due to the ongoing adaptation of man and his antimicrobial weapons and the microbes' powers to block or resist efforts to weaken or annihilate them. For instance, *Staphylococcus* is no longer susceptible to penicillin. Methacillin-resistant *Staphylococcus aureus* (MRSA) is resistant to fluoroquinolones and rifampin. It is expected that MRSA will become resistant to folate inhibitors,

Bactrim, and vancomycin in the near future. Nosocomial *Klebsiella* is no longer sensitive to the penicillins. Staphylococci and gram-positive enterococci account for one half of wound infections and bacteremias that are rapidly becoming resistant. Organisms have the capacity to adapt their physiology to neutralize chemotherapeutic agents; e.g., organisms can produce beta-lactamase, which neutralizes the beta-lactam antibiotics.

Overuse, increased travel, and variation in national policies related to distribution of antiinfectives threaten the twentieth-century miracle of the triumph of the laboratory over infectious diseases. Organisms reproduce themselves thousands of times in a day, multiplying their capacity to change and adapt. Can we outsmart them? It remains to be seen.

Lately we have seen the introduction of protease inhibitors in the war against HIV and the concurrent use of steroids in conjunction with antibiotics for overwhelming infection in immune-compromised patients with bacterial meningitis and *Pneumocystis carinii* pneumonia (PCP). We can expect to see new antibiotics in the future, but the prohibitive costs associated with the development of even one new drug indicate that we may see more development in terms of new usage and new combinations rather than a host of new drugs. However, we must acknowledge the possibility of a paradigm shift away from traditional antibiotics and in the direction of immunologic agents and designer drugs created through polymer chain reactions or DNA synthesis to fight specific organisms.

Antibiotic therapy is directed at causative organisms. When these organisms can be positively identified by culture and an adequate dose of the right drug delivered to the site of infection, curative outcomes are obtained in a patient with an intact immune system. In the real world, antiinfective agents are frequently given on an empirical basis, that is, without positive identification of the specific organism involved. Given the profile of the patient, what agents are most likely to be causing the infection in this anatomic location? Of the antiinfectives available, what is the best choice in this situation? If the patient cannot take the drug of choice (due to allergy, drug availability, or drug-drug interaction), what are the other acceptable choices? Socioeconomic factors influence adherence to therapeutic schedules, and the hunt continues for the magic bullets which are low in cost, have minimal adverse effects, are resistance-proof, and have an effect that can be directly observed after only one dose.

Beta-lactam antibiotics, penicillins, cephalosporins, and macrolides continue to be the first-line drugs in primary care settings, but gram-negative, beta-lactam-resistant organisms such as *Haemophilus influenzae* and *Moraxella catarrhalis* are on the increase in most areas. Treatment with antibiotic agents is associated with allergic reactions, gastric irritation and diarrhea, eighth cranial nerve damage, renal toxicity, and bone marrow depression. Prophylactic antimicrobial agents are recommended for prevention of a variety of conditions, including tuberculosis, endocarditis, rheumatic fever, recurrent cellulitis and lymphangitis in patients with lymphedema, meningococcal meningitis, bite wounds, and herpes virus infection. In addition, prophylactic antimicrobial agents have proved effective in certain surgical procedures, such as a variety of abdominal operations, hysterectomy, and head and neck operations for cancer.

Resources

Hardman JG, Limbird LE, Molinoff PB, et al: *Goodman & Gilman's The Pharmacological Basis of Therapeutics,* 9th ed. New York: McGraw-Hill, 1996. Also available on CD-

ROM. A pharmacology classic, it is available in many clinical areas. It offers clear and concise explanations of pharmacokinetics.

Meyers BR: *Antimicrobial Therapy Guide,* 11th ed. Newtown, PA: Antimicrobial Prescribing, 1996. A small pocket book with excellent explanations and comprehensive coverage of all classes of antimicrobials.

Nurse Practitioners' Prescribing Guide. New York: Prescribing Reference, 1997. A must for any advanced practice nurse or student, this is an up-to-date guide to commonly prescribed pharmaceuticals as well as certain over-the-counter products. It contains specific indications for use and dosage and a checklist of precautions, interactions, and adverse drug reactions. Published 4 times a year, this pocket-sized (big pocket) gem reviews new drugs and new indications over the past 3 months. Distributed free of charge to certified NPs, it is available to students for $32.00 per year.

Sanford JP: *Guide to Antimicrobial Therapy.* Dallas: Antimicrobial Therapy, 1997. A complete guide revised yearly with up-to-date choices and complete indexing.

ISSUES IN DRUG THERAPY

Prescribing Considerations

Viral etiologies are associated with up to 30 percent of eye-ear-nose-throat (EENT) complaints. The use of antibiotics routinely in cases that would otherwise recover spontaneously accomplishes nothing, can cause adverse events, and contributes to the problem of resistant organisms. Infections at other body locations such as the brain, spinal cord, prostate gland, and bones are more likely to require antiinfective agents. Multiple factors contribute to the practice of using antibiotics inappropriately. Many highly stressed people feel that they are entitled to antibiotic therapy to speed recovery. They respond emotionally when given palliative treatment and will shop for a provider with a more liberal policy toward antibiotic treatment. Providers threatened with the loss of the patient may defer to their wishes. To prevent this, it is wise to have attractive office literature explaining the possible adverse effects associated with unnecessary antibiotic treatment and a list of specific interventions for viral infections and allergic conditions for which antibiotics are ineffective. Guidelines should include decongestants, both oral and topical, and general health measures such as hydration and sleep.

Infectious disease control committees are required to gather, maintain, and distribute statistics related to organisms isolated, local sensitivities, resistant organism percentages, and other data contributing to a profile in each site. State health departments issue warnings and bulletins related to the microbial population, resistance profiles, and trends.

Antimicrobial Action

To be a useful antibiotic, a drug should come in contact with susceptible bacteria in sufficient concentration to inhibit the growth of the organism without harming the patient. Bacteriostatic agents slow the growth and cell division of the organism, but the patient's immune system must complete the eradication of the organisms. If the host defenses are not adequate to complete the clearance of the organism, it is advantageous to use a bactericidal agent that will completely kill the organisms (see the discussion below on minimum inhibitory concentrations and minimum bacteriocidal concentrations). Most antibiotics will interfere with the life processes of organisms. The concentration of the drug required to markedly reduce or eradicate the organisms may not be tolerated by the patient. A very high dose of the drug will be necessary and, at such a dose, adverse effects occur to the patient. If the amount of drug required to kill or harm the bacteria would do harm to the patient, the organism is said to be resistant.

Antimicrobial Resistance

Resistance of bacteria to an antibiotic can occur by mutation, adaptation, or horizontal transfer. Changes in the bacterial organism from generation to generation can result in minor or major adaptations which become part of its cell makeup. Such mutations are random events and do not depend on prior exposure to the drug. The organism may adapt itself by changing the cell wall (which will then not bind to the drug) or by developing a highly efficient find-and-eliminate system to move the drug in and out of the cell without harm to itself. Horizontal transfer from another bacterial donor cell occurs by exchanges of genetic material which codes for enzymes that inactivate antimicrobials.[1] Since bacteria are reproducing at a rapid rate compared to humans, one can see the possibilities for the emergence of highly specialized antibiotic resistance techniques. One possibility is that we will be left powerless against infectious diseases that we thought we had conquered.

Identifying the Organism Causing the Infection

Culture of biological material at the site of infection is the only way to really know that the body is colonized with a particular organism. It is also true that colonization is not necessarily infection. Unfortunately, it is not always practical or possible to have a positive identification of a causative microorganism before treating the patient. Serious infections require intervention as soon as possible, particularly when patients are seen on an outpatient basis and could easily be lost to follow-up. Localizing the infection is also important (see Table 12-1); the location of the infection will often determine the choice of drug and route of administration. Certain organisms cause intracellular infections. Quinolones and macrolides achieve better tissue penetration and are concentrated in tissues up to 4 times the serum level. These drugs will work against intracellular infections (i.e., mycoplasma); beta-lactams will not.

Pharmacokinetic Factors

The pharmacokinetic factors that enter into drug therapy selection are as follows:

1. The ability of the drug to concentrate in the target tissues is an important consideration. In addition to choosing the right drug, it is also important to keep antibacterial concentrations at therapeutic levels at the site of infection during the dosing interval. The minimum inhibitory concentration (MIC) represents the lowest

TABLE 12-1

Examples of Common Organisms by Location/Organ Systems

Location	Organism	Class
Meningitis/brain tissue	*Neisseria meningitides*	GNC
Endocarditis/bloodstream	*Streptococcus viridans*	GPC
Liver/pancreas	*Enterobacter*	GNR
Mouth	*Streptococcus*	GPC
Upper respiratory tract	*Haemophilus influenzae*	GNR
Lower respiratory tract	*Streptococcus pneumoniae*	GPC
Hospital-acquired lung infection	*Pseudomonas aeruginosa*	GNR
Skin/soft tissue	*Staphylococcus aureus*	GPC
Bones/joints	*Staphylococcus aureus*	GPC
Genital	*Chlamydia trachomatis*	ATP
Pelvic inflammatory disease	*Neisseria gonorrhoeae*	GNC
Urinary tract	*Escherichia coli*	GNR
Intraabdominal	*Escherichia coli*	GNR

GNC = gram-negative cocci; GPC = gram-positive cocci; GNR = gram-negative rod; ATP = atypical.

amount of the drug that successfully inhibits visible growth in broth after 18 to 24 hours of incubation. The drug to which the organism is most sensitive will have the lowest MIC. It is generally desirable to maintain a serum concentration of the drug equal to or a multiple of the MIC.[1] There are two methods of laboratory measurement that yield information on the MIC. Broth dilution tests give numeric breakpoints for MIC testing and can be used in choosing the appropriate drug as well as monitoring serum levels as indicated in Table 12-2. The disk diffusion method does not yield a specific numeric result. Guidelines from the National Committee for Clinical Laboratory Standards provide "breakpoints" that separate the results of the disk diffusion method into 4 categories—"susceptible," "intermediate," "moderately susceptible," and "resistant." Nurse practitioners should check with their laboratory to determine which of these methods is used.

Minimum bacterial concentration (MBC) is determined by dilution tests that measure inhibition of the growth of target bacteria. The lowest concentration that yields no growth of organisms is considered the MBC. If the MIC and the MBC are the same, the antimicrobial agent is considered bacteriocidal for that organism. If the MBC is much greater than the MIC, the drug is considered bacteriostatic.[2] Depending upon other factors related to pharmacokinetics, drugs with higher MICs may be equally effective in some situations. Remember that MICs and MBCs are determined in test tubes and measure serum concentrations. Tissue concentrations are more important, but laboratory measures are not currently available.

2. The integrity of the blood-brain barrier is diminished during infection but reverses when fever subsides.

TABLE 12-2

Breakpoints for Broth-Dilution MIC Testing of Aerobic Bacteria

Drug	Susceptible (µg/mL)	Moderately Susceptible (µg/mL)	Resistant (µg/mL)
Aminoglycosides			
Amikacin, kanamycin	≤16	32	≥64
Gentamicin,[a] tobramycin	≤4	8	≥16
Netilmicin	≤8	16	≥32
Cephalosporins, cephems, and monobactams			
Cefazolin, cephalothin, cefamandole, ceforanide, cefuroxime, ceftazidime, cefarazil, cefoxitin, loracarbef, aztreonam	≤8	16	≥32
Cefotaxime, ceftizoxime, ceftriaxone, moxalactam	≤8	16–32	≥64
Cefoperazone, cefotetan, cefmetazole	≤16	32	≥64
Clindamycin	≤0.5	1–2	>4
Glycopeptides			
Teicoplanin	≤8	16	≥32
Vancomycin	≤4	8–16	≥32
Imipenem	≤4	8	≥16
Macrolides			
Azithromycin	≤2	4	≥8
Clarithromycin	≤2	4	≥8
Erythromycin	≤0.5	1–4	≥8
Penicillins			
Amoxicillin/clavulanate			
For *Haemophilus* sp., S. aureus	≤4/2	—	≥8/4
Others	≤8/4	16/8	≥32/16
Ampicillin			
For *Haemophilus* sp.	≤2	—	≥4
For Enterobacteriaceae	≤8	16	≥32
Mezlocillin, piperacillin (with or without 4 mg/L of tazobactam), and ticarcillin (with or without 2 mg/L of clavulanate)	≤16	32–64	≥128
For *Pseudomonas aeruginosa*	≤64	—	≥128
For other gram-negative bacilli	≤16	32–64	≥128

TABLE 12-2 *(continued)*

Drug	Susceptible (μg/mL)	Moderately Susceptible (μg/mL)	Resistant (μg/mL)
Nafcillin, oxacillin[b]	≤2	—	≥4
Penicillin G			
For streptococci	≤0.12	0.25–2	≥4
For enterococci	≤8	—	≥16
For pneumococci,			
N. gonorrhoeae	≤0.06	0.1–1	≥2
Quinolones			
Ciprofloxacin	≤1	2	≥4
Ofloxacin, lomefloxacin, floroxacin	≤2	4	≥4
Norfloxacin	≤4	8	≥16
Tetracyclines	4	8	≥16
Trimethoprim-sulfamethoxazole	≤2/38	—	≥4/76

[a]For testing enterococci: susceptible ≤500 mg/L; resistant >500 mg/L.
[b]For testing staphylococci.
SOURCE: Dipiro et al.,[3] p. 1938.

3. Highly protein-bound antimicrobials do not penetrate well.

4. Relatively constant antibacterial activity or high peak concentrations followed by subinhibitory activity characterize different modi operandi of antimicrobial groups. Time-dependent growth inhibition is associated with beta-lactams, penicillins, and cephalosporins, while concentration-dependent growth inhibition is associated with aminoglycosides and quinolones. These features can be used to maximize the effects of the beta-lactams by ensuring administration timed to maintain a peak blood level. This may be achieved by using a long-half-life beta-lactam or a strict dosing schedule. The same principle can minimize the adverse effects of aminoglycosides by giving the maximal dose once a day to spare the kidneys and limit eighth cranial nerve damage.

5. Phase 1 and phase 2 biotransformation reactions occur primarily in the liver by means of genetically determined groups of microsomal enzymes with a high degree of variability from person to person. Phase 1 reactions (oxygenation) produce molecules which are water soluble and equipped to undergo phase 2 reactions (conjugation). The results of this biotransformation account for inactivation of drugs, activation of a pro-drug, and production of toxic metabolites.[4] Interferon production in bacterial infection can impair drug transformation.[5]

6. Significant drug-drug interactions (see Table 12-3) are caused by the variability of the microsomal enzymes in the liver. Ciprofloxacin, enoxacin, norfloxacin,

TABLE 12-3

Antimicrobial Drug Interactions

Antibiotic Drug	Interacting Drug	Effect of Combined Action
Aminoglycosides	Amphotericin B, cyclosporine, cisplatin, NSAIDs, vancomycin	Increased nephrotoxicity
	Penicillins (in patients with renal failure)	Decreased efficacy of parenteral aminoglycosides
	Ethacrynic acid, furosemide	Enhanced potential for ototoxicity
Amoxicillin, ampicillin	Allopurinol	Increased frequency of rash
	Oral beta blockers	Decreased beta-blocker absorption
Clindamycin	Kaolin	Decreased absorption of clindamycin
Macrolides (erythromycin, clarithromycin [Biaxin])	Carbamazepine	Increased toxicity risk for carbamazepine
	Corticosteroids	Increased effects of steroids
	Theophylline	Theophylline-induced toxicity
	Warfarin sodium	Increased risk of bleeding
	Digoxin	Digoxin toxicity
	Ergot alkaloids	Ergot toxicity
	Nonsedating antihistamines (terfenadine, astemizole)	Ventricular arrhythmias
Fluoroquinolones All	Cimetidine, aluminum, calcium, iron, magnesium, zinc, antacids, sucralfate	Increased quinolone levels Decreased absorption of quinolones Decreased quinolone levels
Enoxacin	Fenbufen, theophylline	Seizures, increased theophylline levels

Norfloxacin (Noroxin)	Theophylline	Increased theophylline levels
Ciprofloxacin	Theophylline	Increased theophylline levels
Nitrofurantoin (Furadantin)	Magnesium antacids	Decreased nitrofurantoin absorption
Metronidazole	Warfarin sodium Alcohol	Increased risk of bleeding Disulfiramlike reaction
Sulfonamides	Oral anticoagulants Cyclosporine Methotrexate Phenytoin Sulfonylureas	Increased hypoprothrombinemia Decreased cyclosporine levels Methotrexate toxicity Phenytoin toxicity Increased hypoglycemic risk
Tetracyclines	Aluminum, bismuth, iron Barbiturates, carbamazepine, phenytoin Digoxin	Decreased tetracycline absorption Decreased tetracycline effect Increased digoxin toxicity
Trimethoprim-sulfamethoxazole	Oral anticoagulants Cyclosporine Phenytoin Glipizide Methotrexate	Increased anticoagulant effect Nephrotoxicity Phenytoin toxicity Increased risk of hypoglycemia Bone marrow suppression

NSAIDs = nonsteroidal antiinflammatory drugs.

SOURCE: Gleckman RA, Borrego F: Adverse reactions to antibiotics. *Postgrad Med* 101(4):103, 1997.[6]

rifampin, the azoles, the macrolides, and chloramphenicol result in clinically significant induction and inhibition effects. This explains why some antibiotics will deactivate oral contraceptives and necessitates warnings by the provider to use other methods to prevent unwanted pregnancy.

7. As noted above, the microsomal enzyme system is responsible for most of the biotransformation of lipid-bound drugs to water-soluble agents that can be eliminated by the kidney. Excretion further depends on an intact, functioning kidney. Patients with moderate renal failure may need the antibiotic dose adjusted to prevent toxicity. Men with serum creatinine levels from 1.5 to 2.5 mg/dL and women with 1.1 to 2.0 mg/dL may be presumed to have a moderate impairment and may be treated in primary care and especially geriatric settings. This figure should be adjusted for meat in the diet and muscle mass, both of which elevate the serum creatinine. The methods used are as follows:

   A. The *dose reduction method* in which a percentage of the usual dose is given and the *interval extension method* which prolongs the time between doses based on the glomerular filtration rate.

   B. Estimation of creatinine clearance by the following formula:

$$C_a = \frac{(140 - age) \times (weight\ in\ kg)}{72 \times serum\ creatinine}$$

Multiply above result by 0.85 in females. Tables are available to implement both of these schemes.[7,8]

Host Factors

Factors in patients that can influence drug therapy choices include the following:

1. Inability to mount an immune defense (e.g., HIV, chemotherapy).
2. Absence of phagocytic cells (e.g., bacterial endocarditis, bacterial meningitis).
3. The inability of the drug to make direct, effective contact with the organisms is associated with several common patient situations. Accumulation of the products of phagocytosis can interfere with the ability of the antibiotic to penetrate tissue. The presence of large amounts of pus can act as a barrier to tissue and subsequently to organism penetration. The pH of tissues and an acidic or alkaline influence of infection can neutralize acid- or alkaline-stable drugs; most oral drugs are acid-stable. Abscess formation makes it very difficult for the drug to get into the abscess, which may have thick walls; this is one reason why dental abscesses do not respond well to antibiotics. Any foreign body, including prostheses and even dental implants, will act as a focal point for infection. Incision and drainage or even removal of the focal problem may be necessary in order for the antibiotic to act.
4. Age. Achlorhydria associated with aging results in more effective oral absorption of penicillin G and less effective gastrointestinal absorption of ketoconazole.

Creatinine clearance declines with age, affecting aminoglycoside excretion and increasing the chances of the ototoxic effects of aminoglycosides. Tetracyclines interfere with bone growth and cause discoloration of teeth as well as harm to the tooth enamel. Fluoroquinolones interfere with bone growth, and there are reports of fluoroquinolone-induced bilateral Achilles tendonitis and rupture from Europe, New Zealand, and France.[9]

5. Genetic factors. The cytochrome P-450 system is required for oxidation and conjugation reactions. This is an example of the membrane-bound proteins that biotransform lipophilic drugs to more polar compounds that can be excreted by the kidneys.[1,10] This is known as phase 1 biotransformation. There have been over 12 cytochrome P-450 gene families described. These occur unevenly in the population and are a factor in differences in drug metabolism between individuals and in many drug-drug interactions. Based on this variability of enzyme presence, people can be identified as rapid or slow metabolizers. Slow metabolizers usually have more adverse effects; they "hold on" to the drug. Induction and inhibition potentials of these enzymes determine whether the person will have more or less of the active drug than anticipated. High levels of toxic or even carcinogenic substances also occur. Reversible inhibition occurs with antiinfective agents such as the fluoroquinolones and the macrolides when given with theophylline, thereby causing dangerous levels of theophylline and possibly theophylline-induced seizures. Macrolides may neutralize the cytochrome P-450 system by competitive inhibition, causing dangerous levels of some nonsedating H_2 blockers and ketoconazole.[5] Liver disease, age, and the presence of bacterial infections themselves impair drug biotransformation. Phagocytosis releases a factor that depresses biotransformation.[11]

6. Drug allergy. Anaphylaxis can occur, although most hypersensitivity reactions even after IV administration consist of skin rashes or fever. Allergic reactions are most often associated with the beta-lactam antibiotics (penicillins and cephalosporins). Unfortunately, a family or personal history of IgE-mediated allergic reactions is difficult to obtain. Most patients are unable to distinguish between minor side effects and major problems and will insist they are allergic to penicillin on the basis of nausea or vomiting. Although allergy to penicillin is highly unlikely, by itself, to be associated with isolated nausea and vomiting, caution will prevail; another antibiotic choice will be made, and we will not know if the patient is truly allergic to penicillin. Cases in which urticaria, wheezing, stridor, or shock occur must be treated immediately with epinephrine and constitute a contraindication to further treatment with the drug. Those identified as being at risk should be taught to carry and use EpiPens. Cross-sensitivity with the penicillins or cephalosporins is estimated at from 5 to 16 percent although many say it is much less.[12]

7. Superinfection. Prolonged oral administration of antibiotics and/or an immune-compromised patient may bring about superinfection with resistant organisms. Antibiotic-associated pseudomembranous colitis, caused by *Clostridium difficile*, a toxin-producing organism that requires treatment with metronidazole or oral vancomycin, is a danger when any oral antibiotic is given. This condition is highly associated with clindamycin administration.[13]

8. Noncompliance with antibiotics is a major deterrent to cure. Up to 25 percent of prescriptions will never be filled. This is closely related to cost. Other barriers are prior experience with the drug and perceived seriousness of the condition by the patient.[14] The more frequently the drug is dosed and the longer the patient is directed to take the drug, the less likely that the patient will complete the course. This is true even without considering side effects. Single-dose directly observed therapy prevents nonadherence-related therapeutic failures.

Cost

The advantage of less frequent dosing must frequently be weighed against increased cost. Also, broader-spectrum antibiotics tend to cost more. Although they are effective against more organisms, use of broad-spectrums when a narrow-spectrum would be effective contributes to the problem of antibiotic resistance, a very costly problem for the nation as well as individuals.

HISTORY OF ANTIBIOTICS — 1935–1997

It is difficult for providers to imagine a time when there were no antiinfective agents. The death toll from accidents followed by sepsis was enormous. A brief review of the development of antibiotic agents follows. Early drugs were narrow-spectrum and effective against predominantly gram-positive organisms. Drugs developed later were more likely to be broad-spectrum. The trade-off was a loss of effectiveness against some gram-positive organisms. Science has evolved to the point that now efforts are directed to immunotherapy for prevention of common infections as well as specific action against life-threatening organisms.

1935 Sulfonamides
1940s Penicillin, streptomycin, and chloramphenicol
1950s Tetracycline, erythromycin, vancomycin, and metronidazole
1960s Ampicillin (first semisynthetic penicillin), gentamycin, first-generation cephalosporins, and the antistaphylococcal penicillins (methicillin, oxacillin, nafcillin).
1970s Clindamycin, penicillins with further expanded gram-negative spectrums (carbenicillin, ticarcillin), the aminoglycosides tobramycin and amikacin, and the second-generation cephalosporins cefuroxime and cefoxitin
1980s Penicillins with even further expanded gram-negative spectrums (piperacillin, mezlocillin), third-generation cephalosporins, the quinolones (fluoroquinolones), monobactams, and carbopenims
1990s Continued development of cephalosporins and quinolones plus extended-spectrum erythromycins
2000 Immunotherapy through monoclonal antibody development, especially for gram-negative bacilli-induced septicemia and shock

CLASSIFICATION OF ANTIMICROBIALS

Inhibitors of Cell Wall Synthesis

Beta-Lactam Antibiotics

The beta-lactam antibiotics were introduced in 1940. The first compound was penicillin G, which has been joined by a large number of semisynthetic and extended-spectrum penicillins as well as three to four generations of cephalosporins and other related compounds (see Fig. 12-1). Today these are the most widely used antibiotics in outpatient settings. The earliest penicillins were derived from natural sources and used primarily against infections caused by gram-positive bacteria. All beta-lactams act by inhibition of the cell wall. Since animal cells lack cell walls, humans and animals are not affected by these inhibitors of cell wall synthesis. By 1957 a series of semisynthetic penicillins had evolved. They were rapidly integrated into treatment regimes and prescribed because of increased acid stability (absorbed orally) and their ability to destroy both gram-positive and gram-negative organisms.

Generally speaking, the natural and semisynthetic penicillins have a narrow antibacterial spectrum, a relatively high incidence of allergic and hypersensitivity reactions (i.e., they are the most probable cause of drug-induced anaphylaxis), and penicillin-resistant organisms are all too common. Drug resistance usually occurs for one of the following reasons:

1. A bacterial enzyme inactivates the drug (beta-lactamases).
2. The penicillin is unable to attach to or penetrate into the microbe because of the genetic adaptation of bacterial receptors.
3. The microbe may be inhibited rather than killed because the organism is insensitive to cell wall destruction.
4. The organism may lack cell walls.

Clinical Uses Penicillin G and V are generally indicated for gram-positive organisms, but there is an increasing problem with resistance in some parts of this country and other countries (e.g., Spain, South Africa). Treatment of pneumococcal pneumonia, streptococcal pharyngitis, and syphilis infections still features penicillin as the drug of choice. These drugs may also be used prophylactically in certain cases.

Caution is indicated when using the penicillins in the presence of other medications. For example, aspirin and probenecid may lead to increased blood levels of the drug. Penicillins may be used in conjunction with aminoglycosides for a synergistic effect or to delay microbial resistance to the penicillin, but other drugs are now more likely to be substituted.[7]

Penicillin V is given for infections such as respiratory tract infections, pharyngitis, otitis, and sinusitis, especially in children, and for the treatment of group A beta-hemolytic streptococcal (GABHS) pharyngitis and prophylactically to prevent reinfection. Semisynthetic penicillins such as ampicillin were commonly used for urinary tract infections (UTIs), although the bacterial resistance of *E. coli* is now significant and this is no longer the drug of choice for uncomplicated UTIs.[16] Oral absorption of penicillin G is

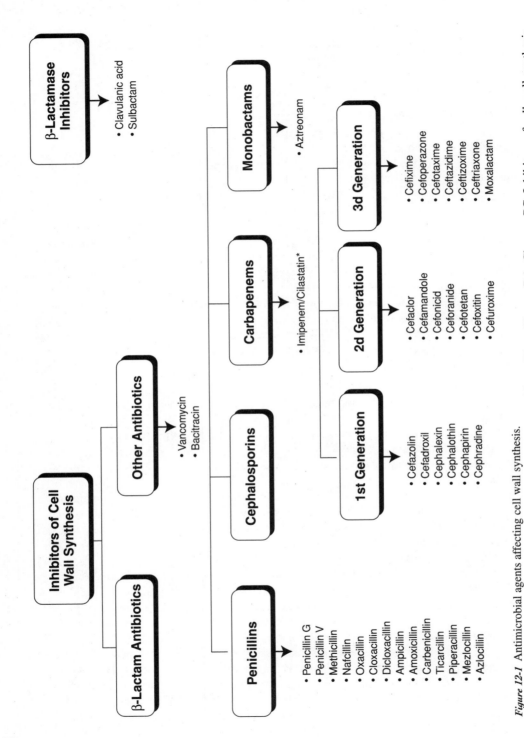

Figure 12-1 Antimicrobial agents affecting cell wall synthesis. (*From* Harvey RA, Champe PC: Inhibitors of cell wall synthesis, in *Lippincott's Illustrated Reviews: Pharmacology.* Philadelphia: Lippincott, 1992.)[15]

*Cilastatin is not an antibiotic but an inhibitor of kidney peptidase.

272

unpredictable; other warnings include avoidance of acidic juices and food (i.e., it should be taken one hour before or after meals). However, parenteral absorption is complete and rapid, and excretion of the drug is quickly and efficiently performed by the kidneys.

Amoxicillin is similar in action, but it is better absorbed in the stomach and has fewer adverse effects. Amoxicillin can be combined with clavulanic acid, which forms a drug combination effective against beta-lactam-resistant organisms. *H. influenzae* meningitis in children may be treated with amoxicillin/clavulanate.

All of the natural and semisynthetic penicillins are pregnancy category B. They are available generically and are inexpensive for a full course of treatment (see Table 12-4). Ninety percent of staphylococci are penicillin-resistant because of the organism's production of penicillinase, which neutralizes the natural and semisynthetic penicillins. The antistaphylococcal penicillins—dicloxacillin, nafcillin, and oxacillin—may still be used because of a chemical alteration which neutralizes the penicillinase. Dosage must be adjusted for a glomerular filtration rate (GFR) less than 60.

Allergic Reactions Anaphylactic shock occurs in 0.05 percent of all recipients with the majority of incidents *following parenteral infusion.* Serum sickness reactions can occur approximately 7 to 12 days following administration; these appear as urticaria, fever joint swelling, angioneurotic edema, intense pruritus, and respiratory difficulties.[17] GI upset, rash, urticaria, vaginitis, superinfection, and anaphylaxis are associated adverse reactions to penicillin.[18]

Cephalosporins

The cephalosporin fungus was first isolated in 1948 off the coast of Sardinia in the sea near a sewer outlet. The drugs were not introduced until the 1960s. Like the penicillins they are beta-lactam antibiotics, share common properties, and have a similar mechanism of action and bacterial spectrum. Cephalosporins are distinguished by three evolutionary waves or generations (see Table 12-5). Generally speaking, the first-generation agents have excellent efficacy against common gram-positive organisms except for methacillin-resistant staphylococci and enterococci. They are effective against skin and skin structure infections and non-hospital-acquired *E. coli,* less so against *Proteus mirabilus* and *Klebsiella,* and ineffective against *Pseudomonas.*

The second generation of drugs includes the cephomycins—cefoxitin, cefotetan, and cefmetazole—but these are not commonly used in the outpatient setting. Second-generation cephalosporins are less active than first-generation against gram-positive bacteria such as *S. aureus* but are more efficacious against gram-negative pathogens. The carbacephem antibiotic loracarbef has a spectrum of activity similar to these agents. They are reliably active against *H. influenzae, M. catarrhalis,* and many strains of *E. coli* (non-hospital-acquired), *Proteus,* and *Klebsiella.*

The third-generation agents are frequently referred to as broad-spectrum since they have wider gram-negative coverage and are able to penetrate the central nervous system. These should be taken on an empty stomach (i.e., at least two hours after meals or one hour before eating). Hypersensitivity is the major adverse effect and is treated the same as with a penicillin allergic reaction. Though rare, rash may be accompanied by eosinophilia. Nausea, vomiting, and diarrhea are the most commonly occurring side

TABLE 12-4

The Penicillins

Drug	Brand Name	Examples of Indications	Recommended Dose	Average Wholesale Cost
Natural and Synthetic Penicillins (available orally)				
Penicillin V	Generic	GABHS, strep pn, URI, otitis, sinusitis, dental & prophylaxis, SBE	250/500 mg qid	$2.00, $4.00
Penicillin G	Generic	Respiratory, skin, soft tissue, erysipelas, scarlet fever, otitis media	1.2 MU IM	$11.00
Ampicillin	Generic	Acute bacterial gastroenteritis	500–1000 mg q 6 h	$7.00
Amoxicillin	Generic	Otitis media, respiratory, urinary tract, skin, uncomplicated gonorrhea	250/500 mg tid	$5.00, $10.00
Dicloxacillin	Generic	Penicillinase-producing staph	250/500 mg qid	$15.00
Nafcillin	Nafcil, Unipen	Penicillinase-producing staph	500–1000 mg q 4–6 h	$238.00
Oxacillin	Bacticil, Prostaphlin	Penicillinase-producing staph	500–1000 mg q 4–6 h	$77.00
Extended-Spectrum Penicillins (available orally)				
Amoxicillin/ potassium clavulanate	Augmentin	Otitis media, resp, skin, UTI, sinusitis, beta-lactamase- producing strains	250–500 mg PO tid	$44.55

GABHS = group A beta-hemolytic strep; URI = upper respiratory infection; SBE = subacute bacterial endocarditis; strep pn = streptococcal pneumonia.

TABLE 12-5

The Cephalosporins

Drug	Brand Name	Examples of Indications	Recommended Dose	Average Wholesale Cost
First-Generation Cephalosporins (available orally)				
Cefadroxil	Duricef, Ultracef	UTI, skin, pharyngitis, tonsillitis, impetigo	500–1000 mg bid	$62.00, $116.00
Cephalexin	Keflex	Otitis media, skin, bone, respiratory, or GU inf.	250–500 mg bid	$20.00, $35.00
Second-Generation Cephalosporins (available orally)				
Cefaclor	Ceclor	Mild to moderate resp., skin	250–1000 mg q 8 h	$55.00, $110.00
Cefprozil	Cefzil	Pharyngitis, tonsillitis, ABECB, acute sinus, skin, OM	250–500 mg bid	$55.00, $107.00
Cefuroxime axetil	Ceftin	Pharyngitis, tonsillitis sinusitis, skin UTI, GC	250–500 mg bid	$63.00, $122.00
Loracarbef	Lorabid	OM, skin, ABECB	200–400 mg bid	$60.00, $76.00
Third-Generation Cephalosporins (available orally)				
Cefixame	Suprax	Pharyngitis, tonsillitis, ABECB, OM, UTI, uncompli. GC	200–400 mg qd	$31.00, $61.00
Cefpodoxame proxetil	Vantin	OM, ABECB, CAP, pharyngitis, tonsillitis, skin, uncompli. GC	100–200–400 mg bid	$63.00, $126.00
Third-Generation Cephalosporins (intramuscular)				
Ceftriaxone	Rocephin	LRI, UTI, skin, bone joint, GYN	1000–2000 mg IM q12–24 h	$36.98 per IM injection

ABECB = acute bacterial exacerbation of chronic bronchitis; CAP = community-acquired pneumonia; GC = gonorrhea; LRI = lower respiratory infection; OM = otitis media; UTI = urinary tract infection.

effects. Administration of the medication may cause superinfection, an allergic reaction, or occasionally nephrotoxicity. Dosage requires adjustment for GFR less than 60.

The compatibility of this drug with other prescribed medications should be assessed, especially with those that enhance its effects, for example, loop diuretics, gentamicin, and probenecid. Tetracycline should not be given with beta-lactams. The beta-lactams require growing organisms to act and tetracycline interferes with cell reproduction.

Clindamycin and lincomycin inhibit cell wall synthesis in gram-positive organisms, *Bacteroides,* and other anaerobes. Lincomycin is rarely used and will not be considered here. Clindamycin is used as a second-line drug in penicillin allergy and in bacterial vaginosis caused by *Gardnerella vaginalis.* Adverse effects include pseudomembranous colitis, diarrhea, GI upset, rash, anaphylaxis, renal dysfunction, blood dyscrasias, polyarthritis, and superinfection. It is only used in serious infections and does not need to be adjusted for moderate renal failure.

Vancomycin also acts by affecting cell wall synthesis. It is effective oral therapy against *C. difficile* since it is not systemically absorbed and acts in the GI tract. Given intravenously, it is active against MRSA. It can be ototoxic and nephrotoxic, and the dosing schedule requires adjusting in moderate renal failure. Rapid intravenous infusion can cause flushing, rash, and a sudden fall in blood pressure caused by histamine release. The clinical picture is known as "red man syndrome."

Bacitracin is severely nephrotoxic and is rarely used systemically. In outpatient settings it is used in topical and ophthalmic applications to treat surface infections of the skin and mucous membranes. The possibility of hypersensitivity reactions does exist, but it is rare.

Metronidazole has long been used for the treatment of protozoal disease, but it is also strongly active against most anaerobic bacteria. It is particularly effective against amebic dysentery, amebic liver abscesses, and mixed intra-abdominal and GYN infections, including peritonitis due to *B. fragilis* and *Clostridium* species. Serious skin infections, septicemia, and bone and joint, CNS, and lower respiratory tract infections and endocarditis due to *B. fragilis* and *Clostridium* species are sensitive to metronidazole. Mixed infections with aerobic and anaerobic causative organisms must be treated with the appropriate aerobic coverage. It is pregnancy category B and is used only if essential in the first trimester. Adverse effects include convulsive seizures and paresthesias of an extremity. Patients on prolonged therapy should be screened for symptoms and the drug stopped if they appear. GI distress, ataxia, metallic taste, and skin rash are possible as are neutropenia and thrombocytopenia. A disulfiram effect may occur when metronidazole is taken with ethanol.

Inhibitors of Protein Synthesis
Aminoglycosides

The first type of aminoglycoside was streptomycin, discovered in 1943. Over time its potential for toxicity has decreased; however, there has been an increase in microbial resistance toward the drug. Gentamicin is the drug of choice in hospitals, and amikacin is generally used when the invading bacteria is resistant to gentamicin. The medication acts on the organism by absolutely preventing it from synthesizing protein (i.e., it acts on the bacterial ribosome in such a way as to cause specific misreading of the genetic code so that amino acids cannot be strung together to form peptide chains).

These antibiotics are primarily used against gram-negative infections, especially those caused by aerobic organisms such as hospital-acquired *E. coli* and *Pseudomonas aeruginosa.* They are often used in combination with other antibiotics to achieve broad-spectrum coverage. Their use is limited because they require parenteral administration and there is *a high risk of toxic reaction,* particularly in the presence of renal impairment. They are poorly absorbed when given orally. The elderly and those who are dehydrated experience the most serious adverse effects. Ototoxicity, nephrotoxicity, and, with high doses, neuromuscular blockade may occur. Minor toxicities include fever and a skin rash. The half-life is about one half hour to two hours; that time increases to 24 hours for patients with renal insufficiency. The drug is metabolized and excreted relatively unchanged in urine primarily through glomerular filtration. Since they are commonly used only on an inpatient basis, they will not be discussed further.

Polymixins have similar action. They interfere with bacterial cell wall membrane transport and osmotic regulation. They are bactericidal. They are extremely nephrotoxic and should not be used by the nurse practitioner.

Tetracyclines

This medication was isolated in 1948 and was introduced in 1950. Its mechanism of action is similar to that of the aminoglycosides. It prevents protein synthesis, and it is bacteriostatic. Tetracyclines served as the prototype for the first truly broad-spectrum antibiotics. They are used to treat mixed infections such as peritonitis and chronic bronchitis or bronchitis and sinusitis. They are effective against chlamydiae and are the drug of choice against rickettsial infections. Central nervous system penetration is poor for doxycycline but good with minocycline (a second-generation tetracycline).

They are readily but incompletely absorbed in the GI tract on an empty stomach. Their action is inhibited by food, milk or milk products (except for minocycline and doxycycline), and by the concurrent administration of antacids. The drug has an affinity for and binds to calcium; consequently, it is deposited in newly forming bones and teeth. Discoloration of teeth and depression of bone growth may occur in the young. The drugs are able to cross the blood-brain barrier and placenta, and they are also excreted in breast milk. Therefore, these drugs should not be administered during pregnancy nor to children under the age of 8 years.

The most common adverse effects are GI disturbances and include nausea, vomiting, steatorrhea, and diarrhea. With long-term therapy superinfections are a problem and delayed blood coagulation is also reported. Reactions reported with intense exposure to sunlight or artificial ultraviolet light are associated with tetracycline, but this reaction is rare with doxycycline and minocycline.[19] Large dosages are known to cause liver impairment and kidney damage. There is a real danger in taking outdated prescriptions because the drug decomposes with age, light, extreme heat, and humidity and then becomes toxic when ingested.[12]

Social implications are an important consideration because these drugs are often administered widely and indiscriminately since they are effective against a broad range of organisms. The drug is used primarily for respiratory infections, urinary tract infections, pneumonias, and acne (see Table 12-6); consequently, the organisms may quickly develop resistance. Organisms have learned to seek and destroy the drug by eliminating it intact through excretion. Sometimes aminoglycosides are given in conjunction with this drug to discourage this adaptive transformation in the bacteria.

Chloramphenicol

Chloramphenicol has similar actions to tetracycline (i.e., a potent inhibitor of protein synthesis, bacteriostatic, and broad-spectrum). Because of its serious and sometimes fatal toxic effects, it is used only as a last resort in life-threatening infections such as (1) severe typhoid fever, (2) rickettsial infections that are resistant to other antibiotics, (3) *Haemophilus influenzae* meningitis, (4) anaerobic or mixed infections in the central nervous system, such as a brain abscess, or (5) life-threatening sepsis originating in the lower bowel.

The side effects are infrequent but *severe* when they do occur. Hematologic effects include aplastic anemia that may be fatal, bone marrow depression, and leukopenia. In newborns toxicity is often fatal. It is labeled "gray baby" syndrome since systemic vasomotor collapse is the cause of death. These drugs are also known to increase the half-lives of warfarin, phenytoin, tolbutamide, and chlorpropamide.

Considering that the drug has severe toxic effects and that it is absorbed into the central nervous system and cerebrospinal fluid, it is essential that blood is drawn frequently to ascertain whether there is a potential or an actual toxicity problem. It is appropriate to admit the patient into the hospital for continual surveillance while the drug is administered. It should not be used by nurse practitioners in an outpatient setting.

Erythromycins

Erythromycin is the first of a class of antiinfectives known as macrolides. These drugs were introduced in 1952; they are both bacteriostatic and bacteriocidal (in high doses), and their mechanism of action is similar to the aminoglycosides in that they inhibit

TABLE 12-6

Commonly Used Tetracyclines

Drug	Brand Name	Examples of Indications	Recommended Dose	Average Wholesale Cost
Doxycycline	Generic	Rickettsia, plague, Lyme disease, URI, CAP (X Klebs.), STD, animal bites, malaria	100–200 mg q 12–24 h (loading dose × 72 h)	$14.00
Minocycline	Minocin	MRSA, Lyme disease, Legionella, CNS, Acne V. mycoplasma, CAP (X Klebs.)	100–200 mg q 6–12 h	$52.00

STD = sexually transmitted diseases; X = except; CAP = community-acquired-pneumonia.

protein synthesis. They are highly effective against gram-positive cocci such as streptococci, pneumococci, and corynebacteria as well as gram-positive bacilli such as *C. perfringens*. They are the drugs of choice in the treatment of Legionnaires' disease, mycoplasmal pneumonia, and diphtheria. They are also useful as a penicillin substitute in those patients who are allergic to penicillin. Strains of streptococci that are resistant to erythromycin may be on the rise, and local statistics should be known before prescribing. It should not be used for serious staphylococcal infections, and it does not diffuse into the brain and spinal cord.

Clarithromycin and azithromycin are newer semisynthetic derivatives of erythromycin with broader spectra of activity particularly against *H. influenzae*. They are readily absorbed in the GI tract, but since these drugs are destroyed by gastric acid they are packaged in enteric-coated tablets. Commonly, the GI side effects (nausea, vomiting, and diarrhea) are the major cause of discontinuation of the drugs, leading to a poor compliance profile. The newer macrolides are associated with less GI upset, although clarithromycin causes a metallic taste in the mouth that is disturbing to some patients. GI symptoms decrease when the drug is administered with food.

Bioavailability of azithromycin is diminished by food, and it is better taken on an empty stomach if tolerated. It has wide tissue distribution and reaches high and long-lasting concentrations in the cell, even in phagocytes. Only clarithromycin requires dosage adjustment for moderate renal failure.[8]

These drugs are known as the safest antibiotics, but rare allergic reactions and hepatotoxicity can occur. Clarithromycin is pregnancy category C and must not be used when there is a possibility of pregnancy. Azithromycin has recently been approved for use in children and is pregnancy category B, as is erythromycin. Its high tissue concentrations and short dosing period improve compliance. It was at first very expensive but several cost reductions have occurred. Erythromycin is still an extremely good choice for many infections (see Table 12-7). Its cost is about one third of the newer macrolides and its

TABLE 12-7

Macrolide Antibiotics

Drug	Brand Name	Examples of Indications	Recommended Dose	Average Wholesale Cost
Erythromycin	Generic	URI, LRI, chlamydia, simple skin	250–500 mg q 6 h	$10.00
Clarithromycin	Biaxin	URI, LRI, skin, Legionella, H. jejunum, GERD	250–500 mg bid	$63.00
Azithromycin	Zithromax	URI, LRI, chlamydia, skin	500 mg day 1, 250 mg days 2–5	$36.00

GERD = gastroesophageal reflux disease; LRI = lower respiratory infection; URI = upper respiratory infection.

narrow spectrum prevents resistance when used appropriately. A one-dose 1-g azithromycin treatment of chlamydia in females is indeed a magic bullet for this disease. Problems with high blood levels of terfenadine have caused deaths from QT prolongation with ventricular tachycardia. Astemazole, corticosteroids, digoxin, terfenadine, theophylline, valproate, and warfarin are some of the drugs which may be potentiated by the macrolides through interference with the P-450 enzyme system. These drugs are excreted in the bile and urine.

Folate Antagonists
Sulfonamides

Sulfonamides were introduced in 1935 as the first antibiotic agents. They were the only defense against bacterial infections before the availability of penicillins. Now there are as many as 150 variants of the drug on the market at any given time. The broad applicability of these drugs to many infections, as well as their relatively low cost, has made them very popular in developing areas of the world. Unfortunately, uncontrolled distribution has led to widespread resistance. Sulfonamides competitively inhibit synthesis of essential metabolites required for folate synthesis which is necessary for survival. They are primarily bacteriostatic in their actions (see Table 12-8).[12]

The usefulness of these drugs as a single entity is limited due to this potential for bacterial acquired resistance, but this response can be reduced if the drug is used in combination with other antibiotics. Trimethoprim is a nonsulfonamide agent that also inhibits bacterial folate metabolism.[1]

Combinations of these drugs produce a synergistic effect. They are not to be used in pregnancy category C. Sulfonamides are absorbed in the GI tract (do not administer with antacids as this will decrease absorption), distributed systemically, and excreted by the kidney. Adverse effects include GI disturbances (anorexia, nausea, and vomiting), with the potential to cause crystalluria-induced nephrotoxicity. It is necessary to encourage increased fluid intake (at least 3 quarts) to ensure a minimum of 1200 mL of urinary output in 24 hours to avoid renal toxicity. The dose must be adjusted for a glomerular filtration rate of less than 50.[8] Liquids and vitamins that produce acidic urine should be avoided.

Quinolones

Quinolones are synthetic analogues of nalidixic acid that were introduced in 1963 for the treatment of urinary tract infections caused by coliform infections. Resistance developed quickly and the original product currently has very limited use. All quinolones are potent inhibitors of bacterial DNA synthesis. The fluoroquinolones are active against a variety of gram-negative bacteria including *H. influenzae, M. catarrhalis,* and most enteric bacilli. Ciprofloxacin has good activity against *Pseudomonas aeruginosa.*

Much higher doses are required to treat gram-positive infections, and staphylococcal and streptococcal resistance is rapidly emerging. Quinolones are easily absorbed in the GI tract and rapidly excreted in the urine. Norfloxacin, lomefloxacin, and enoxacin have no significant systemic antibacterial action since they concentrate mainly in the GI and GU tract. Other members of the class, ofloxacin and levofloxacin, achieve wide tissue penetration and are active intracellularly.

TABLE 12-8

Sulfonamides

Drug	Brand Name	Examples of Indications	Recommended Dose	Average Wholesale Cost
Silver sulfadiazine	Silvadine	Burns	Topical cream applied with dressing change	$2.50 per tube
Sulfacetamide	Bleph 10, Sodium sulamyd	Infections of conjunctiva and cornea	2 gtts q 2 h of 30% ophthalmic solution	$1.00 per bottle (15 cc)
Trimethoprim with Sulfamethoxazole	Bactrim, Septra	Acute otitis media, UTI, chronic bronchitis, PCP prophylaxis, traveler's diarrhea prophylaxis	1 single-strength tablet q 12 h to 2; double-strength tablets q 6 h	$0.10 per single- or double-strength tablet
Sulfasalazine	Azulfidine	Ulcerative colitis	Treatment: 1000 mg q 4–8 h after meals Maintenance: 500 mg q 4–8 h	$0.15 per 500-mg tablet
Sulfinpyrazone	Anturane	Chronic or intermittent gouty arthritis	200–400 mg bid with food	$0.26 per 200-mg tablet

Diarrheal illnesses respond very well to these drugs. They are reasonable first-line drugs for prostatitis in older men, prolonged serious bacterial diarrheas, complicated urinary tract infections, diabetic foot ulcers, and single-dose therapy for gonorrhea together with doxycycline 500 mg bid for seven days (see Table 12-9).

A number of side effects have been reported: hyperglycemia and glycosuria, GI disturbances, skin rash, photosensitivity, visual disturbances, and CNS stimulation leading to seizures. Quinolones increase theophylline levels through inhibition of the P-450 cytochrome system and should never be given with theophylline. Isolated cases of Achilles tendon rupture have occurred, and musculoskeletal complaints must be taken seriously. These drugs are not currently approved for pregnancy, lactation, or in those under 18 years of age. They are expensive and should not be used as first-line choices for any but the most serious urinary and GI tract infections, serious gram-negative pneumonias, and bone, soft tissue, and skin infections.[20]

Antituberculous Agents

Antituberculous agents have markedly improved the prognosis for those with tuberculosis. The most significant reasons for ineffective drug therapy are bacterial resistance and the patient's lack of self-administration. Resistant strains of this bacteria have been

TABLE 12-9

Fluoroquinolones

Drug	Brand Name	Examples of Indications	Recommended Dose	Average Wholesale Cost
Ciprofloxacin	Cipro	LRI (not strep pn), skin, joint, and bone infection, UTI, STDs, Inf. diarrhea	250, 500, 750 mg bid	$54.00, $62.00, $110.00
Ofloxacin	Floxin	Same as above and prostatitis	200, 300, 400 mg bid	$59.00, $70.00, $73.00
Norfloxacin	Noroxin	STDs, prostatitis, UTI	400 mg bid	$51.00
Lomefloxacin	Maxaquin	Same as norfloxacin	400 mg qd	$64.00
Enoxacin	Penetrex	Same as norfloxacin	200, 400 mg bid	$63.00
Levofloxacin	Levaquin	Sinusitis, chronic bronchitis, CAP, UTI	500 mg qd	$7.00 each

reported in patients with immunosuppression, especially in those who have HIV infection. Problems are encountered in self-administration of medicine over a long period of time (up to 2 years) and the number of drugs that must be taken because of patterns of resistance. Four-drug therapy is recommended (see Table 12-10). Streptomycin was the first drug available to treat tuberculosis. It is now rarely used and not regularly available.

Isoniazid

This drug interferes with cell wall synthesis in acid-fast organisms. Its main use is for *Mycobacterium tuberculosis.* Resistance develops quickly since the drug does not accumulate in the organisms. Missed doses or incomplete therapy allows the organism to become resistant. It is readily absorbed orally but must not be taken with aluminum-containing antacids. The dose must be adjusted for slow acetylators and for those with a GFR less than 10.

The most severe adverse effect is hepatitis, the incidence of which increases with age. Those receiving the drug should be questioned monthly and the drug discontinued if clinical evidence of hepatitis exists. Routine monitoring of liver enzymes is recommended for those over 35 years of age. Elevations of up to three times of transaminase levels without symptoms do not constitute an indication to stop therapy. Alcohol consumption should be monitored.[21]

Other adverse effects include peripheral neuritis caused by neutralization of vitamin B_6. Vitamin supplementation is advised in malnutrition and in pregnancy or lactation. Optic neuritis has also occurred. Overdose or accumulation of drug in slow acetylators can be life-threatening and is eliminated by hemodialysis.

Rifampin

Rifampin is used in combination with other drugs for the treatment of tuberculosis. It is bacteriocidal due to its ability to block RNA synthesis in selected organisms but not in animals. It also has been used prophylactically in those exposed to meningitis and *H. influenzae* and as adjunct therapy with a macrolide against *Legionella.*

Adverse effects include flu-like symptoms when used less than twice per week or in very large doses; hepatic effects, skin rash, GI effects, and overdose toxicity occur rarely. The drug is not readily eliminated by dialysis. The drug turns body fluids orange and will ruin clothing and contact lenses. Rifampin is a potent inducer of hepatic enzymes and can shorten the half-lives of most drugs including Coumarin.[12]

Pyrazinamide

Pyrazinamide is an orally effective bacteriocidal antitubercular agent used for short-term therapy with isoniazid and rifampin. About 1 to 5 percent of patients taking these three drugs will experience liver dysfunction. Urate retention may occur, precipitating a gouty attack.[15]

Ethambutol

Ethambutol is an orally active bacteriostatic drug effective against *M. tuberculosis* and *M. kansasii.* It concentrates in erythrocytes. Adverse effects include exacerbation of gouty arthritis and reversible optic neuritis. Loss of visual acuity and red-green color

TABLE 12-10

Drugs for the Treatment of Mycobacterial Disease in Adults[a]

Commonly Used Agents	Available Strengths of Oral Tablets or Capsules (mg)	Dosage			Most Common Side Effects	Tests for Side Effects	Drug Interactions[b]
		Total Once Daily Dose	Twice Weekly Dosage	Three Times Weekly Dosage			
Isoniazid[c]	100, 300	5–10 mg/kg up to 300 mg PO or IM	15 mg/kg PO or IM	15 mg/kg up to 900 mg PO or IM	Peripheral neuritis, hepatitis, hypersensitivity	Aminotransferases (not as a routine)	Carbamazepine: increased toxicity, both drugs; Disulfiram: psychosis, ataxia; Phenytoin: toxicity increased
Rifampin	600	10 mg/kg up to 600 mg PO	10 mg/kg up to 600 mg PO	10 mg/kg up to 600 mg PO	Hepatitis, febrile reaction, purpura (rare)	Aminotransferases (not as a routine)	May reduce the effect of the following drugs due to increased hepatic metabolism: oral contraceptives, quinidine, corticosteroids, anticoagulants, disopyramide, diazepam, barbiturates, methadone, digitoxin, digoxin, oral hypoglycemics; p-aminosalicyclic acid may interfere with absorption of rifampin
Streptomycin		15–20 mg/kg up to 1 g IM	25–30 mg/kg up to 1 g IM	25–30 mg/kg up to 1 g IM	Eighth nerve damage, nephrotoxicity	Vestibular function, audiograms; blood urea nitrogen and creatinine	Neuromuscular blocking agents—may be potentiated to cause prolonged paralysis
Pyrazinamide	500	15–30 mg/kg up to 2 g PO	50–70 mg/kg PO	50–70 mg/kg up to 3 g PO	Hyperuricemia, hepatoxicity	Uric acid, aminotransferases	
Ethambutol	100, 400	15–25 mg/kg PO	50 mg/kg PO	25–30 mg/kg up to 2.5 g PO	Optic neuritis (reversible with discontinuation of drug; very rare at 15 mg/kg), skin rash	Red-green color discrimination and visual acuity,[d] difficult to test in a child under 3 years	

[a]Adapted from American Thoracic Society: Treatment of tuberculosis and tuberculosis infection in adults and children. *Am Rev Respir Dis* 134:355, 1986; and *MMWR* 42:2, 1993.
[b]Reference should be made to current literature, particularly on rifampin, because it induces hepatic microenzymes and therefore interacts with many drugs.
[c]With pyridoxine 25 mg daily for poorly nourished or pregnant patients, to prevent peripheral neuropathy.
[d]Initial examination should be done at start of treatment.

blindness are signs which should be monitored. Dosage must be adjusted in moderate renal failure. All of the antituberculous drugs can cause hypersensitivity reactions but such an occurrence with ethambutol is rare (less than 0.1 percent).[12]

Antiviral Agents

Many antiviral drugs have been approved for specific indications in the United States since the FDA adopted a fast-track approval process for treatment of AIDS. The protease inhibitors in combination with nucleoside analogues and other drugs have brought about a revolution in the treatment of AIDS and in the life expectancy and quality of life of AIDS patients.

Treatment of Respiratory Virus Infections

Influenza A and the respiratory syncytial virus (RSV) are sometimes weakened by amantadine and rimantidine. They can be given orally at the first sign of illness or exposure, and they are variably effective as prophylactic agents. Ribavirin is used as an aerosol inhalation for children with RSV; the aerosol must not be inhaled by pregnant women as it is pregnancy category X. Ribavirin is used in treating infants and children infected with severe RSV infections. It is available by aerosol as well as orally and intravenously. It is contraindicated in pregnancy.

Treatment of Herpes Virus Infections

Vidarabine is an ophthalmic solution for the treatment of herpes simplex keratitis. Acyclovir is a nucleoside analogue and is widely used, again with variable effect, in shingles and genital herpes infections. Acyclovir has now been approved for treating chickenpox infections. It is recommended at the first sign of chickenpox in those over 2 years old.

Treatment of HIV Infections

Zidovudine (AZT), didanosine (ddI), and zalcitabine (ddC) are the old standbys. They are still effective, especially when given in combination. Due to increased research efforts and a fast-track FDA approval process, the selections have multiplied and treatment options are complex and evolving. The latest official directive as referred to by the CDC is a July 10, 1996, article summarizing the recommendations of an international panel.[22] The article recommends initiation of therapy based on CD4+ cell counts, plasma HIV RNA level (viral load), or clinical status. "Preferred initial drug regimens include nucleoside combinations; at present protease inhibitors are best reserved for patients at higher progression risk."[2]

Antiretroviral therapy should be initiated (see Table 12-11) in all patients with symptomatic HIV disease (e.g., recurrent mucosal candidiasis; oral hairy leukoplakia; chronic or otherwise unexplained fever, night sweats, or weight loss).[22]

Verticle transmission of HIV from mother to child has been reduced by approximately two thirds, from 24.9 to 7.8 percent. Perinatal prophylaxis with AZT is recommended for all HIV-infected women as is treatment for the newborn regardless of whether the mother is treated.[22])

TABLE 12-11

When to Initiate Therapy in HIV Disease

Status	Recommendation
Symptomatic HIV disease*	Therapy recommended for all patients
Asymptomatic, CD4$^+$ cell count <0.500 × 10^9/L	Therapy recommended†
Asymptomatic CD4$^+$ cell count >0.500 × 10^9/L	Therapy recommended for patients with >30,000–50,000 HIV RNA copies/mL or rapidly declining CD4$^+$ cell counts
	Therapy should be considered for patients with >5000 to 10,000 HIV RNA copies/mL

*Symptomatic human immunodeficiency virus (HIV) disease includes symptoms such as recurrent mucosal candidiasis, oral hairy leukoplakia, and chronic and unexplained fever, night sweats, and weight loss.

†Some would defer therapy in a subset of patients with stable CD4$^+$ cell counts between 0.350 and 0.500 × 10^9/L and plasma HIV RNA levels consistently below 5000 to 10,000 copies/mL.

SOURCE: Carpenter CCJ, Fischl MA, Hammer SM, et al. Antiretroviral therapy for HIV infection in 1996: Recommendations of an international panel. JAMA 276, 1996.[22]

Alternating therapy is well accepted, due to:

- Better antiretroviral activity
- Improved drug toxicity
- Less drug resistance
- Availability of recombinant human erythropoietin which is better than transfusions for drug-related anemia

Table 12-12 summarizes key information regarding currently available antiretroviral agents. New and investigational drugs continue to appear at rapid rates. Many providers on the forefront of research are investigating the effect of very early combination drug therapy. Cases are reported of treatment with combination therapy (nucleosides, non-nucleosides, reverse transcriptase inhibitors, and protease inhibitors) where viral load was reduced to nondetectable levels.

Newer protease inhibitors including nelfunavir (Viracept) and VX-478 are in clinical trials. Nevirapine (Viramune) and delaverdine (in clinical trial) are non-nucleoside reverse transcriptase inhibitors (NNRTIs). Resistant virus emerges rapidly when NNRTIs are given as monotherapy; they should always be given with at least one other antiretroviral agent.

Unfortunately, protease inhibitors are effective in only 50 percent of AIDS cases and recently a number of cases of adult onset diabetes mellitus have been reported. All the

TABLE 12-12

Antiretroviral Agents at a Glance

Drug	Key Uses*	Daily Dosage	Major Toxicities
Nucleoside analogues Zidovudine, AZT (Retrovir) Capsules, syrup, IV injection	Treatment of adults with HIV infection and CD4 cell count ≤500/μL Treatment of children >3 mo of age with HIV-related symptoms or laboratory evidence of significant HIV-related immunosuppression	500–600 mg PO (typically 200 mg PO tid) Children 3 mo–12 yr: 180 mg/m² q 6 h, not to exceed 200 mg q 6 h	Bone marrow suppression Severe anemia Granulocytopenia Symptomatic myopathy, myositis (with prolonged use)
Didanosine, ddl, (Videx) Chewable tablets, buffered powder for oral solution, powder for oral solution (pediatric)	Treatment of adults with advanced HIV infection who have received prolonged prior AZT therapy Treatment of all patients >6 mo of age with advanced HIV infection who show intolerance to AZT or clinical or immunologic deterioration while taking AZT	Two 100-mg tablets bid (≥60 kg) One 100-mg tab plus one 25-mg tab bid (<60 kg) Powder: 250 mg bid (≥60 kg) 167 mg bid (<60 kg)	Pancreatitis Peripheral neuropathy Liver failure Retinal depigmentation and change in vision (in children)
Zalcitabine, ddC (Hivid) Tablets	Combination therapy with AZT in selected patients with advanced HIV disease (CD4 cell count ≤300/μL) who have experienced significant clinical or immunologic deterioration Monotherapy for adults with advanced HIV disease who cannot tolerate AZT or experience disease progression while taking AZT	0.75 mg PO tid (0.375 mg PO tid for patients <30 kg) 0.75 mg PO tid	Severe peripheral neuropathy Pancreatitis Esophageal ulcers Cardiomyopathy/congestive heart failure Anaphylactoid reaction

(continued)

TABLE 12-12

Antiretroviral Agents at a Glance (continued)

Drug	Key Uses*	Daily Dosage	Major Toxicities
Stavudine, d4T (Zerit) Capsules	Treatment of adults with advanced HIV infection who cannot tolerate other approved therapies with proven clinical benefit or who experience significant clinical or immunologic deterioration while taking those therapies or for whom such therapies are contraindicated	40 mg PO bid (≥60 kg) 30 mg PO bid (<60 kg)	Delayed peripheral neuropathy Hepatotoxicity Anemia (but decreased bone marrow toxicity in comparison to zidovudine)
Lamivudine, 3TC (Epivir) Tablets, oral solution	Combination therapy with AZT	150 mg PO bid (>50 kg) with AZT 2 mg/kg PO bid (<50 kg) with AZT	Headache, insomnia, fatigue, peripheral neuropathy, myalgia
Protease inhibitors Saquinavir mesylate (Invirase)	Monotherapy, or combination therapy with a nucleoside analogue	600 mg PO tid	All are generally well-tolerated
Ritonavir (Norvir) Indinavir (Crixivan)		600 mg bid 800 mg tid	

Note: Drugs that produce similar toxicities should not be used in combination (e.g., didanosine and zalcitabine, both of which have a risk of peripheral neuropathy and pancreatitis).

*Some drugs may not be FDA-approved for the specific uses listed.

SOURCE: Davey RT, Goldschmidt, RH, Sande MA: Antiretroviral agents at a glance. *Patient Care* 3(9)–66, 1996.[23]

antivirals are accompanied by adverse effects which range from nausea, fatigue, headaches, and insomnia to hematologic abnormalities, myopathy, neuropathy (see Table 12-12), and Stevens-Johnson syndrome. Often these adverse effects diminish with time and in the case of Viramune rash may be avoided by a 14-day lead-in period of low-dose therapy.

Antifungals

Many fungi are resistant to antifungal agents. Relapse is a big problem; sometimes life-long therapy is needed. Unfortunately, fungal infections are diseases of the immune-compromised host, and they are on the increase due to cancer chemotherapy, AIDS, and steroid use. They occur endemically in the southwestern part of the United States in California, Arizona, and Texas.

Amphotericin B is the original antifungal agent for serious deep fungal infections. It is currently only available for IV administration. It has serious adverse effects, including chills and fever, bronchospasm, hypotension, arrhythmias, shock, nephro- and hepatotoxicity, anaphylaxis, respiratory, cardiac, and neurological disorders, malaise, tinnitis, visual impairment, hearing loss, diarrhea, and others. It is not a drug to be used by nurse practitioners without consultation.

Azoles are a new category of antifungals that can be administered orally. There are two classes of azoles: the immutazoles include miconazole and ketoconazole, and the triazoles include fluconazole and itraconazole (see Table 12-13). They are not without adverse effects, including fatal hepatic toxicity and anaphylaxis, and can never be used in combination because of cytochrome P-450 activity which increases toxicity. Ketoconazole (Nizorol) cannot be given with cisapride, terfenadine, or astemizole.

TABLE 12-13

Treatment of Mycoses

Deep Mycoses	Drugs	Superficial Mycoses	Drugs
Aspergillosis, invasive		**Candidiasis**	
Immunosuppressed	Amphotericin B	Vulvovaginal	Topical
Nonimmunosuppressed	Amphotericin B, itraconazole		Butoconazole
			Clotrimazole
			Miconazole
Blastomycosis			Nystatin
Rapidly progressive or CNS	Amphotericin B		Terconazole
			Tioconazole
Indolent, non-CNS	Itraconazole, ketoconazole	Oral	Fluconazole

(continued)

TABLE 12-13

Treatment of Mycoses (continued)

Deep Mycoses	Drugs	Superficial Mycoses	Drugs
		Candidiasis *(continued)*	
Coccidioidomycosis		Oropharyngeal	Topical
Rapidly progressing	Amphotericin B		Clotrimazole
Indolent	Itraconazole, ketoconazole, fluconazole		Nystatin
			Oral (systemic)
Meningeal	Fluconazole, inthrathecal amphotericin B		Fluconazole
			Ketoconazole
Cryptococcosis		Cutaneous	Topical
Non-AIDS and initial AIDS	Amphotericin B ± flucytosine		Amphotericin B
			Clotrimazole
Maintenance, AIDS	Fluconazole		Ciclopirox
Histoplasmosis			Econazole
Chronic pulmonary	Itraconazole		Ketoconazole
Disseminated			Miconazole
Rapidly progressing or CNS	Amphotericin B		Nystatin
Indolent, non-CNS	Itraconazole	**Ringworm**	Topical
Maintenance, AIDS	Itraconazole		Clotrimazole
Mucormycosis	Amphotericin B		Ciclopirox
Pseudallescheriasis	Itraconazole, IV miconazole		Econazole
			Haloprogin
			Ketoconazole
Sporotrichosis			Miconazole
Cutaneous	Iodine, itraconazole		Naftifine
Extracutaneous	Amphotericin B		Terbinafine
			Undecylenate
		Systemic	Griseofulvin
			Itraconazole
			Terbinafine

SOURCE: Hardman JG, Limbird LE, Molinogg PB, et al: *Goodman & Gilman's The Pharmacological Basis of Therapeutics*, 9th ed. New York: McGraw-Hill, 1996.[1]

PRESCRIBING VARIABLES

Patient Variables

Advanced age and infirmity make it difficult for patients to follow instructions in regard to food intake and frequency and duration of dosing.

Many antimicrobial agents are pregnancy categories C, D, and X. Careful questioning of the patient is necessary to determine the possibility of pregnancy. Some would go so far as to eliminate tetracyclines and quinolones from their formulary in vulnerable populations (e.g., college health).

Chronic use of antacids can produce problems when antibiotics are acid-stable. They need an acid environment to be absorbed from the stomach.

In cases of renal dysfunction, either the dose and/or the frequency of antibiotic administration may need to be decreased. This is particularly true in the elderly where considerable kidney function can be lost before creatinine clearance is affected.

Drug Variables

We have dealt mostly in this chapter with oral medications. Interactions with other drugs have been described under each section.

Drug Selection

Choosing the right drug for the right organism and location in the body is only half the battle. If the drug is too expensive or requires frequent dosing, the patient may not buy the drug or even if it is provided, may not take the drug as prescribed. See each section for the most cost-effective choices. Limited information has been provided here. The current *Nurse Practitioner Prescribing Reference* must be consulted for particular prescribing information. Current pricing may be referenced in *The Red Book Update*.[24]

REFERENCES

1. Hardman JG, Limbird LE, Molinoff PB, et al: *Goodman & Gilman's The Pharmacological Basis of Therapeutics,* 9th ed. New York: McGraw-Hill, 1996.
2. Rosenblatt JE: Laboratory tests used to guide antimicrobial therapy. *Mayo Clin Proc* 66: 942–948, 1991.
3. Dipiro JT, Talbert RL, Yee GC, et al: *Pharmacotherapy: A Pathophysiologic Approach,* 3d ed. Stamford, CT: Appleton & Lange, 1997.
4. Sweeney G: *Clinical Pharmacology: A Conceptual Approach.* New York: Churchill Livingstone, 1990, 22–29.
5. Meyer JM, Rodvold KA: Drug biotransformation by the cytochrome P-450 enzyme system. *Infect Med* 13(6):463–464,523, 1996.
6. Gleckman RA, Borrego F: Adverse reactions to antibiotics. *Postgrad Med* 101(4):103, 1997.
7. Meyers BR: *Antimicrobial Therapy Guide.* Newtown, PA: Antimicrobial Prescribing, 1996.
8. Bennett WM, Aronoff GR, Golper TA, et al: *Drug Prescribing in Renal Failure: Dosing Guidelines for Adults,* 3d ed. Philadelphia: American College of Physicians, 1994.
9. Ribard P, Audisio F, Kahn MF, et al: Achilles tendonitis including 3 complicated by rupture during fluoroquinolone therapy. *J Rheumatol* 19:1479–1481, 1992.
10. Spatzenegger M, Jaeger W: Clinical importance of hepatic cytochrome P450 in drug metabolism. *Drug Metab Rev* 27:397–417, 1995.

11. May DG: Genetic differences in drug disposition. *J Clin Pharmacol* 34:881–897, 1994.
12. Katzung B: *Drug Therapy,* 2d ed. Norwalk, CT: Appleton & Lange, 1991, p 139.
13. Chambers HF, Sande MA: Antimicrobial agents: General considerations, in Hardman JG, Limbird LE, Molinoff PB, et al: *Goodman & Gilman's The Pharmacological Basis of Therapeutics,* 9th ed. New York: McGraw-Hill, 1996, p 1036.
14. Wood CA, Bosker G: Antibiotic update 1996: Cost effective treatment guidelines for bacterial infections managed in the ED. *Emerg Med Rep* 17(1):2, 1996.
15. Harvey RA, Champe PC: Inhibitors of cell wall synthesis, in *Lippincott's Illustrated Reviews: Pharmacology.* Philadelphia: Lippincott, 1992.
16. Stamm WE, Hooton TM: Management of urinary tract infections in adults. *N Engl J Med* 329(18):1328–1333, 1993.
17. Kaiser HB, Kaliner MA, Scott JL: Anaphylaxis: When routine turns nightmare. *Patient Care* 15:16–52, 1991.
18. *Nurse Practitioners' Prescribing Guide.* New York: Prescribing Reference, 1997, p 131.
19. Cunha BA: New uses for older antibiotics. *Postgrad Med* 10(4):73, 1997.
20. Fitzgerald MA: The fluoroquinolones. *J Am Acad Nurse Pract* 6(9):449, 1994.
21. Tierney JR, McPhee SJ, Papadakis MA: *Current Medical Diagnosis and Treatment.* Stamford, CT: Appleton & Lange, 1997.
22. Carpenter CCJ, Fischl MA, Hammer SM, et al: Antiretroviral therapy for HIV infection in 1996: Recommendations of an international panel. *JAMA* 276, 1996.
23. Davey RT, Goldschmidt RH, Sande MA: Antiretroviral agents at a glance. *Patient Care* 3(9):66, 1996.
24. *1995 Red Book.* Montvale, NJ: Medical Economics Data Production Company.

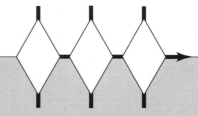

Chapter 13

CARDIAC DRUG THERAPY IN AMBULATORY PATIENTS

Susan K. Chase

Understanding the use of cardiac drugs in clinical practice is made complex by two factors. First, the large number of cardiac drugs are daunting to learn. Even when drugs are grouped together by category, there are many categories of drugs. Secondly, for any given cardiac condition, there are a number of possible drug groups that could be used. Similarly, any one group of cardiac drugs can be used for a number of different cardiac conditions. This presents the clinician with a kind of matrix of cardiac and related conditions and of drugs from which to choose for their management. The choice of drug to use is determined both by the drug's intended effects and by the pattern of side effects it may cause, considering patients' related conditions. This matrix is represented in Table 13-1.

In order to simplify this complex pattern for the reader, this chapter will be organized by drug group. However, within the discussion of each drug group will be a separate consideration of the group's use for each of the several conditions for which it is recommended. In this way, the reader can easily find all drug groups that are useful for the management of a given condition, such as hypertension.

TABLE 13-1

Cardiac and Related Conditions and Indications for Drug Therapy

Condition	Beta blockers	Calcium channel blockers	Diuretics	ACE inhibitors	Alpha blockers	Vaso-dilators
Hypertension	+	+	+	+	+	
Angina	+	+				−
CHF	−	−	+	+	+	+
Lipid disorders	−	+	−	+	+	

(continued)

293

TABLE 13-1

Cardiac and Related Conditions and Indications for Drug Therapy (continued)

Condition	Beta blockers	Calcium channel blockers	Diuretics	ACE inhibitors	Alpha blockers	Vasodilators
Asthma	–	+	+	+		
PVD	–	+		+		
Sexual dysfunction	–	+	–	+	+	
Depression	–	+	+	+	–Reserpine	
DM	–	+	–	+		
Renal failure	+	+	+	±		+
Pregnancy			–	–	+Methyldopa	

+ = helpful; – = potential negative effects.
CHF = congestive heart failure; PVD = peripheral vascular disease; DM = diabetes mellitus.

OVERVIEW OF CARDIOVASCULAR PHYSIOLOGY AND DRUGS

Electrophysiology

Cardiac muscle cells are unique in that they can initiate their own action potentials; that is, they do not require external innervation to initiate an action potential and subsequent contraction. Cells in different areas of the heart possess different underlying rates of depolarization, the fastest being the sinoatrial (SA) node, which depolarizes at an average rate of 60 to 100 times per minute. The SA node normally controls the electrical activation of the heart. The heart has backup systems that allow for some cardiac function even if the SA node fails to fire or is blocked. The atrioventricular node tissue depolarizes at about 30 to 40 times per minute, and the ventricular cells depolarize at 30 times per minute. Therefore, if the conduction system of the heart were completely blocked, an underlying ventricular rhythm of 30 times a minute could sustain life.

The action potential of the cardiac cell membrane occurs in four phases, including depolarization and repolarization, which will be described in brief because certain cardiac drugs act at certain phases of depolarization. The cell membrane is polarized at rest in that there are more positive ions lined up outside the cell membrane than inside because the cell membrane is more permeable to potassium ion outflow than sodium ion inflow. In phase 0, the fast sodium channels of the cell membrane open allowing sodium ions to rush into the cell, carrying with them their positive electrical charge. This "depolarizes" the membrane. During phase 1 of partial repolarization, the fast sodium channels close and a slow leak of potassium out of the cell begins the return to a more polarized state. Phase 2, plateau, occurs when the slow calcium channels open and allow positively charged calcium ions to enter the cell. During the plateau phase, the net effect of K^+ leaving and Ca^{++} entering results in very little change in the polarity of the membrane. Phase 3, repolarization, occurs as the calcium channels close and potassium leaves the cell, returning the electrical potential to near baseline. The sodium-potassium pump is an important mechanism for returning the proper baseline concentration of ions across the cell membrane. For every three sodium ions pumped out against the concentration gradient, two potassium ions are returned inside the cell. This imbalance helps to repolarize the cell membrane and prepare it for the next action potential.

As a result of depolarization, the sarcoplasmic reticulum that fills the cardiac muscle cell also depolarizes, releasing stored calcium ions into the sarcoplasm. Calcium is required by the actin-myosin system for coupling to occur. The coupling of actin and myosin results in muscle contraction. Electrical events precede but do not guarantee mechanical events. Appropriate electrolyte concentrations as well as sufficient energy substrates are required for mechanical work.

Contractility, Preload, and Afterload

Cardiac output is determined by heart rate multiplied by stroke volume. The force of contraction of the ventricle or contractility can be modified by several factors including sympathetic tone, serum electrolyte levels, and quality of blood supply to the myocardium. *Preload* is a concept related to the volume of the ventricle at the end of filling or diastole. This represents availability of blood to be pumped out with the next systole. Low preload can result from dehydration, hypovolemia, or vasodilation, which allows fluid to remain in the periphery. High preload can result from high intravascular volume. *Afterload* is the resistance that the heart must pump against during systole. High afterload can result from restricted aortic outflow, from high peripheral arteriolar resistance, or from arteriosclerotic arterioles. Low afterload can result from arteriolar dilatation. Pumping against high afterload increases the workload of the heart.

Autonomic Nervous System

The autonomic nervous system is a portion of the peripheral nervous system consisting of the sympathetic system and the parasympathetic system. The sympathetic nervous system is associated with the fight-or-flight response of the body to a threat. With sympathetic challenge, the body responds by releasing neurotransmitters from sympathetic nerves. The sympathetic neurotransmitters epinephrine and norepinephrine cause several responses that could be seen as beneficial in a physical challenge. The heart rate

TABLE 13-2

Effects of Selected Sympathetic Receptor Activation

Alpha$_1$	Alpha$_2$	Beta$_1$	Beta$_2$
Vasoconstriction	Inhibits	Tachycardia	Vasodilation
Increases PVR	norepinephrine	Increases lipolysis	Decreases PVR
Increases BP		Increases cardiac	Bronchodilation
Inhibits insulin		contractility	Glycogenolysis
release			Release of glucagon
Closes bladder			Relaxes uterine
sphincter			smooth muscle

PVR = peripheral vascular resistance.

increases, the blood pressure increases, blood is shunted away from the intestinal system to the vital organs and muscles, bronchioles dilate as do pupils, renal blood flow is reduced, and less urine is produced. These responses are termed *adrenergic* responses. The sympathetic system responds in seconds to perceived threats.

In contrast, the parasympathetic system uses acetylcholine as its neurotransmitter. Acetylcholine slows the rate of firing of the SA node, increases the amount of delay of conduction at the atrioventricular (AV) node, allows arterioles to relax, and promotes digestion and bladder emptying. There is a dynamic balance of parasympathetic and sympathetic influence over most bodily functions. Sympathetic neurotransmitter receptors are classified as either alpha or beta receptors. A summary of alpha and beta receptor function is illustrated in Table 13-2.

Renin-Angiotensin System

When the kidneys receive reduced blood flow or sense a reduction in blood volume, a hormone called *renin* is released from the juxtaglomerular apparatus near the afferent arterioles of the kidneys. Renin causes the release of angiotensin I from the substrate angiotensinogen of the liver. Angiotensin I is converted to angiotensin II in the lungs by the action of an angiotensin-converting enzyme (ACE). Angiotensin II is a powerful vasoconstrictor, resulting in higher vascular resistance and blood pressure. Angiotensin II also causes the release of aldosterone, which causes sodium and water retention by the kidneys.

OVERVIEW OF MAJOR CARDIOVASCULAR CONDITIONS AND APPROACHES TO THERAPY

Atherosclerosis

Lipoproteins of various sizes circulate in the blood. Macrophages circulating near the endothelial layer of the blood vessels attempt to phagocytose lipid particles, causing the development of fatty streaks. This initiates an inflammatory response inside the blood vessels that activates fibroblasts. These fibroblasts create plaques inside the vessels that contain lipids and fibromuscular layers, causing a narrowing of the vessel lumen. If these plaques enlarge to the point of rupture, the endothelial lining of the blood vessels is interrupted, initiating platelet aggregation and clot formation. This can initiate a thrombotic event. Therapeutics are aimed at decreasing the absorption or reabsorption of cholesterol or bile or decreasing the production of cholesterol.

Angina

When an insufficient blood supply reaches the myocardium through the coronary arteries because of atherosclerotic changes, there can be an imbalance of energy demand and supply. Muscle cells that do not receive sufficient oxygen must utilize anaerobic metabolism, which is inefficient and results in localized acidosis and pain. This pain is usually exertion-related and is experienced as angina. This pain most frequently is felt in the substernal area, but especially in women the pain can be felt in the neck area or occipital region. Angina pain is relieved by rest. Unstable angina is more severe and is not exertion-related. Goals of therapy are to control pain, allowing for energy to conduct the activities of daily living. Drug therapy is aimed at vasodilation to decrease preload and afterload.

Hypertension

In the United States, 50 million people have hypertension, causing 20 percent of all white and 30 percent of African-American deaths from cardiovascular causes. Hypertension can be classified in stages according to severity and is related to cardiac mortality and morbidity unless it is properly controlled. There are usually no symptoms related to hypertension, but after years of poor control, target organ damage such as retinal changes or renal function test changes can be recognized. Goals of therapy are to control blood pressure, preferably below 140/90 (slightly higher in the elderly), to prevent target organ damage, and to reduce the risk of cardiovascular mortality. Drug therapy is aimed at reducing blood volume (e.g., diuretics, ACE inhibitors), decreasing cardiac output (e.g., beta blockers), and/or increasing arteriolar dilation (ACE inhibitors, beta blockers). Specific drugs are chosen based upon other medical conditions and in some cases on ethnicity of the patient.

More than 90 percent of hypertension is primary or essential. Significant causes of secondary hypertension include renal disease and various endocrine disorders. Patients who do not respond to management of hypertension should be evaluated for these conditions.

Heart Failure

Heart failure affects 2.5 million Americans and can be the result of previous muscle damage from long-standing hypertension or from myocardial infarction or other myocardial damage. It can also result from cardiac valvular disorders. Systolic dysfunction results from inefficient contraction of the ventricles. Diastolic dysfunction results from the inability of the myocardium to relax. The body attempts to compensate for low cardiac output by retaining water and by elevating the blood pressure, resulting in increased afterload. Overall and pharmacologic goals of therapy for congestive heart failure are to decrease cardiac workload by eliminating edema, supporting cardiac function by reducing afterload.

Resources on Pharmacology of Cardiac Drugs

Books

Agency for Health Care Policy Research. *Diagnosing and Managing Unstable Angina.* AHCPR Publication No. 94-0603. Rockville, MD: The Agency, 1994.

Agency for Health Care Policy Research. *Heart Failure: Evaluation and Care of Patients with Left Ventricular Systolic Dysfunction. Clinical Practice Guideline No. 11.* AHCPR Publication No. 94-0612. Rockville, MD: The Agency, 1994.

National Institutes of Health. *The Fifth Report of the Joint National Committee of Detection, Evaluation and Treatment of High Blood Pressure.* NIH Publication No. 93-1088. Bethesda, MD: The Institutes, 1993.

National Institutes of Health. Report of the Expert Panel on Population Strategies for Blood Cholesterol Reduction. NIH Publication No. 93-3046. Bethesda, MD: The Institute, 1993.

Computer/Internet

PharmInfo Net Home Page (http://pharminfo.com)

ISSUES IN DRUG THERAPY

Nitrates

Prescribing Considerations

Angina   Nitrates are a group of drugs used to promote coronary artery vasodilation to support increased blood flow to the myocardium. Nitrates also decrease both arterial and venous tone, resulting in a decrease in preload and afterload. Both of these effects are positive for a heart whose own blood supply is insufficient to meet the demands of its workload. By decreasing the work of the heart, nitrates decrease the oxygen demand on the heart. Nitrates can also be used prophylactically before exertion to prevent angina pain. If no response to three doses of nitrates is obtained, immediate emergency care should be sought, as this may indicate unstable angina or impending myocardial infarction. In unstable angina, nitrates can be given intravenously in the hospital. In this case, continuous arterial blood pressure (BP) monitoring is required. There is no evidence (as there is with beta blockers) that the use of nitrates improves long-term survival for those using these drugs following myocardial infarction. Nevertheless, nitrates are often useful to decrease cardiac pain and offer a better quality of life for angina sufferers.

Other interventions for angina to be used in addition to these drugs are planned activity and rest periods. Losing weight can also decrease cardiac workload.

Prescribing Variables

Patient Variables   Patients develop a tolerance to effects of nitrates when used over the long term. For patients who are using transdermal nitrates, the paste or patch should be removed at bedtime when cardiac demand is low so that the nitrate can be cleared for a period of time. In the morning, reapplication of the device will result in a greater beneficial effect. Nitrates are listed as pregnancy category C.

Patients for whom precautions must be taken include those with acute myocardial infarction (MI), volume depletion, hypotension heart failure, and hypertrophic cardiomyopathy. Nitrates are potentiated by alcohol and vasodilators. Adverse reactions include headache, dizziness, flushing, orthostatic hypotension, tachycardia, increased angina, nausea, and rash. Nitrates should not be used in the following situations: nitrate allergy, severe anemia, congestive heart failure, left ventricular hypertrophy, bleeding, hemorrhage, and low blood pressure.

Drug Variables   The treatment of choice for angina pain is sublingual nitroglycerin in 2.5-mg tablets. The sublingual form avoids first-pass liver metabolism. Given in this form, nitroglycerin acts in 1 to 2 min. If relief is not obtained, the dose can be repeated in 3 to 5 min. These drugs are listed as pregnancy category B. They interact with calcium channel blockers, producing hypotension. Nitrates have a short half-life, and several methods have been developed to extend the duration of action. These include extended-release oral doses and transdermal patches. A buccal spray form is also available. This form has the advantage of being convenient to carry and not requiring manual dexterity in maneuvering the small nitroglycerin tablets. This form is also more stable over time.

Drugs in Category   Rapid-acting nitrates:

Nitroglycerin lingual aerosol spray (Nitrolingual) is the buccal aerosol form of the drug. Patients should be instructed not to inhale the spray.
Nitroglycerin sublingual tablets (Nitrostat) may be repeated in 15 min for persistent pain and can be used prophylactically 5 to 10 min before activity.

Long-acting nitrates include oral sustained-release capsules to be used to prevent angina but not for acute attacks:

Isosorbide dinitrate (Isordil, Dilatrate-SR).
Isosorbide mononitrate (Ismo, Monoket, Imdur, Sorbitrate).

Topical preparations include the following:

Nitroglycerin transdermal adhesive films and patches (Deponit, Minitran, Nitro-Dur, Nitrodisc, Transderm-Nitro) are most effective if used 12 to 14 hours a day.
Nitroglycerin ointment (Nitro-Bid, Nitrol) contains lanolin. Precautions should be taken in patients with severe anemia, narrow-angle glaucoma, and orthostatic hypotension. This drug is potentiated with alcohol and calcium channel blockers.

Contextual Issues   Drugs should be replaced every six months since the tablet form is very unstable. Tablets should be stored in a cool, dark, dry place. If tablets are carried in a pocket, they should be replaced at least every six months. Tablet forms are more economical than spray or patch forms of delivery. Blood pressure, pulse, and electrocardiogram should be monitored over time. Do not discontinue suddenly; taper doses to avoid rebound angina pain.

Calcium Channel Blockers

Prescribing Considerations

Angina   Calcium channel blockers are a group of drugs that differ from each other more than most other drugs that are found in the same class. They can control angina by decreasing myocardial oxygen requirements and by causing coronary and peripheral artery vasodilation. With vasospasm associated with angina, calcium channel blockers are the drug of choice. By decreasing blood pressure, calcium channel blockers can decrease left ventricular wall stress. Following MI, verapamil and diltiazem can prevent reinfarction in non-Q-wave infarcts. On the other hand, calcium channel blockers exacerbate congestive heart failure. With nitrates, diltiazem or verapamil can be used in unstable angina for patients who cannot take beta blockers.

Arrhythmia   Calcium channel blockers are useful for arrhythmias because they decrease calcium entry across the cell membrane, resulting in a decreased rate of phase 4 spontaneous depolarization. They slow conduction in the AV node. Verapamil and diltiazem selectively block channels in frequent use, thereby having greater effects during tachycardic episodes than when heart rates are normal. Calcium channel blockers are particularly effective in atrial arrhythmias.

Hypertension   This group of drugs is also useful for hypertension. All drugs in this group cause smooth muscle cell relaxation and vasodilation and also have a natriuretic effect. These drugs are good for patients for whom other antihypertensives are contraindicated, such as asthmatic, diabetic, angina, and peripheral vascular disease patients. Along with thiazide diuretics, they are especially effective in controlling hypertension among African-American patients.

Prescribing Variables

Patient Variables When used for angina, contraindications for all calcium channel blockers include aortic stenosis, severe obstructive coronary artery disease, and heart failure. These drugs are classified as pregnancy category C and are not recommended for nursing mothers or for children.

Drug Variables Common adverse reactions include peripheral edema, hypotension, headache, flushing, dizziness, fatigue, constipation, muscle cramps, rash, and exacerbation of heart failure or angina. Verapamil and diltiazem are absorbed from the GI tract with significant first-pass metabolism by the liver. The short half-life of these drugs requires multiple daily dosing or extended-release forms of the drug for hypertension.

Nifedipine is a potent vasodilator. It is most powerful in reducing blood pressure. Mild to moderate reflex tachycardia can occur after dosing. An increase in cardiac-related deaths was initially reported with the use of short-acting forms of nifedipine. Longer-acting forms now available are not associated with increased mortality. Calcium channel blockers do not adversely affect plasma lipids, glucose metabolism, or uric acid retention. Verapamil and diltiazem are less often used for hypertension because they can cause bradycardia and decreased force of ventricular contraction. These drugs should be used with caution for patients also taking beta blockers. They can precipitate cardiac failure more often than nifedipine or amlodipine.

Drugs in Category Diltiazem (Cardizem, Dilacor XR) should be taken in the morning on an empty stomach and should not be crushed or chewed. This drug is contraindicated for sick sinus syndrome, second- or third-degree AV block or hypotension. Precautions include impaired hepatic or renal function. While on this drug, patients' liver function should be monitored. Interactions with digoxin and beta blockers may lead to AV block. Serum propranolol and carbamazepine levels may be increased. Diltiazem is potentiated by cimetidine. Adverse reactions include asthenia, first-degree AV block, and liver abnormalities. Diltiazem decreases resting heart rate and exercise heart rate and causes less reflex tachycardia than verapamil, but can cause ischemia in congestive heart failure patients.

Verapamil (Calan, Isoptin, Covera-HS) is useful in controlling atrial flutter or atrial fibrillation. Patients with moderate to severe heart failure, AV conduction or neuromuscular transmission disorders, and hepatic or renal dysfunction should be observed closely. Patients on long-term therapy should have their liver function monitored. Drug interactions occur with beta blockers and other antihypertensives, neuromuscular blockers, digitalis, flecainide, carbamazepine, and cyclosporine, which are all potentiated. Monitor theophylline and lithium levels. This drug is antagonized by rifampin and phenobarbital. Adverse reactions include impaired AV conduction, bradycardia, constipation, nausea, dyspnea, elevated hepatic enzymes, and paralytic ileus. Verapamil decreases resting heart rate and causes less reflex tachycardia than other drugs in the class, but does increase the risk of AV block and heart failure as well as ischemia for patients with congestive heart failure.

Nifedipine (Adalat, Procardia XL) is useful in the control of hypertension but should be used with care as it is a potent vasodilator. Nifedipine can cause dizziness, flushing, tachycardia, and edema. Blood pressure should be monitored closely when initiating therapy. Interactions include the potentiation of antihypertensives and digoxin. When used with beta blockers nifedipine can cause angina and heart failure. Avoid short-acting forms of nifedipine as they have been associated with increased cardiac-related deaths. Nifedipine is potentiated by cimetidine. Oral anticoagulants and quinidine should be monitored while using nifedipine.

Nicardipine (Cardene) must be used carefully with hepatic or renal impairment. When initiating therapy, measure BP 1 to 2 h and 8 h after initial dose. Potential drug interactions include potentiation by cimetidine and increased serum levels of cyclosporine and possibly digoxin. Adverse reactions include increased angina, hypotension, flushing, headache, pedal edema, asthenia, dizziness, tachycardia, and somnolence.

Amlodipine (Norvasc) must be used cautiously with patients with severe obstructive coronary disease or hepatic impairment. Adverse reactions include palpitations, GI upset, and drowsiness. Amlodipine causes less negative inotropic effects than other drugs in the class.

Bepridil (Vascor) is contraindicated with ventricular arrhythmias, sick sinus syndrome, and second- or third-degree AV block unless paced, and should be used cautiously with recent MI, bundle branch block, and hepatic or renal dysfunction. With the elderly, potassium should be monitored. Drugs with which bepridil interacts include quinidine, procainamide, antiarrhythmics, and tricyclic antidepressants. When used with potassium wasting diuretics, hypokalemia may produce torsades de pointes, a ventricular tachycardia. When used with digoxin, bepridil can increase AV block. Adverse reactions include gastrointestinal upset, nervousness, tremor, drowsiness, dyspnea, dry mouth, anorexia, ventricular tachycardia, uterine hypotonia and elevated liver enzymes.

Isradipine and felodipine are not approved in the United States for angina. Felodipine has a less negative inotropic effect than other calcium channel blockers.

Contextual Issues   Nifedipine is one of the most commonly prescribed drugs in the United States. Calcium channel blockers are more expensive than diuretics and some beta blockers, which can also be used to control hypertension.

Beta Blockers

Prescribing Considerations

Angina   Beta blockers as a group have several beneficial effects for cardiac patients. One effect is to decrease oxygen demands of the myocardium, thereby preventing angina. Beta blockers accomplish this by decreasing heart rate, contractility, and afterload. Beta$_1$ blockers inhibit the receptors of the heart and are called *cardioselective*. They have fewer side effects outside the cardiovascular system unless used in high doses. Beta$_2$ blockers inhibit peripheral vascular receptors and those in the bronchi, pancreas, kidney, and liver. In general, beta blockers decrease heart rate, force of contraction, cardiac output, and renin secretion. Beta blockers with intrinsic sympathomimetic activity (ISA) are less likely to cause bradycardia and peripheral constriction. Research has demonstrated a positive benefit in longer life for post–myocardial infarction patients who are placed on beta blockers early postinfarction. Beta blockers are front-line drugs for hypertension. They are useful for hypertensives who also have angina or arrhythmias.

TABLE 13-3

Beta Blockers

Name	Protein binding, %	Metabolism/ excretion	Cardio-selectivity	Intrinsic sympatho-mimetic activity	Membrane stabilizing	Lipid solubility
Acebutolol	25	Hepatic/renal	++	+	+	Low
Atenolol	10	Biliary/fecal	+			Low
Betaxolol	50	Renal	+			Low
Bisoprolol		Hepatic/renal	+			Low to medium
Carteolol	30	Hepatic/renal		+		Low
Labetalol	50	Hepatic/renal			+	Medium
Metoprolol	12	Hepatic/renal	+			Medium
Nadolol	30					Low
Penbutolol	80	Hepatic/renal		+		Medium
Pindolol	40	Hepatic/renal		+	+	Medium
Propranolol	90	Hepatic/renal			+	High
Timolol	10	Hepatic/renal				Medium

+ = presence of attribute.

Beta blockers are considered first-line therapy for angina. Beta blockers decrease instances of ventricular fibrillation post–myocardial infarction. All beta blockers appear to be effective clinically in decreasing angina attacks, except pindolol, which has some sympathomimetic activity. Recent research has shown that many patients who would benefit from beta blocker therapy, that is, patients who have had a myocardial infarction or who have unstable angina, are not receiving the drug. Clinicians should consider placing all patients at risk for recurrent MI on beta blockers unless there are contraindications in that patient.

In unstable angina, beta blockers are especially useful if there is a tachycardic response to the condition. The goal of treatment is to keep the heart rate between 60 to 70 and BP between 100/70 to 120/80. This can be accomplished using oral or IV esmolol.

For hypertension, other interventions to use in lieu of or in conjunction with drug therapy include reducing modifiable risk factors such as overweight, smoking, and sedentary lifestyle.

Prescribing Variables

Patient Variables   Beta blockers are contraindicated in patients with bronchospasm because of the block of sympathomimetic responses that maintain open airways. They are also contraindicated with bradycardia because of the direct effect of the drugs on heart rate, second- or third-degree AV block, and heart failure caused by a decrease in contractility. Precautions must be taken for patients with ischemic heart disease, COPD, renal or hepatic dysfunction, diabetes mellitus, or hyperthyroidism. These drugs are classified as pregnancy category C unless otherwise indicated. They are not recommended for nursing mothers. Adverse reactions include bradycardia, dizziness, fatigue, cold extremities, heart failure, heart block, bronchospasm, GI upset, rash, and pruritus. They are not recommended for children. Beta blockers are the best antihypertensive medications for young patients. They are less effective in African-Americans and the elderly.

Drug Variables   There are many beta blockers available for prescription. Clinicians are advised to select one or two with which to become familiar and to use as front-line drugs. Side effect patterns might indicate a change in drug therapy. Table 13-3 summarizes the features of selected beta blockers. Cardioselective preparations select to beta$_1$ receptor sites and therefore have less effect on such tissues as bronchioles and peripheral vascular tissue and are less likely to cause hypoglycemia. Preparations with ISA have fewer cardiac suppressive and bronchoconstricting effects. They also do not increase triglycerides and can decrease HDL cholesterol. Non-ISA beta blockers, such as metoprolol or propranolol, are the type that are associated with decreased cardiac mortality. Membrane-stabilizing activity is beneficial in the treatment of some arrhythmias. Lipid solubility allows the drug to easily enter CNS tissue and cause mental changes. All beta blockers over time will have some CNS effects. For all beta blockers, monitor blood pressure, heart rate, CBC, EKG, eye pressure, renal and liver function studies, as well as glucose. For patients with renal failure, use metoprolol, timolol, propranolol, and labetalol for hypertension. For patients who have liver abnormalities, use atenolol or nadolol.

Drugs in Category Acebutolol (Sectral) is cardioselective and less apt to cause extremity coldness. It has less effect on resting heart rate and cardiac output than propranolol.

Atenolol (Tenormin) is cardioselective, but still has adverse effects on triglycerides and HDL cholesterol. It has low lipid solubility and therefore fewer CNS effects than drugs with higher lipid solubility. Lower doses should be used with the elderly or for patients with renal impairment. Trough blood pressure, which can be low for those not hypertensive, should be monitored. Take precautions when prescribing beta blockers with a lack of ISA for patients with peripheral vascular disease. This can lead to peripheral constriction. Atenolol has additive effects with prazosin. Concurrent use of digoxin can cause conduction abnormalities. Calcium channel blockers can interact to cause heart block.

Labetalol (Normodyne, Trandate) antagonizes both alpha and beta receptors and therefore is not recommended for asthmatic hypertensives. Labetalol is more effective than the other beta blockers in treating hypertension in African-Americans, probably because of its mixed alpha-adrenergic blocking activity. Because it has alpha-blocking effects, it can cause postural hypotension. It has interactions with catecholamine-depleting drugs and can potentiate hypotension and bradycardia. It can increase the cardiac effects of calcium channel blockers and digitalis. It is antagonized by NSAIDs. There may be a need to adjust antidiabetic medications, and it may interfere with glaucoma screening tests. Because it has alpha-blocking activity, it may block epinephrine needed for emergency treatment. Labetalol is good for Raynaud's disease and for those with liver damage.

Metoprolol tartrate (Lopressor) is potentiated by felodipine and antagonized by barbiturates and rifampin. Its adverse effects include depression, diarrhea, dyspnea, cold extremities, palpitations, peripheral edema, hypotension, and heart block. Metoprolol is more cardioselective than propranolol, but still has adverse effects on triglycerides and HDL cholesterol.

Metoprolol succinate (Toprol XL) is a cardioselective beta blocker that requires precaution in prescribing for hepatic dysfunction and can potentiate hypotension with prazosin, reserpine, hydralazine, cimetidine, and antithyroid drugs. It can increase the cardiac effects of verapamil and lidocaine. It has decreased effectiveness with Indocin, barbiturates, and rifampin. Adverse reactions include depression, cold hands and feet, CHF, edema, syncope, chest pain, and angina.

Nadolol (Corgard) is a noncardioselective form of beta blocker. It is therefore contraindicated in asthma, peripheral vascular disease, and diabetes.

Pindolol (Visken) is noncardioselective and because of intrinsic sympathomimetic activity, less apt to cause extremity coldness. It has less effect on resting heart rate and cardiac output than propranolol.

Propranolol HCl (Inderal) is the oldest form of beta blocker. It is noncardioselective and therefore has the adverse effects of hypotension and depression. In addition, it can produce peripheral ischemia, CNS disturbance, bronchospasm, CHF, and reduced exercise tolerance, adversely affect plasma lipids, and decrease liver glucose metabolism. It can cause agranulocytosis. Despite this side effect profile, it has been shown to decrease mortality for patients following myocardial infarction in the ISIS-I study.[1] It is also useful for subaortic stenosis. Its use should be avoided in Wolff-Parkinson-White syndrome. It is potentiated by alcohol, CNS depressants, other antihypertensives, antithyroid drugs, haloperidol, chlorpromazine, and cimetidine; it is antagonized by barbiturates, rifampin, and phenytoin. It may increase the effects of lidocaine and potentiate theophylline.

Timolol (Blocadren) is noncardioselective, but is useful for hypertension.

Contextual Issues   Early versions of beta blockers such as propranolol are available in a cheaper generic form, which might be important for patients. Abrupt cessation of beta blockers should be avoided. Beta blockers can decrease exercise tolerance for some patients. This information should be included in patient teaching. For patients who need both beta blockers and diuretics to control hypertension, combined dosage forms are available. The use of these forms should not be initiated until proper doses of individual drugs are determined. Also consider that the combined form of drug might be more expensive than two separate generic forms.

Inotropes

Prescribing Considerations

Digitalis derivatives are often used to treat congestive heart failure. In the past, digitalis derivatives were considered the first-line therapy. Recently, ACE inhibitors have been replacing digitalis as the first-line drug to treat congestive heart failure. Digitalis increases inotropic response by increasing intracellular calcium, which is needed to support the actin and myosin movement that supports muscle contraction. Calcium enhances actin and myosin cross-bridging. Digitalis bonds to the sodium-potassium ATPase enzyme, inhibiting the sodium pump. This increases intracellular sodium and facilitates the exchange of sodium and calcium. Digitalis also enhances the cardiac effects of the parasympathetic nervous system, which slow the rate of SA node impulse generation and increase the block of impulses at the AV node. This makes the AV node refractory to conduct fast atrial impulses such as those found in atrial fibrillation. This causes a decreased ventricular response to supraventricular arrhythmias such as atrial fibrillation and flutter. It also decreases SA node automaticity. In high doses, digoxin can increase ventricular excitability. One limitation of the use of digoxin therapy is the fact that toxic effects are increased with low serum potassium and high serum calcium. Toxic levels of the drug are close to therapeutic levels.

Prescribing Variables

Digoxin is the most commonly used glycoside. When a patient is started on digoxin, initial doses are higher. A full digitalizing dose is 0.5 mg daily for 3 days. Once the patient is digitalized, maintenance levels can be achieved with 0.25 to 0.125 mg a day. Digoxin has a half-life of 36 to 48 hours and is primarily excreted by the kidneys. Elderly patients are prone to toxicity if their kidneys have a decreased creatinine clearance rate. Absorption of digoxin is decreased by bile acid sequestrants, broad-spectrum antibiotics, and antacids. Serum digoxin levels can be increased with concomitant use of quinidine, verapamil, amiodarone, and propafanone. This can move a patient from therapeutic to toxic levels of digoxin. There is a narrow therapeutic index resulting in frequent toxicities. Toxic signs are anorexia, headache, disorientation, AV conduction delays, SA arrest, premature ventricular contractions, and Mobitz type I blocks.

ACE Inhibitors

Prescribing Considerations

Angiotensin-converting enzyme (ACE) inhibitors are the drugs of choice in congestive heart failure. They work in two ways to improve patient response to the condition. First, by blocking the conversion of angiotensin I to angiotensin II, they prevent the vasoconstrictive effects of angiotensin II. This decreases blood pressure and afterload, decreasing the workload of the heart. Furthermore, by blocking angiotensin II, one powerful stimulant for aldosterone is blocked. Blocking aldosterone results in excretion of sodium by the kidneys; this results in less edema. At the same time, potassium is preserved. In addition, ACE inhibitors block the degradation of bradykinin, which increases the production of vasodilating prostaglandins. Indirectly, ACE inhibitors inhibit the sympathetic nervous system.

Post–myocardial infarction heart function can be improved by using captopril. Studies have shown decreased incidence of heart failure and mortality with this drug begun 3 to 16 days following infarction.[2]

Prescribing Variables

Patient Variables   ACE inhibitors are useful antihypertensive agents for patients with heart failure, diabetes, asthma, and peripheral vascular disease. They are contraindicated in pregnancy (category D) because they can cause renal changes in the fetus during the second and third trimesters. They can cause taste disturbances and rash. ACE inhibitors are not as effective in hypertension for African-Americans as they are for whites. They are, however, good for diabetic patients. In diabetics ACE inhibitors have been shown to reduce proteinuria and to slow the progression of nephropathy. Preliminary studies have also shown that they decrease insulin resistance.

Drug Variables   The most frequent side effect of the use of ACE inhibitors is a dry cough. This cough is persistent and requires a change to a different drug category. Renal function should be monitored. ACE inhibitors can precipitate acute renal failure and can cause hyperkalemia with renal insufficiency. Potassium-sparing diuretics and potassium supplementation should be avoided during ACE inhibitor therapy.

Drugs in Category   Drugs in this group include those shown in Table 13-4.

TABLE 13-4

ACE Inhibitors

Drug	Trade Name	Comment
Benazepril	Lotensin	Given in pro-drug form, good for elderly
Captopril	Capoten	Short-acting, more likely to cause rash
Enalapril	Vasotec	Longer half-life, fewer doses than captopril
Fosinopril	Monopril	Eliminated by both renal and hepatic routes; good for elderly
Lisinopril	Prinivil, Zestril	Once-daily dosing
Moexipril	Univasc	
Quinapril	Accupril	Most potent
Ramipril	Altace	Once-daily dosing
Trandolapril	Mavik	

Contextual Issues   For patients with both congestive heart failure and hypertension, ACE inhibitors are an excellent drug choice. For hypertension alone, ACE inhibitors are more expensive than simple thiazide diuretics or beta blockers.

Angiotensin II Receptor Antagonists

A new drug, losartan (Hyzaar), acts by blocking receptor sites for angiotensin II; it does not prevent angiotensin II production. It should be avoided in pregnant women and is not as useful for hypertension in African-American patients as it is in whites.

Antiarrhythmics

Prescribing Considerations

The causes of any arrhythmia must be considered when choosing drug therapy. Classes of disorders require different classes of drugs. General groups of disorders include problems with (a) automaticity, that is, ectopic beats fire when not expected, (b) sinoatrial node arrest results in a lack of normal impulse generation, requiring backup systems to fire or resulting in loss of cardiac impulses, or (c) reentry arrhythmia occurs when some small section of myocardium is selectively refractory to impulse transmission. As these areas eventually are able to transmit, they regenerate a new impulse. Serious arrhythmias require cardiologist evaluation. These are not conditions that nurses in advanced practice manage independently. General information is given here for patients in a general practice who happen to be receiving antiarrhythmic therapy. Advanced practice nurses in a cardiology setting will acquire specialized knowledge in this area.

Prescribing Variables

Patient Variables   Drugs that patients currently use, legal and illegal, as well as alcohol ingestion can contribute to arrhythmia development. As always, a good history is essential to good clinical care.

Drug Variables   Antiarrhythmic drugs are grouped in several different classes, depending upon which phase of depolarization they affect.

Class I drugs are sodium channel blockers. Class Ia drugs slow the rate of rise of action potential and prolong the duration of the action potential. They decrease phase 0 depolarization. They are useful for supraventricular tachycardia, ventricular tachycardia, ventricular fibrillation, and symptomatic ventricular premature beats (PVCs). They slow conduction of impulses and increase refractoriness of cells to transmit new impulses. This helps to prevent reentry phenomena because all cells are made refractory to match the underlying refractory area. This results in a normal, orderly transmission of impulses.

Class Ib drugs shorten action potential and repolarization and have no effect on conduction. They are useful for ventricular tachycardia (VT), ventricular fibrillation, and symptomatic PVCs. Class Ic drugs prolong action potential rate of rise, decrease phase 0 depolarization, and slow repolarization more than Class Ia drugs.

Class II antiarrhythmics are the beta blockers discussed in detail elsewhere. They work to decrease arrhythmias by decreasing automaticity and prolonging AV conduction, making them a good treatment for supraventricular tachycardia. They also may prevent ventricular fibrillation.

Class III antiarrhythmics are potassium blockers that prolong repolarization, widen the QRS wave, prolong the QT interval, and increase refractoriness. They are useful for refractory VT and supraventricular tachycardia and can prevent VT and ventricular fibrillation.

Class IV drugs are the calcium channel blockers discussed earlier in this chapter. They work as antiarrhythmics by decreasing automaticity and decreasing AV conduction and are useful for supraventricular tachycardia.

Some sources classify digoxin as a Class V antiarrhythmic and include adenosine in this category as well.

Ironically, all antiarrhythmic drugs can actually promote arrhythmias. This is a major side effect of antiarrhythmic drug therapy.

Drugs in Category   Table 13-5 summarizes antiarrhythmic drugs by group.

Disopyramide (Norpace) has anticholinergic effects which can cause urinary retention in affected individuals, as well as worsening glaucoma. It can also cause decreased cardiac output, confusion, delirium, and memory problems in the elderly.

Procainamide (Pronestyl) can cause systemic lupus erythematosus symptoms in some individuals. Patients should be monitored for joint pain and renal function. In general, however, it has fewer side effects than quinidine. CBC, EKG, BP, liver enzymes, and ANA titers should be monitored.

TABLE 13-5

Antiarrhythmic Drugs

Class	Drugs and Actions	Types of Arrhythmias

Class Ia
  Sodium channel
  blockers
	Quinidine, procainamide;
	  slow phase 0
	  depolarization
		Atrial flutter,
		  atrial fibrillation,
		  AV nodal and
		  ventricular arrhythmias

Ib	Lidocaine, tocainide,
	  mexiletine; shorten
	  phase 3 repolarization
		Ventricular arrhythmias

Ic	Encainide, flecainide,
	  others; markedly slow
	  phase 0 depolarization
		Severe ventricular
		  arrhythmias

Class II
  Beta blockers
	Propranolol, others;
	  suppress phase 4
	  depolarization
		Atrial flutter,
		  atrial fibrillation,
		  AV nodal reentry

Class III
  Potassium channel
  blockers
	Amiodarone, bretylium;
	  prolong phase 3
	  repolarization
		Ventricular tachycardia
		  fibrillation

Class IV
  Calcium channel
  blockers
	Verapamil, diltiazem,
	  others; shorten action
	  potential
		Paroxysmal supraventricular
		  tachycardia, atrial flutter,
		  atrial fibrillation

Tocainide (Tonocard) can cause nausea, vomiting, dizziness, tremor, confusion, bone marrow depression, hepatitis, and lung inflammation. The patient's EKG, CBC, CXR, and liver enzymes should be monitored.

Mexiletine (Mexitil) slows the heart rate. Patients should be monitored for bleeding tendencies, EKG, and liver enzymes with long-term therapy.

Contextual Issues   Patients with serious arrhythmias will need emotional support from the nurse practitioner.

Vasodilators

Prescribing Considerations

Hydralazine and minoxidil decrease peripheral vascular resistance by dilating the arterioles and can be used as adjuncts in hypertension therapy. They are not considered first-line drugs. They decrease afterload but do not have some of the side effects of alpha blockers, such as postural hypotension, sexual dysfunction, or weakness. These drugs can have a rebound effect that stimulates the heart and therefore should not be used with angina patients. Patients on long-term therapy should be monitored for chest pain. These drugs can increase plasma renin, decrease sodium excretion, and cause edema. Vasodilators should be combined with diuretics and/or beta blockers in treating hypertension. This will decrease fluid retention and reflex tachycardia which can accompany vasodilator therapy.

As with other antihypertensives, nonpharmacologic measures of weight loss, sodium restriction, regular exercise, and avoidance of stress are recommended.

Prescribing Variables

Patient Variables   In general, avoid using vasodilators in patients with CHF and coronary artery disease. Side effects include postural hypotension. Patients develop a tolerance to these drugs, and when discontinuing these drugs a gradual tapering of dosage and timing is required to prevent rebound hypertension. In patients using vasodilators for hypertension, heart rate, blood pressure, ANA titers, CBC, and direct Coomb's test should be monitored.

Drug Variables   Hydralazine can cause systemic lupus erythematosus (SLE). Patients should be monitored for joint pain. ANA titers can be drawn for patients for whom SLE is suspected.

Drugs in Category   Hydralazine (Apresoline) is contraindicated with severe renal impairment, and patients should be monitored for lupus-like syndromes. Minoxidil (Loniten) should be used with beta blockers and diuretics, not alone. It can cause pericardial effusion and hirsutism.

Contextual Issues   This group of drugs is not to be used for first-line therapy for hypertension. They can be useful when therapy with beta blockers and diuretics is not effective.

Adrenergic Antagonists

Prescribing Considerations

Drug Variables   Alpha$_1$ receptor blockers include prazosin (Minipress), terazosin (Hytrin), and doxazosin (Cardura). As with other antihypertensives, nonpharmacologic measures of weight loss, sodium restriction, regular exercise, and avoidance of stress are recommended. Alpha$_1$ receptor blockers are selected as adjunctive blood pressure medications. Alpha blockers dilate both arterioles and venules and therefore are useful for hypertensive patients with concurrent congestive heart failure. They are most effective when combined or added to beta-blocker therapy. This group of drugs is useful for hypertensive patients with asthma, heart block, and peripheral vascular and renal disease. Alpha blockers can cause postural hypotension, and tolerance to these drugs develops. First-dose syncope has been reported, and therefore first doses should be low and taken at bedtime. Sexual dysfunction and nightmares have been reported. For all these drugs, standing blood pressure should be monitored.

Peripheral adrenergic antagonists must be used with caution. Reserpine in high doses has been associated with depression and suicide. Guanethidine can cause decreased cardiac output, decreased systolic blood pressure, and exertional hypotension.

Centrally acting alpha$_2$ agonists stimulate receptors in the central nervous system that inhibit sympathetic activity centrally and indirectly block sympathetic activation. Methyldopa has been used safely for both mother and fetus in pregnant women, but has side effects of dry mouth and sedation. It can also cause hepatotoxicity and autoimmune disorders. Clonidine can cause rebound hypertension if discontinued suddenly. It comes in a patch form that can be left on for a week. Guanabenz and guanfacine are also in this group of drugs.

Hypolipidemics

Lowering serum cholesterol through the use of antihyperlipidemic drugs has been shown to reduce deaths due to coronary heart disease.

Prescribing Considerations

Hyperlipidemia is a cluster of conditions. Clinicians should carefully evaluate the pattern of hyperlipidemia before beginning therapy. Fasting lipid panels are required for accurate assessment of the lipid disorder. Some cases of hyperlipidemia are due to a familial tendency to overproduce cholesterol. Other cases are related to both genetic and dietary influences. Secondary hyperlipidemia can result from diabetes mellitus, alcohol intake, thyroid disturbance, or liver cirrhosis. Secondary disorders require the control of the underlying problem as well as consideration of treating the hyperlipidemia. Before prescribing medications, patients should be instructed in changing their diets to reduce saturated fats, mostly animal fats, to increase dietary fiber, and to increase aerobic exercise.

Prescribing Variables

Patient Variables   Types of hyperlipidemia are summarized in Table 13-6. Type I, familial hyperchylomicronemia, is a genetic disorder that is rare in clinical practice. There is no increased risk of coronary artery disease and no drug treatment is recommended, but dietary control is sometimes recommended. Types IIa, familial hyperbetalipoproteinemia, and IIb, familial mixed hyperlipidemia, are the most common forms of the condition. Dietary control of fatty foods and increased fiber and exercise are recommended. Type III, familial dysbetalipoproteinemia, is frequently associated with xanthomas and is rare. It is associated with increased coronary artery disease. In addition to the dietary changes recommended above, patients should limit alcohol intake. Type IV, familial hypertriglyceridemia, is common and is associated with increased risk of coronary artery disease. This group of patients should also restrict alcohol consumption. Type

TABLE 13-6

Categories of Hyperlipidemia

Type	Cholesterol	VLDL	LDL	HDL	Triglycerides	Useful Drugs
I	normal				highly elevated	None
IIa	elevated		elevated		normal	statin, BAS, or NA
IIb	elevated	elevated	elevated		elevated	BAS plus NA
III	elevated	elevated	elevated		elevated	NA, gem, or clo
IV	normal and elevated	elevated			elevated	NA or gem
V	elevated	elevated	decreased		highly elevated	NA and/or clo

statin = HMG CoA reductase group; BAS = bile acid sequestrant; NA = nicotinic acid; gem = gemfibrozil; clo = clofibrate.

V, familial mixed hypertriglyceridemia, is rare. The dietary recommendation is a high-protein, low-fat, low-carbohydrate diet with no alcohol.

Overall goals of therapy in hyperlipidemia are to keep LDL cholesterol below 160 mg/dL with no more than one cardiac risk factor, or below 130 mg/dL with two or more cardiac risk factors.

Drug Variables Fibric (isobutyric) acid derivatives such as clofibrate (Atromid-S) and gemfibrozil (Lopid) lower both VLDL cholesterol and triglycerides. In some patients they raise HDL cholesterol. These drugs are contraindicated with hepatic impairment and should not be used with the HMG CoA reductase drugs (statins). Side effects include gastrointestinal distress, headache, and myalgia. Gallbladder disease is possible with clofibrate.

Bile acid sequestrants such as colestipol (Colestid) and cholestyramine (Questran Light) are used in conjunction with control of dietary fats and with the promotion of exercise. This group of drugs acts as an exchange resin that is not absorbed systemically but acts locally in the GI tract to trap bile acids and carry them out with the stool. This prevents recycling of the bile and necessitates liver production of bile, causing a loss of LDL cholesterol and triglycerides. Additionally, with long-term use, the liver becomes more efficient in removing cholesterol from the blood.

During therapy, digoxin, propranolol, and the lipid panel should be monitored. Patients may need fat-soluble vitamin supplementation. Drug interactions include reduced absorption of thiazides, furosemide, tetracycline, penicillin G, and gemfibrozil. Because of the binding capacity of these drugs, they should not be taken within one hour of other drugs. Adverse reactions include constipation, impaction, and hemorrhoids. Patients should be instructed to take these drugs with adequate fluids.

Drugs in Category HMG CoA reductase inhibitors interfere with an enzyme necessary for the body to produce cholesterol. Drugs in this group are used as an adjunct to a total program of lipid control including dietary reduction of saturated fats and exercise. They are contraindicated in active liver disease and unexplained elevated serum transaminase. They should not be prescribed for women who might be pregnant; these drugs are listed as pregnancy category X. Liver function, especially for alcoholics, should be monitored; discontinue with myopathy or elevated CPK. Interaction effects are found with gemfibrozil and clofibrate, immunosuppressive agents, nicotinic acid, and erythromycin. Patients who are taking oral anticoagulants or digoxin should be monitored closely. Adverse effects include GI upset and rhabdomyolysis. When following patients, question them about muscle pains or inflammation. Liver toxicity is a possibility with this drug group and liver function tests should be given every 6 weeks. HMG CoA reductase inhibitors should never be given with gemfibrozil. This combination can cause muscle and kidney damage. If taken with cholestyramine, HMG CoA reductase inhibitors should be taken one hour before or four hours after the cholestyramine to ensure proper absorption of the drug from the GI tract.

For patients on fluvastatin (Lescol), monitor for endocrine dysfunction. Lovastatin (Mevacor) slows progression of coronary atherosclerosis. Adverse effects include blurred vision and pruritus. Lovastatin is lipid soluble.

Pravastatin (Pravachol) must be used with caution with ketoconazole, spironolactone, and cimetidine. Adverse reactions include headache, myalgia, rash, chest pain, fatigue, cough, and influenza symptoms. Pravastatin is less lipid soluble than lovastatin.

Simvastatin (Zocor) is another member of this group.

Niacin (Nicolar) decreases liver production of triglycerides. This prevents VLDL synthesis. It is used as adjunctive therapy for hyperlipidemia. Nicotinic acid derivatives do everything that antihyperlipidemic drugs should do. They lower LDL cholesterol and triglycerides while increasing HDL cholesterol. Their usefulness is limited by side effects that many patients find intolerable, notably flushing and a feeling that the skin is burning hot. This can be minimized by taking 120 to 300 mg of aspirin 30 min prior to the niacin dose.

Patients should be instructed to take this drug with food. This drug is contraindicated with liver dysfunction, active peptic ulcers, or arterial bleeding. Precautions should be taken for patients with gallbladder disease or a history of jaundice, liver disease, gout, or diabetes. Liver function and glucose should be monitored. This drug can potentiate antihypertensives. Patients should be monitored for myopathy if concurrently taking HMG CoA reductase inhibitors. Adverse effects include arrhythmias, flushing, glucose intolerance, peptic ulcer, abnormal liver function tests, jaundice, GI upset, dry skin, hyperuricemia, pruritus, toxic amblyopia, hypotension, and headache. Patients can premedicate with aspirin or ibuprofen as a precaution against flushing. The dosage should be started low and gradually increased as patients tolerate the drug.

Contextual Issues   Patient compliance with the prescribed regimen can be an important factor with antihyperlipidemics. Side effects are more bothersome in the short term for patients than the asymptomatic condition. Frequent monitoring and open feedback on progress can help to motivate patients. Inquire about side effects and work as a team with the patient and family to minimize side effects while encouraging staying on the prescribed regimen. Nicotinic acid is the cheapest drug regimen available for hyperlipidemia.

Diuretics

Prescribing Considerations

Diuretics are useful in relieving moderate to severe congestive heart failure. They are needed even when other drugs such as ACE inhibitors are in use. In addition they are useful as monotherapy for the management of hypertension. Dietary sodium restriction is useful in the control of hypertension and edema. Patients should be instructed about appropriate sodium restriction.

Prescribing Variables

Patient Variables   Thiazide diuretics can elevate serum uric acid levels and exacerbate gout. Diuretics are a good first choice for stage 1 and 2 hypertension. They are particularly useful for African-American patients and the elderly.

Drug Variables   Several groups of diuretics exist. Thiazide diuretics are the usual first-line choice for hypertension. They have the benefit for the elderly of preventing calcium loss from bone. They have been used safely for many years and are available in economic generic forms and can be given in single daily doses. However, they can cause elevated serum uric acid, glucose, cholesterol, and triglycerides. They can deplete potassium, magnesium, and sodium. Thiazide diuretics inhibit sodium and chloride reabsorption in the ascending loop of Henle, which causes a mild diuresis.

Loop diuretics are stronger than thiazides and can be used in patients with borderline renal function. They can cause dehydration and loss of potassium, sodium, magnesium, and calcium. They can cause metabolic alkalosis and a rise in serum glucose and uric acid. They can also lead to blood dyscrasias. High doses of loop diuretics can be nephrotoxic and ototoxic.

When using potassium-sparing diuretics, check the full list of medications patients are taking. They should not be used in conjunction with potassium supplements or with ACE inhibitors.

Drugs in Category   Table 13-7 summarizes the types of diuretics.

Contextual Issues   Thiazide diuretics are excellent choices for first-line hypertension management. They are inexpensive, but costs of monitoring serum electrolytes need to be considered in overall management cost estimates. For patients who require both thiazides and beta blockers or calcium channel blockers, several combination formulations are available. These may be more expensive than single preparations, but the convenience and possible better adherence to the therapeutic regimen might be justified for some patients.

TABLE 13-7

Diuretics

Drug	Trade Name
Thiazides	
Chlorothiazide	Diuril
Hydrochlorothiazide	Esidrix, HydroDiuril, Oretic
Indapamide	Lozol
Methyclothiazide	Enduron
Metolazone	Mykrox, Zaroxolyn
Loop Diuretics	
Bumetanide	Bumex
Ethacrynic acid	Edecrin
Furosemide	Lasix
Potassium-Sparing Diuretics	
Amiloride	Midamor
Spironolactone	Aldactone
Triamterene	Dyrenium

REFERENCES

1. ISIS-1 First International Study of Infarct Survival Collaborative Group: Randomised trial of intravenous atenolol among 16,027 cases of suspected acute myocardial infarction: ISIS-1. *Lancet* 2(8498):57–66, 1986.
2. Rutherford JD, Pfeffer MA, Moye LA, et al: Effects of captopril on ischemic events after myocardial infarction: Results of the Survival and Ventricular Enlargement trial (SAVE). *Circulation* 90:1731–1738, 1994.

SELECTED BIBLIOGRAPHY

Alderman MH: Which antihypertensive drugs first—and why! *JAMA* 267:2786–2787, 1992.
Ciccone CD: Current trends in cardiovascular pharmacology. *Phys Ther* 76:481–497, 1996.
Collins R, Peto R, MacMahon S, et al: Blood pressure, stroke and coronary heart disease. Part 2: Short term reductions in blood pressure: Overview of randomised drug trials in their epidemiological context. *Lancet* 335:827–838, 1990.
Goldszer R: Hypertension in the elderly. *Prim Care Newsletter* 2(6):4–6, 1991.
Harvey RA, Champe PC: *Lippincott's Illustrated Reviews: Pharmacology,* 2d ed. Philadelphia: Lippincott, 1996.
Kaplan NM: *Clinical Hypertension.* Baltimore: Williams & Wilkins, 1994.
Kayser SR: Pharmacology news: Antiarrhythmic drug therapy. Part 1: General principles of drug selection. *Prog Cardiovasc Nurs* 11(2):33–37, 1996.

Koda-Kimble MA, Young LY (eds): *Applied Therapeutics,* 5th ed. Vancouver: Applied Therapeutics, 1992.

Lubsen J, Tijsenn JG: Efficacy of nifedipine and metoprolol in the early treatment of unstable angina in the coronary care unit: Findings from the Holland Interuniversity Nifedipine/metoprolol Trial (HINT). *Am J Cardiol* 60(2):18A–25A, 1987.

Miller MM: Current trends in the primary care management of chronic congestive heart failure. *Nurse Pract* 19(5):64–72, 1994.

Morgensen CE: Angiotensin converting enzyme inhibitors and diabetic nephropathy: Their effects on proteinuria may be independent of their effects on blood pressure. *Br Med J* 304:327–328, 1992.

National Institutes of Health. *The Fifth Report of the Joint National Committee of Detection, Evaluation and Treatment of High Blood Pressure.* NIH Publication No. 93-1088. Bethesda, MD: NIH, 1993.

Porsche R: Hypertension: Diagnosis, acute antihypertension therapy, and long term management *AACN Clin Issues* 6:515–525, 1995.

Porterfield LM, Porterfield JG: Understanding cardiovascular drug interaction. *Focus Crit Care.* 17:412–416, 1990.

RISC Group. Risk of myocardial infarction and death during treatment with low dose aspirin and intravenous heparin in men with unstable coronary artery disease. *Lancet* 336:827–830, 1990.

SHEP Cooperative Research Group. Prevention of stroke by antihypertensive drug treatment in older persons with isolated systolic hypertension. *JAMA* 265:3255–3264, 1991.

Skillings J: Improving survival in congestive heart failure: The role of ACE inhibitors. *Phys Assist* July:26–45, 1995.

Tierney LM, McPhee SJ, Papadakis MA, Schroeder SA: *Current Medical Diagnosis and Treatment,* 36th ed. Stamford, CT: Appleton & Lange, 1997.

Woodhead GA: The management of cholesterol in coronary heart disease risk reduction. *Nurse Pract* 21(9):45, 48, 51, 1996.

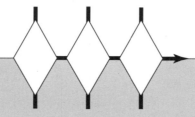

Chapter 14

DRUG THERAPY IN PEPTIC ULCER DISEASE AND GERD

Laurel A. Eisenhauer

OVERVIEW OF DRUG THERAPY AND PATHOPHYSIOLOGY

Peptic ulcer disease had long been considered to be the result of excess production of hydrochloric acid, which then results in gastric distress and ulceration of the gastric and duodenal mucosa. More recently the pathophysiology has come to be seen as a multi-causal imbalance between gastric acid and mucosal integrity—a breakdown in mucosal defenses from excess acid production, inhibition of prostaglandin protection of the mucosa, and impairment of the mucosal integrity.

Drug therapy is now directed primarily toward suppression of acid production through H_2 blockers (cimetidine, ranitidine, famotidine, and nizatidine) and proton pump inhibitors (omeprazole) or enhancement or protection of mucosal integrity (sucralfate, misoprostol, and antibiotics to control *Helicobacter pylori* infection). Antacids continue to be used, primarily for the control of pain; although they can promote healing of ulcers, they are inconvenient due to the multiple doses (e.g., seven times per day) required throughout the day. A prostaglandin analogue (misoprostol) is sometimes given with NSAIDs to replace the prostaglandin in the stomach mucosa; however, dosages that are considered to be therapeutic also produce considerable side effects such as abdominal cramping, diarrhea, and uterine contractions.

Gastroesophageal reflux disorder (GERD) is a result of dysfunction of antireflux mechanisms, resulting in a reflux of gastric contents containing acid, pepsin, bile, and pancreatic enzymes into the lower esophagus. It is aggravated by hiatal hernia and other conditions (e.g., pregnancy, obesity) in which abdominal pressure is increased; it can lead to esophagitis and the formation of strictures. It has also been associated with acute episodes of asthma—GERD may provoke asthma, and asthma may promote GERD.[1] Drug therapy is similar to that for peptic ulcer disease. In addition, prokinetics such as cisapride may be used to increase lower esophageal sphincter (LES) tone and to promote gastric emptying.

Selected Bibliography

Fay M, Jaffe PE: Diagnostic and treatment guidelines for *Helicobacter pylori. Nurse Pract* 21(7):28, 30, 33–34, 38, 1996.

Helicobacter pylori in peptic ulcer disease—interim draft statement. *NIH Consensus Statement Online* 12(1), Jan. 7–9, 1994.

Soll AH: Practice Parameters Committee of the American College of Gastroenterology. Medical treatment of peptic ulcer disease practice guidelines. *JAMA* 275(8):622–629, 1996. [Published erratum appears in *JAMA* 275(17):1314, 1996.]

Sullivan CA, Samuelson WM: Gastroesophageal reflux: A common exacerbating factor in adult asthma. *Nurse Pract* 21(11):82, 84, 93–94, 96, 1996.

ISSUES IN DRUG THERAPY

Prescribing Considerations

Peptic ulcer disease occurs as a result of multiple factors. In some individuals stress and emotional responses can increase the production of HCl and gastric symptoms; in these individuals the use of relaxation techniques and other stress-reducing strategies may help to prevent or treat peptic ulcers. Diet adaptations to avoid foods that cause symptoms of gastric distress are recommended but are individualized to those affecting the individual patient. Although various foods (e.g., spicy foods, caffeine beverages, milk) are known to increase the production of gastric acid and produce dyspepsia, they have not been shown to cause gastric ulcers. Alcohol can result in mucosal damage and bleeding, but its role in causing peptic ulcer disease is not clear. Cigarette smoking should be discouraged because of its association with the occurrence of peptic ulcer disease, delay in healing of peptic ulcers, and recurrence rate.[2]

Ulcerogenic drugs should be considered as a potential cause of gastric irritation; certain oral antibiotics (e.g., tetracycline, erythromycin) and aspirin and other NSAIDs cause gastric irritation. Glucocorticosteroids are thought to contribute to ulcer formation through their inhibition of prostaglandin.

Aspirin and NSAIDs are considered to be ulcerogenic. More than three aspirins a day may result in a sixfold increase in the risk of gastric ulcer.[3] In addition, aspirin and NSAIDs through their effects on platelets can contribute to bleeding of ulcers or other lesions. The effects of one aspirin on platelets may last up to 10 days, and the effects of one dose of an NSAID up to 3 days.

About 10 percent of patients taking NSAIDs will have an active ulcer. Gastric or duodenal bleeding from aspirin and NSAIDs occurs more frequently in elderly patients (over 60 years) and can occur without symptoms of gastric distress (e.g., epigastric pain).

Initial treatment for GERD consists of lifestyle alterations. The patient should be taught not to lie down for at least three hours after eating or at least a half hour after taking medications, to eat small low-fat protein-rich meals, to lose weight (if appropriate), to raise the head of the bed at least 6 inches (or use a wedge to keep the upper body in an equivalent position), and to stop smoking. Foods that should be avoided include peppermint, citric juices, onion, alcohol, chocolate, coffee and other caffeine-containing foods, and tomatoes. Drugs that might lower the LES pressure should also be avoided if possible. Such drugs are calcium channel blockers, morphine, nitrates, theophylline, sedatives, progesterone, ethanol, nicotine, and estrogen.

Patient Variables

An assessment of measures initiated by the patient is important. Since H_2 blockers and antacids are available over the counter, patients may have been taking these drugs before consulting a clinician. Home remedies such as baking soda (sodium bicarbonate) may also have been tried by patients.

Renal function is important to consider since the dosages of H_2 blockers may need to be decreased. Also, patients with renal insufficiency may experience side effects of antacids (see below). Patients who are pregnant should not receive misoprostol since this stimulates uterine contractions. Patients with CHF or with fluid and electrolyte imbalances may have complications from certain antacids (e.g., those containing sodium).

Allergies, especially to antiinfectives or aspirin, are important to determine since this could influence choice of drugs for treating *H. pylori* infection. Assessment of patient potential to comply with complex drug regimens is of particular importance in antiinfective therapy for *H. pylori* infection where three to four doses of several drugs over a 2-week period is usually involved. Antacid therapy with the goal of peptic ulcer treatment (rather than just pain relief) requires frequent dosing during the day (e.g., seven to eight doses).

Drug Variables

Drug Selection

Goals of therapy for both peptic ulcer disease and GERD are relief of symptoms, prevention or healing of any ulcers, and prevention of complications and reoccurrence. Pain relief usually occurs in 7 to 10 days with gastric ulcers and somewhat longer for duodenal ulcers.

Drug therapy in the presence of peptic ulcer should be viewed in relation to a time line for treatment. Most peptic ulcers (65 to 90 percent) can be healed with pharmacologic agents in 6 to 12 weeks, with gastric ulcers requiring a longer healing time than duodenal ulcers. Pain usually is relieved in the first 7 to 10 days.

Therapy with omeprazole has been considered to be time-limited (4 weeks) because of concerns that it may produce cancer, although this has only been demonstrated in rats and not in humans to date. Safety beyond 4 weeks has begun to be demonstrated.

Maintenance therapy may be necessary in patients who continue to experience recurrence, e.g., patients on NSAID therapy, patients with a history of bleeding or perforated ulcer, elderly patients (over 60 years), and smokers. Maintenance therapy usually is an H_2 blocker at bedtime for a year.

Treating **H. pylori** *Infection*   The recognition that a microorganism may play a major role as the cause of peptic ulcer disease has been revolutionary but also somewhat controversial despite an NIH consensus statement. *H. pylori* is a gram-negative spiral organism that infects only the gastric epithelium. Its incidence increases with increasing age; an estimated 60 percent of people over 60 years have *H. pylori*. Not everyone who has *H. pylori* infection has a peptic ulcer; however, an estimated 90 percent of persons with peptic ulcer have *H. pylori* infection.[2] Thus *H. pylori* infection is not the sole causative factor in peptic ulcer disease. Because of this some clinicians have been reluctant to use antibiotic therapy that would unnecessarily expose the patient to risks of side effects, as well as possibly contribute to the development of resistant strains of microorganisms. However, treatment protocols for *H. pylori* infection in peptic ulcer disease have been successful in achieving healing in 10 to 12 days of treatment.

Antiinfectives for treating *H. pylori* infections ideally are initiated only with confirmation of the infection. The gold standard for this is the gastric biopsy for histology and also for culture and sensitivity. However, two less invasive tests are now available: a breath test which detects urease in stomach (but may produce false negatives shortly after treatment) and a serum ELISA test to detect IgG and IgA antibodies to *H. pylori*.

H_2 Blockers   Currently there are four H_2 blockers available in the United States: cimetidine (Tagamet), ranitidine (Zantac), famotidine (Pepcid), and nizatidine (Axid). All are now available OTC; OTC preparations and recommended doses are half of the prescription dose.

All H_2 blockers are considered to be equally effective, with the main differences being in side effects and drug interactions. Healing rates are 75 to 90 percent at 4 to 8 weeks for duodenal ulcers and 65 to 90 percent at 8 to 12 weeks for gastric ulcers.[2] Cimetidine inhibits activity of the cytochrome P-450 pathway in the liver, resulting in potentially slower metabolism of other drugs metabolized by this mechanism. Higher serum levels and possible toxic effects of these other drugs (e.g., benzodiazepines, warfarin, propranolol, theophylline) may occur particularly in patients with decreased renal function or other conditions that may affect elimination of these drugs from the body. Generally the clearance of these drugs will be reduced by 20 to 30 percent.[4] The other three H_2 blockers have little or no effect on the P-450 system. Cimetidine and ranitidine inhibit renal excretion of procainamide and its metabolite by competing for renal tubular secretion.

H_2 blockers may affect the absorption of other drugs. By raising the pH of the GI tract, cimetidine has been shown to slow the dissolution of ketoconazole. Cimetidine, ranitidine, and nizatidine may increase ethanol absorption by inhibiting gastric alcohol dehydrogenase; however, this has not been confirmed by other research.[4]

Cimetidine was the first H_2 blocker on the market; therefore, it has the longest history of use and more known side effects that may or may not occur with the other H_2 blockers as they are used more widely and over longer periods of time. Cimetidine side effects include GI discomfort, CNS symptoms (e.g., confusion, drowsiness, headache), muscular aches, and gynecomastia and impotence from antiandrogenic effects. Initially, cimetidine dosing was four times a day; now all H_2 blockers are usually considered to be effective for most patients with once-a-day dosing at night.

Proton Pump Inhibitors   Proton pump inhibitors (omeprazole and lansoprazole) are potent inhibitors of acid secretion and can produce healing in 4 weeks in up to 90 to 100 percent of patients with peptic ulcers. They are given once daily in the morning. They are useful in treating patients with GERD. Use beyond 8 weeks is not recommended because of concerns about its prolonged achlorhydria and potential for carcinogenesis. Dosage adjustments in patients with renal dysfunction or mild liver dysfunction usually are not indicated. These drugs bind with certain subcomponents of the cytochrome P-450 system and thus do not affect all drugs metabolized by the P-450 system. Omeprazole slows the metabolism of diazepam, phenytoin, tolbutamide, and warfarin. Lansoprazole may increase the clearance of theophylline; the absorption and bioavailability of lansoprazole can be delayed by coadministration with sucralfate. Their effect on gastric pH could affect the absorption of drugs affected by gastric pH (e.g., digoxin).

Antacids   Although antacids can produce ulcer healing with multiple doses per day, their use has been supplanted by other agents that are more convenient for patients to take. Currently most antacids are used on a PRN basis for the relief of pain.

Antacids differ from each other primarily in their strength (acid-neutralizing capacity, or ANC) and the ingredients which cause different side effects. Magnesium and sodium ingredients tend to produce diarrhea, while calcium and aluminum ingredients tend to cause constipation. Many antacid preparations have more than one ingredient, usually in an attempt to "balance" these GI effects. When high doses of magnesium-aluminum combinations are used, diarrhea will usually predominate.[4] A patient experiencing diarrhea or constipation with one type of antacid may need to take a different one with the ingredients that cause more of the opposite effects. The ANC refers to the strength of the antacid in neutralizing hydrochloric acid; the higher the number, the stronger the antacid. Other considerations in selection of an antacid include the amount of sugar and/or sodium and the formulation. Tablets should be chewed before swallowing in order to have more immediate effects. Liquids are more difficult to carry but are already in liquid form and are faster-acting.

A combination antacid product, Gaviscon, is often used to treat GERD. Gaviscon contains alginic acid, aluminum hydroxide, magnesium trisilicate, and sodium bicarbonate. Alginic acid forms a highly viscous solution that is believed to impair reflux mechanically or by protecting the esophageal mucosa.

Drug interactions with antacids need to be considered in selecting drugs and/or in the dosing schedule. Tetracycline absorption may be inhibited by calcium-containing antacids. Other drugs whose absorption may be reduced by antacids are digoxin, ciprofloxacin, isoniazid, quinidine, H_2 blockers, phenytoin, ferrous sulfate, NSAIDs, theophylline, and warfarin.

Side effects of antacids also need to be considered. Most antacids are not absorbed to any great degree except, of course, baking soda (sodium bicarbonate), which is a systemic antacid often used as a home remedy. Sodium bicarbonate should not be used on a long-term basis because of its metabolic effects (systemic alkalosis) and potential fluid and electrolyte imbalances. Sodium bicarbonate may be an ingredient in some antacid preparations.

Chronic use of nonsystemic antacids can cause systemic problems, however. Antacids with calcium can cause hypercalcemia, renal impairment, alkalosis, and milk-alkali syndrome. Milk-alkali syndrome, also known as Burnett's syndrome, occurs with hypercalcemia secondary to high intake of milk or antacids. From 4 to 60 g per day of calcium carbonate is estimated to produce the syndrome. Signs and symptoms include shortening of the QT interval (usually at serum calcium levels above 13 mg/dL), weakness, renal failure, dizziness, and confusion; serum calcium levels in these patients may be further elevated by use of thiazide diuretics. All calcium-containing drugs and thiazide diuretics should be discontinued; treatment consists of intravenous administration of saline solution and the use of loop diuretics.[5]

Aluminum-containing antacids can cause osteomalacia, osteoporosis, and phosphate depletion. In patients with chronic renal failure, the binding of aluminum hydroxide antacids with phosphates in the GI tract can help to reduce hyperphosphatemia. Chronic use of magnesium-containing antacids can cause hypermagnesia, especially in patients with renal disease.

Other Drugs   Sucralfate (Carafate) works in several ways. It forms a protective barrier on the ulcerated mucosa and thereby protects it from the further effects of acid. Other actions of sucralfate include binding of bile salts, augmenting of prostaglandin secretion or gastric mucous production, and inhibition of pepsin. Healing rates equivalent to H_2 blockers have been demonstrated by a dosage regimen of a 1-g tablet four times a day between meals.[2] Constipation is its main side effect (sucralfate is an aluminum hydroxide salt of sucrose octasulfate). Sucralfate is available in liquid or tablet form. Tablets are large and may be a problem for individuals who have difficulty in swallowing. Sucralfate should be taken on an empty stomach and should not be taken within one half hour before or an hour after antacids. Sucralfate may affect absorption of phenytoin, tetracycline, fluoroquinolones, and fat-soluble vitamins.

Although not approved for this use, bismuth preparations such as bismuth subsalicylate (Pepto-Bismol) can be effective in treatment of peptic ulcers. Bismuth may act by inhibiting *H. pylori* and also may have a role in providing protection to gastric mucosa. Bismuth subcalicylate dissociates in the GI tract to bismuth and salicylate. Two bismuth salicylate tablets yield 204 mg salicylate that results in plasma levels comparable to 204 mg of aspirin. Therefore, it should be used cautiously in patients who are allergic to aspirin, who are on anticoagulant therapy, or have coagulation problems. Patients and clinicians should be aware that the patient's tongue may become black and furry in texture and that the stools will become black in color.

Antiinfective therapy has been shown to be effective in the healing of peptic ulcers believed caused by *H. pylori* infection. Therapy is usually over a 12- to 14-day period and requires good compliance since usually three different drugs are taken 3 to 4 times per day. Combinations usually used have been bismuth, metronidazole, and tetracycline. Amoxicillin and clarithromycin have also been in other regimens. An acid inhibitor (omeprazole or ranitidine) sometimes has been used. Triple-therapy regimens have resulted in eradication of peptic ulcers in the range of 70 to 90 percent compared to about 20 percent with monotherapy or 40 to 50 percent with dual therapy.

Misoprostol (Cytotec) is a prostaglandin E_1 analogue that can be used prophylactically in patients on NSAIDs. It presumably replaces the prostaglandins and thereby provides protection to the gastric mucosa. It also inhibits acid secretion and had been used to heal duodenal ulcers. However, because of its side effects (e.g., diarrhea, abdominal cramping) it is not well tolerated. It should not be used in pregnant women because it also causes uterine contractions.

Prokinetics in GERD Prokinetics are drugs which increase LES tone and/or promote gastric emptying. Currently, these are metoclopramide (Reglan), bethanechol (Urecholine), and cisapride (Propulsid). Metoclopromide commonly causes extrapyramidal side effects that make it difficult to use, especially in the elderly. Bethanechol can produce cholinergic side effects such as abdominal cramps, diarrhea, blurred vision, and urinary frequency; relative contraindications are peptic ulcer disease, asthma, and COPD. Cisapride does not cause extrapyramidal side effects; however, its use concurrently with ketoconazole, miconazole, itraconazole, or troleandomycin may prolong the QT interval and result in ventricular arrhythmias.[6]

Monitoring and Evaluation

Monitoring of the patient's degree of comfort or discomfort is important; however, pain is not a reliable indicator of healing or of the presence of ulceration, especially in the elderly. If pain continues beyond 7 to 10 days, there is a need to reevaluate diagnosis and treatment.

Testing stool for blood should be done; a UGI series may be indicated. If the patient is on cimetidine, he or she should be monitored for toxic effects of other drugs metabolized by the P-450 cytochrome system.

CONTEXTUAL ISSUES

A patient's lifestyle may interfere with taking antacids, especially liquid forms. Therefore antacids are not commonly used as monotherapy. H_2 blockers can be purchased OTC by the patient; these preparations are in lower dosage than prescription formulation. Patients will not be able to be reimbursed for OTC formulations; prescription strengths of H_2 blockers may be covered by some third-party plans.

Generic cimetidine is the least costly H_2 blocker. Omeprazole is the most expensive acid suppressor. Typical costs for a 30-day supply of standard-dose therapy are shown in Table 14-1.

Increased competition among drug manufacturers has resulted in some hospitals and managed care organizations agreeing to carry only certain brands in a class of drugs such as H_2 blockers. In these settings, the organizations may have been given a reduced price by the drug manufacturer. The clinician needs to be aware of the policies related to both generic substitution (substitution of a different brand of the same drug) and/or

TABLE 14-1

Typical Drug Costs

Drug	Amount/Strength		Typical Costs
H$_2$ Blockers			
cimetidine	60	400 mg tablets	$23.72 (generic); Tagamet $92.60
famotidine	30	20 mg tablets	$46.22
nizatidine	60	150 mg tablets	$92.31
ranitidine	30	300 mg capsules	$86.99
Proton Pump Inhibitors			
lansoprazole	30	15 mg capsules	$97.51
omeprazole	30	20 mg capsules	$108.90
Prokinetic Agents			
bethanecol	100	10 mg tablets	$2.48 (generic); Urecholine $66.61
cisapride	100	10 mg tablets	$62.94
metoclopramide	100	10 mg tablets	$25.88 (generic); Reglan $64.79

SOURCE: Mosby.[7]

therapeutic substitution (substitution of a drug in a different pharmacologic group used for the same therapeutic indication).

REFERENCES

1. Sullivan CA, Samuelson WM: Gastroesophageal reflux: A common exacerbating factor in adult asthma. *Nurse Pract* 21(11):82, 84, 93–94, 96, 1996.
2. Katz PO: Peptic ulcer disease, in Barker LR, Burton JR, Zieve PD (eds): *Principals of Ambulatory Medicine,* 4th ed. Baltimore: Williams & Wilkins, 1994, pp 456–469.
3. Allison JE, Feldman R, Tekawa IS, et al: Hemoccult screening in detecting colorectal neoplasm: sensitivity, specificity, and predictive value. *Ann Intern Med* 112:328, 1990.
4. Smith CJ: Upper gastrointestinal disorders, in Young LL, Koda-Kimble MA (eds): *Applied Therapeutics: The Clinical Use of Drugs,* 6th ed. Vancouver, WA: Applied Therapeutics, 1995, pp 23–1 to 23–24.
5. Newmark K, Nugent P: Milk-alkali syndrome. A consequence of chronic antacid abuse. *Postgrad Med* 93(6):149, 1993.
6. Williams DB, Welage LS: Gastroesophageal reflux disease, in DiPiro JT, Talbert RL, Yee GC, et al (eds): *Pharmacotherapy. A Pathophysiological Approach,* 3d ed. Stamford, CT: Appleton & Lange, 1997.
7. *Mosby's Complete Drug Reference. Physician's GenRx,* 7th ed. St. Louis: Mosby, 1997.

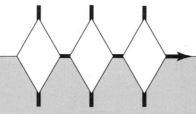

Chapter 15

STEROID DRUG THERAPY

Laurel A. Eisenhauer

OVERVIEW

The term *steroid* refers to a particular chemical structure; the human body has many different steroids. Steroid drug therapy usually refers to the use of adrenocorticosteroids as replacement therapy in case of insufficient adrenal function or at pharmacological levels to decrease the inflammatory response in a variety of conditions.

This chapter will address general principles and considerations for the use of steroid therapy at pharmacological (supraphysiologic) levels given to treat the more commonly encountered conditions in ambulatory care settings (e.g., conditions based on inflammatory and/or allergic responses).

Terms
Adrenocorticosteroids = Corticosteroids: refers to 3 types of steroids produced by adrenal cortex: glucocorticosteroids, mineralocorticosteroids, and sex hormones
Glucocorticosteroids = glucocorticoids: hydrocortisone (cortisol) is the main glucocorticoid produced by the adrenal glands
Mineralocorticosteroids = mineralocorticoids = aldosterone

Adrenal steroids are produced by the adrenal cortex in response to stimulation by the ACTH produced by the pituitary gland. Its production is regulated by a negative feedback loop called the *hypothalamic-pituitary-adrenal* (HPA) axis. The level of adrenocorticosteroids in the blood fluctuates according to the circadian cycle; the highest levels of adrenocorticosteroids in the blood are in the early morning hours, e.g., 2 to 8 A.M., and the lowest levels are 4 P.M. to midnight.

Adrenocorticosteroids may be used as replacement therapy in patients with insufficient adrenal cortex function (e.g., Addison's disease), adrenalectomy, or insufficient ACTH stimulation from hypophysectomy or other conditions causing an incomplete HPA axis. These patients usually need a steroid with high mineralocorticoid activity in order to maintain fluid and electrolytic balance; their dosage is aimed to be at "usual" physiological levels and is regulated according to the patient's activity and stress levels. Signs and symptoms of Addisonian crisis (which also would be signs of adrenal atrophy in a patient who had been on high dose or prolonged steroid therapy) are fatigue, nausea, anorexia, dyspnea, hypotension, hypoglycemia, myalgia, malaise, fever, arthralgia, dizziness, fainting, and desquamation of the skin.

PATIENT VARIABLES

Drugs that enhance the clearance of steroids include aminoglutethimide, mitotane, phenobarbital, phenytoin, rifampin. Diseases increasing clearance include hyperthyroidism and renal disease (dexamethasone only). Those that decrease clearance are ketoconazole, estrogens, and estrogen-containing oral contraceptives. Clearance may also be decreased by liver disease, hypothyroidism, renal disease (prednisolone only), malnutrition, anorexia nervosa, pregnancy, and age (over 65).[1]

Liver or renal diseases may affect steroid metabolism and excretion since metabolism occurs in both the liver and kidney. Glucocorticoids should not be used in patients with systemic fungal infections.

DRUG VARIABLES

Glucocorticosteroids have as their primary function the protection of the body from its own defense mechanisms.[2] Glucocorticosteroids are used for their antiinflammatory effects in arthritis and rheumatic disorders, allergic reactions, asthma, and other autoimmune conditions. Therapy with supraphysiological levels is not curative; i.e., it controls only the immediate consequences of the body's inflammatory response.[3]

Glucocorticosteroids have a number of other effects, and many produce serious side effects that must be monitored or treated. Untoward effects become increasingly common when doses are in the range of two to three times the daily replacement equivalent.[3] Some of these effects, however, also can be the basis for prescribing a steroid for an intended therapeutic effect. The suppression of lymphatic tissue and lymphatic function can be an adverse effect in increasing the susceptibility of a patient to infection; however, this is a basis for steroid use in cancer chemotherapy regimens. Delayed wound healing, usually considered a negative effect, can be beneficial in slowing down wound healing in a patient with a tendency for excessive scar formation.

Other side effects may require adjustments in the dosages of other drugs or the use of other drugs to treat the side effects. Patients who are diabetic may require an increase in their oral agents or insulin since glucocorticosteroids increase blood sugar levels. Patients who are hypertensive may have an increase in blood pressure and may need an increase in antihypertensive drug therapy because of the retention of sodium and water produced by steroid therapy. The use of antacids and/or other agents to prevent or treat peptic ulcer may be necessary. Since glucocorticosteroids produce potassium loss, hypokalemia can be a concern, especially if the patient is also on a diuretic that also may tend to produce hypokalemia; this is of special concern if the patient is on digoxin because of the increased potential for digoxin toxicity that can occur in hypokalemia.

Immunizations should not be done with immunosuppressed patients; live vaccines must not be used. Anticoagulant doses may need to be adjusted.

Some glucocorticoids have overlapping mineralocorticoid effects because they may interact with mineralocorticoid receptors as well as glucocorticoid receptors.

The pharmacokinetics of a steroid depends on the route and the particular agent. Most oral agents are well absorbed. When given intramuscularly, water-soluble preparations are absorbed more rapidly than fat-soluble. A daily dose (400 µg) of beclomethasone (2 puffs every 6 hours) is equivalent therapeutically to 7.5 mg of prednisone daily; less systemic absorption of an inhaled steroid occurs if a spacer is used.[2] Steroids are highly protein bound. Therefore, there is a potential for increased toxicity when used in patients receiving other highly bound drugs or who have low serum albumin levels.

Glucocorticoids can be differentiated according to their half-life: short, intermediate, and longer. However, their half-life does not necessarily correlate with the pharmacodynamic effects on tissues; i.e., therapeutic effects may extend beyond those expected based on half-life.

When applying glucocorticoids to the skin, systemic absorption can occur and is enhanced by use after a bath (increased four to five times), on inflamed or abraded skin, on thin skin (eyelids, forehead, scrotum), or when occluded by plastic (increased 10 times).[2] Adverse effects include thinning of skin, flushing, icthyosis-like changes, abnormal pigmentation, acne, superficial infections, rosacea-like dermatitis, perioral dermatitis, purpura, telangiectasis, photosensitivity, delayed wound healing, and false scars. Glaucoma and cataracts may be associated with topical ophthalmic use. Fluorinated glucocorticoids (e.g., betamethasone, dexamethasone, triamcinolone) should not be used on the face or other areas of thin skin because of skin atrophy.[2]

Selecting a Steroid

In choosing a glucocorticosteroid, both the necessary therapeutic effect to treat the underlying condition as well as the characteristics of the patient must be considered. Glucocorticoids and steroids differ in their relative amounts of glucocorticoid and mineralocorticoid activity as well as their route of administration. Glucocorticoids with mineralocorticoid effects may need to be avoided in patients with conditions that have or are sensitive to sodium and fluid retention (e.g., CHF, edema, renal failure). Other conditions of the patient that could alter hepatic metabolism and therefore prevent activation of pro-drugs should be assessed. Conditions such as liver disease or renal insufficiency that may impact on pharmacokinetics may influence the choice of glucocorticoids or the dose used. Most preparations are active drugs; however, two are pro-drugs and need to be metabolized before they are active drugs. Prednisone converts to prednisolone, and cortisone converts to cortisol.

The therapeutic goal and parameter to evaluate should be determined based on the underlying condition being treated (e.g., peak expiratory flowrate (PEFR) in asthma, decrease in sedimentation rate). Subjective evaluation may be confounded by the mood changes (e.g., euphoria) that steroids produce in many patients. Other drug therapy should be considered prior to consideration of steroid therapy or in conjunction with

TABLE 15-1

Glucocorticoid Equivalencies, Potencies, and Half-Life

Glucocorticoid	Approximate Equivalent Dose (mg)	Relative Antiinflammatory (Glucocorticoid) Potency	Relative Mineralo-corticoid Potency	Plasma (min)	Biologic (hrs)
Short-acting					
Cortisone	25	0.8	2	30	8–12
Hydrocortisone	20	1	2	80–118	8–12
Intermediate-acting					
Prednisone	5	4	1	60	18–36
Prednisolone	5	4	1	115–212	18–36
Triamcinolone	4	5	0	200+	18–36
Methylprednisolone	4	5	0	78–188	18–36
Long-acting					
Dexamethasone	0.75	20–30	0	110–210	36–54
Betamethasone	0.6–0.75	20–30	0	300+	36–54

SOURCE: © 1997 by Facts and Comparisons. Used with permission from *Drug Facts and Comparisons.* 1997 ed. St. Louis, MO: Facts and Comparisons, a Wolters Kluwer Company.[3]

steroid therapy; the latter may have the advantage of having a steroid sparing effect, i.e., reducing the steroid dosage needed. Table 15-1 illustrates the relative potency of the various preparations.

Dosing

When possible, the least dose for the shortest time period, preferably given in the morning, should be used. Alternate-day therapy should be used whenever possible if use is long term (Table 15-2). The clinician should consult the literature about the underlying condition to evaluate the appropriateness of alternate-day therapy for that condition. Giant-cell arteritis requires more frequent dosage scheduling to ensure adequate control.[4]

Topical Steroids

Topical steroids for treating skin conditions are available at OTC strength or in prescription strength. Usually their effect is suppression of inflammation at the local level. Systemic absorption could occur, however, with prolonged use on inflamed or denuded skin. Continued use also can lead to a thinning of skin.

Other Drugs   Table 15-3 delineates the common side effects of glucocorticosteroid therapy and the implications for patient care and monitoring of steroid therapy.

TABLE 15-2

Scheme for the Conversion to an Alternate-Day Regimen for Glucocorticoids (Initial dose prednisone 60 mg/day)

Day	Dose (mg)	Day	Dose (mg)
A. Reduce dosage by 5 mg every 3 days until a dose of prednisone 20 mg is reached:			
1	55	13	35
2	55	14	35
3	55	15	35
4	50	16	30
5	50	17	30
6	50	18	30
7	45	19	25
8	45	20	25
9	45	21	25
10	40	22	20
11	40	23	20
12	40	24	20
B. Reduce dosage by 2.5 mg on alternate days every 3 cycles until no prednisone on alternate days:			
25	20	49	20
26	17.5	50	7.5
27	20	51	20
28	17.5	52	7.5
29	20	53	20
30	17.5	54	7.5
31	20	55	20
32	15	56	5
33	20	57	20
34	15	58	5
35	20	59	20
36	15	60	5
37	20	61	20
38	12.5	62	2.5
39	20	63	20
40	12.5	64	2.5
41	20	65	20
42	12.5	66	2.5
43	20	67	20
44	10	68	0
45	20	69	20
46	10	70	0
47	20	71	20
48	10	72	0

SOURCE: Shlom ES: Adrenocortical dysfunction and clinical use of steroids, in Herfindel ET, Gourley DR (eds): *Clinical Pharmacy and Therapeutics*, 6th ed. Baltimore: Williams & Wilkins, 1996. Used with permission.[2]

TABLE 15-3

Side Effects and Monitoring in Systemic Long-Term Glucocorticosteroid Therapy in Adults

Monitor for:	Comments/Implications
Infection	Usual signs and symptoms of infection and inflammation are suppressed; monitor for any indication of decline in well-being; patients should avoid persons with infections; incidence of infection decreased by use of alternate-day therapy
Weight* (fluid retention, enhanced appetite); edema	Possible need for dietary control and/or use of diuretics
Blood pressure (hypertension from sodium and fluid retention)	May need to increase dosage of any antihypertensive; decrease sodium intake
2-hr postprandial glucose, FBS (elevated blood glucose, glucose intolerance*)	May need to add or increase dosage of antidiabetic agents; monitor also for hypertriglyceridemia
Serum electrolytes (e.g., potassium, sodium)	May need to encourage increased potassium in diet or use of potassium supplement; monitor closely if patient on digitalis preparation
Tests for occult blood in stool/ peptic ulcer/perforation	Antacids, H_2 blockers, and sucralfate have been used for prevention and treatment; avoid use of NSAIDs or aspirin
Impaired wound healing; skin atrophy	
Muscle weakness/atrophy	
Ophthalmic exams for cataracts, glaucoma	Increased risk with ophthalmic use but can occur with systemic therapy and inhalation therapy
Body image changes: hirsutism, acne, moonface, buffalo hump, central obesity	
Thromboembolism or fat embolism; arrhythmias	If patient on anticoagulant therapy, may need to adjust dosage
Osteoporosis (bone loss tends to occur in trabecular bones (e.g., ribs and vertebrae rather than long bones); aseptic necrosis of femoral and humeral heads	Can occur with 7.5 mg/day prednisone equivalent. Encourage increased calcium intake; if long-term therapy should take calcium and vitamin D (plus estrogen supplement for postmenopausal women); use of etidronate or calcitonin may become necessary

Monitor for:	Comments/Implications
Amenorrhea, postmenopausal bleeding, and other menstrual abnormalities	
Negative nitrogen balance	Encourage protein intake
Steroid psychosis, mood changes,* emotional lability, insomnia, increased intracranial pressure, convulsions, euphoria	Steroid psychosis (rare if dose under 40 mg prednisone/day, 18% of patients receiving > 80 mg prednisone daily)†
Suppression of growth	Monitor growth of young adults/ adolescents

*Most common early side effects occurring.
†Boston Collaborative Drug Surveillance Program.[5]

Prevention of Adrenal Atrophy

The potential for developing adrenal atrophy or suppression of the HPA axis due to the exogenous use of steroids is a major concern and a limiting factor in the prolonged use of adrenal steroids. Usually there is little danger of HPA axis suppression in patients on short-term therapy of less than 20 mg prednisone (or equivalent) per day for less than 3 weeks.

Signs and symptoms of steroid withdrawal are similar to adrenal insufficiency and include arthralgia, fatigue, weakness, nausea, hypotension, and dizziness. HPA suppression is more likely to occur with longer-acting steroids, such as dexamethasone. The degree of suppression increases with continued therapy. Patients may require supplementation with steroids if they experience surgery or stress for up to 12 to 18 months after steroids have been discontinued.

Prevention is best done by avoiding the unnecessary use of steroids and limiting the dosage or duration if at all possible. When these limitations are not possible because of the nature of the condition being treated, there are some dosing variations that can help to decrease the development of adrenal atrophy:

1. Giving all or most of the drug in the morning. This means that the exogenous dose joins the natural high serum levels at a time when the HPA is normally suppressed. This results in less adrenal suppression than when steroid doses are given in the evening. Usually, antiinflammatory effects last longer than suggested by serum levels so this dosing regimen may be possible in many patients. Recent data, however, suggest an increased incidence of asthma in the evening and at night; this may mean that the administration of system systemic steroids for some asthma patients might need to be later in the day.

2. Use of alternate-day therapy is done using twice the daily dose every other morning using intermediate-acting steroids. The therapeutic effects are believed to last beyond the first day yet the decrease in serum levels on the off day will stimulate the HPA axis (see Table 15-2).

TABLE 15-4

Tapering from Glucocorticosteroid Therapy

- During the tapering process, consider not only the issue of suppression of HPA axis but possible exacerbation of underlying condition for which the steroid therapy was prescribed
- Monitor patient for indications of adrenal insufficiency (iatrogenic Addison's disease): anorexia, fluid and electrolyte disturbance, malaise, lethargy, myalgia, nausea, vomiting, fever
- Patients may experience symptoms if stressed during tapering and for 12 to 18 months after tapering
- Symptoms of adrenal insufficiency usually occur when the daily dose of glucocorticosteroid is decreased below the physiological replacement level (e.g., 5 mg of prednisone or 20 mg of cortisol or equivalent)
- No tapering schedule is appropriate for all patients and conditions; alternate-day therapy may be tried; reductions of 5 mg of cortisol (or equivalent) every 2 to 3 weeks after 2 months at level of physiological replacement may be tried

SOURCE: Barker et al.[6]

Tapering

Tapering a patient from steroid therapy needs to be done carefully and gradually (see Table 15-4). During the taper, the patient needs to be monitored for both signs and symptoms of adrenal insufficiency and of exacerbation of the condition being treated. When a tapering dose reaches the range of 20 to 30 mg per day, the taper should be slowed and the patient's HPA axis checked. Since the normal adult, on average, produces 20 to 30 mg of cortisol per day with a peak around 8 A.M., exogenous amounts below that should trigger the patient's own production of cortisol.[1]

Evaluating Patient for Adrenal Insufficiency

The patient can be monitored for signs and symptoms of steroid withdrawal as the steroid is tapered. Tests available for assessment of the HPA axis/adrenal atrophy are insulin-induced hypoglycemia, metapyrone, lysine-vasopressin, and ACTH stimulation. The last test involves measurement of serum cortisol levels before and after administration of ACTH (cosyntropin).[7(p42-8)]

CONTEXTUAL ISSUES

The use of enteric-coated preparations of oral products may decrease the rate but not the extent of absorption; however, the extent is decreased if these are also given with food. Therefore, enteric-coated preparations should not be taken with food.[2(p301)]

Cost containment may necessitate initial trials of tapering patients off steroid therapy while monitoring symptoms, before using the more expensive laboratory tests of the HPA axis.

In many patients with chronic conditions, steroid therapy relieves pain or other symptoms and discomfort as well as perhaps producing euphoria and a sense of well-being. This makes some patients want to continue with steroid therapy, sometimes resulting in the difficult situation of needing to wean the patient off therapy for both psychological and physiological reasons in order to prevent the many adverse effects of chronic use.

Because of the dangers that could occur from abrupt discontinuation of steroid therapy, patients need to be sure that they have an adequate supply (and a renewal prescription if necessary) in the event of weather or other emergencies when the patient may not be able to get to the pharmacy or contact the prescriber.

REFERENCES

1. Gums JG, Wilt VM: Disorders of the adrenal gland, in DiPiro JT, Talbert RL, Yee GC, et al (eds): *Pharmacotherapy. A Pathophysiological Approach,* 3d ed. Stamford, CT: Appleton & Lange, 1997, pp 1547–1564.

2. Shlom ES: Adrenocortical dysfunction and clinical use of steroids, in Herfindel ET, Gourley DR (eds): *Clinical Pharmacy and Therapeutics,* 6th ed. Baltimore: Williams & Wilkins, 1996, pp 285–308.

3. *Drug Facts and Comparisons.* St. Louis: Facts and Comparisons, 1997.

4. Ontjes DA: Adrenal corticosteroids, corticotropin releasing hormone, adrenocorticotropin, and antiadrenal drugs, in Munson PL (ed): *Principles of Pharmacology. Basic Concepts and Clinical Applications.* New York: Chapman and Hall, 1995.

5. Boston Collaborative Drug Surveillance Program: Acute adverse reactions to prednisone in relation to dosage. *Clin Pharmacol Therap* 13:694–698, 1972.

6. Barker LR, Burton JR, Zieve PD (eds): *Principles of Ambulatory Medicine*, 4th ed. Baltimore: Williams & Wilkins, 1995.

7. Small RE, Cooksey LJ: Connective tissue disorders: The clinical use of corticosteroids, in Young LY, Koda-Kimble MA (eds): *Applied Therapeutics: The Clinical Use of Drugs,* 6th ed. Vancouver, WA: Applied Therapeutics, 1995, pp 42–1 to 42–11.

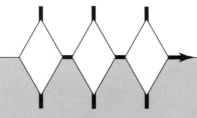

Chapter 16

PSYCHOTROPICS IN PRIMARY CARE

*Judith A. Shindul-Rothschild and
Anthony J. Rothschild*

OVERVIEW OF PSYCHOPHARMACOLOGY AND PATHOPHYSIOLOGY FOR THE TREATMENT OF MAJOR DEPRESSION AND ANXIETY DISORDERS

One American in three experiences some disability from a diagnosable mental illness during his or her lifetime.[1] Yet only a third of individuals suffering from mental illness will receive appropriate and timely treatment.[2] In 1996 the U.S. Congress designated the last decade of the twentieth century as the "Decade of the Brain" in acknowledgment of the dramatic breakthroughs in the diagnosis and treatment of mental illness.[3] The field of psychopharmacology in particular has witnessed an explosion of new medication treatments over the past 10 years that have had a significant impact on the quality of life for millions of Americans.

To increase the nursing profession's awareness of the great strides in neurobiologic research and psychopharmacology, the National Institute of Mental Health (NIMH) and the American Nurses' Association (ANA) jointly sponsored the Psychiatric Mental Health Nursing Psychopharmacology Project. Early in its deliberations, the ANA Task Force on Psychopharmacology recognized the urgent need for advanced practice nurses to have solid expertise in the area of clinical psychopharmacology. The aspects of clinical psychopharmacology that are essential for advanced practice nurses to administer and monitor psychiatric medications appropriately are listed in Table 16-1.[4]

TABLE 16-1

ANA Guidelines for Nursing Education in Psychopharmacology

1. Pharmacokinetics and pharmacodynamics
2. Target symptoms
3. Stages and progression of illness
4. Factors affecting medication choice
5. Development of treatment plans
6. Medication effect variables
7. Drug interactions and side effects
8. Monitoring
9. Psycho-education
10. Quality of life
11. Discontinuation
12. Relapse prevention
13. Continuing education

SOURCE: Reprinted with permission from the Psychiatric Mental Health Nursing Psychopharmacology Project, copyright 1994. American Nurses' Association.[4]

Mental illness is one of the least discussed, yet most prevalent illnesses treated by primary care providers. In primary care settings, it is estimated that 6 to 8 percent of all outpatients have a major depressive disorder.[2] Surveys show that 70 percent of suicide victims have seen a primary care provider within two months preceding their death.[5]

Advanced practice nurses, regardless of specialty or practice setting, are likely routinely to encounter patients who have been diagnosed with major mental illness. Major mental illness may be classified in three broad categories: mood disorders, anxiety disorders, and psychotic disorders. The most severe and debilitating mental illnesses—major depression, panic disorder, schizophrenia, and manic-depressive or bipolar disorder—affect approximately 11.4 million Americans with about half experiencing a chronic or persistent course.

It has become increasingly important for primary care providers to be thoroughly familiar with the signs and symptoms of mental illness, appropriate treatment modalities, and criteria for referral. In primary care settings the presenting symptoms often are masked by physical complaints such as headaches, body aches, gastrointestinal distress, fatigue, or sexual dysfunction. Any client who verbalizes feelings of sadness or exhibits signs and symptoms of depression should be asked directly if they have ever had suicidal thoughts, had a family member or friend attempt suicide, or have attempted suicide in the past. Pharmacologic treatment or consultation should be considered for any patient exhibiting a marked change in neurovegetative signs (especially sleep or appetite), fatigue, cognitive symptoms that impair normal daily activities, marked changes in mood, psychosis, or suicidal tendencies.

In this chapter, mood and anxiety disorders that are commonly diagnosed by primary care providers will be reviewed. There are certain clinical presentations that clearly warrant referral to psychiatric clinical specialists. Although managed care has sought to severely curtail the referrals of patients to specialists, indications for referral to psychiatric specialists will be described in detail, as well as specific psychotherapy modalities.

Recommended References

American Psychological Association: *Diagnostic and Statistical Manual of Mental Disorders,* 4th ed. Washington, DC: American Psychiatric Press, 1994.

Depression in Primary Care. Vol 1 (Diagnosis and Detection); vol 2 (Treatment of Major Depression). Rockville, MD: The Agency for Health Policy Research, 1993.

Gitlin MJ: *The Psychotherapist's Guide to Psychopharmacology,* 2d ed. New York: The Free Press, 1996.

Laraia MT, Beeber LS, Callwood GB, et al: Psychiatric Mental Health Nursing Psychopharmacology Project. Washington, DC: American Nurses' Association, 1994.

Long PW: *Mental Illness in America.* National Institute of Mental Health. *Internet Mental Health* (www.mentalhealth.com), 1997.

National Institute of Mental Health: *Decade of the Brain-Medications.* Washington, DC: National Institutes of Health, 1995, Pub. no. 95-3929.

Oakley LD, Potter C: *Psychiatric Primary Care.* St. Louis: Mosby, 1997.

Schatzberg AF, Nemeroff CB (eds): *The American Psychiatric Press Textbook of Psychopharmacology.* Washington, DC: American Psychiatric Press, 1995.

Sederer LI, Rothschild AJ (eds): *Acute Care Psychiatry: Diagnosis and Treatment.* Baltimore: Williams & Wilkins, 1997.

ISSUES IN DRUG THERAPY

Prescribing Considerations

Prior to administering any psychotropic drug, advanced practice nurses should either perform a thorough physical assessment or assume responsibility for ensuring that the patient receives a proper medical workup.[6] The physical examination should include routine vital signs, a neurological examination, and a complete mental status examination. A physical examination within the past year is important for several reasons: (1) ruling out other possible medical disorders and drug-drug interactions (see Table 16-2), (2) ensuring that liver, cardiac, and renal functions are within normal limits, (3) ensuring that women of childbearing age are not pregnant, and (4) assessing for any evidence of trauma.

Routine laboratory tests and medical procedures as well as those recommended to rule out specific mental conditions are listed in Table 16-3.[7] Costly and less frequently used tests and procedures to properly differentiate dementia and other neurological disorders from major mental illnesses include: neuropsychologic testing, single photon emission computed tomography (SPECT) and positron emission tomography (PET) scans, sleep deprived electroencephalograms (EEG), or EEG with nasopharyngeal leads.

TABLE 16-2

Medications and Medical Disorders That May Cause Depressive Symptoms

Cause	
Most Common	**Examples**
Neurologic disorders	Parkinson's disease
Endocrine disorders	Hypothyroidism, diabetes, Cushing's disease, Addison's disease
Substance abuse and withdrawal	Alcohol, amphetamines, cocaine, steroids
Cancer	Pancreatic carcinoma, primary cerebral tumor, cerebral metastasis
Infectious disease	Mononucleosis, acquired immune deficiency syndrome (AIDS)
Less Common	**Examples**
Neurologic disorders	Alzheimer's disease, multiple sclerosis, Huntington's disease, postconcussion syndromes, chronic subdural hematoma
Endocrine disorders	Hyperthyroidism, hyperparathyroidism, hypoparathyroidism, hypoglycemia
Cancer	Lung cancer
Infectious disease	Syphilis, hepatitis, tuberculosis, influenza, Lyme disease
Medications	Barbiturates, opiates, antihypertensives, sedatives, digitalis, oral contraceptives
Toxins	Lead, manganese, mercury
Nutritional deficiencies	Iron, folate, vitamins B_{12}, B_2, B_1

TABLE 16-3

Guidelines for the Laboratory and Radiologic Diagnosis of Depression

Recommended Baseline Laboratory Studies

Complete blood count with differential
Electrolytes
Chemistry panel including glucose, blood urea nitrogen/creatinine, liver function tests, calcium, and phosphorus

TABLE 16-3 *(continued)*

Recommended Baseline Laboratory Studies

Comprehensive serum and/or urine toxic screen, particularly if substance use/abuse is suspected

Thyroid-stimulating hormone and thyroxine, especially when considering lithium treatment or if thyroid problem suspected

Electrocardiogram in patients with cardiac disease, taking cardiotoxic medication, and/or older than 40 years

Beta human chorionic gonadotropin in female patients of childbearing age

Special Laboratory Studies

Serum B_{12} and folate

Erythrocyte sedimentation rate

Antinuclear antibody

Serum ceruloplasmin

Tuberculosis skin test

Lumbar puncture

Radiologic studies (only if neurologic disorder suspected or if moderate to severe cognitive deficits are present)

   Computed tomography and/or magnetic resonance imaging

   Single photon emission computed tomography or positron emission tomography

Diagnostic studies

   Dexamethasone suppression test

   Thyroid stimulating test

   Polysomnography

SOURCE: Grady TA, Sederer LI, Rothschild AJ: Depression, in Sederer LI, Rothschild AJ (eds). *Acute Care Psychiatry: Diagnosis and Treatment.* Baltimore: Williams & Wilkins, 1997, pp 83–121. Used with permission.[7]

Biology

Mood Disorders Biochemical hypotheses of the etiology of depression have focused on dysregulation of central nervous system (CNS) neurotransmitters.[8,9] Monoamines (norepinephrine and serotonin) are the primary neurotransmitters implicated in classic biochemical hypotheses of major depressive illness. The original amine hypothesis was derived from clinical research with a number of centrally active medications. In experiments with reserpine, norepinephrine and serotonin were depleted. The monoamine oxidase inhibitor (MAOI) isoniazid was shown to increase CNS catecholamines. The tricyclic antidepressants (TCAs) delayed inactivation of neurotransmitters via reuptake blockade. Lithium produced an increase in the reuptake of catecholamines, thereby decreasing the availability of these transmitters. Electroconvulsive therapy (ECT) resulted in an increase in norepinephrine levels.

The amine hypothesis of depression postulated a deficiency of monoamines (norepinephrine and serotonin) in the neurosynaptic junction. Antidepressants were thought to alleviate depression by correcting the deficiency, which they achieved by inhibiting uptake or decreasing catabolism once uptake had occurred.[10,11] More recent investigations of specific neurotransmitters in mood disorders does not support completely the original monoamine hypothesis of depressive illness. Evidence suggests that other neurotransmitter systems such as acetylcholine and gamma-aminobutyric acid (GABA) also may play a role. Another focus of recent research has been on receptor sensitivity. Findings point to a decrease in the number of postsynaptic beta-adrenergic receptors by almost all antidepressants. The decrease in the receptors has been termed "down-regulation."

Other areas under investigation with regard to potential biologic hypotheses of major depression are neuroendocrinology and circadian rhythms, including neurohormonal hypotheses that focus on the regulation and functional properties of neurohormones within the hypothalamic-pituitary-adrenal (HPA) and hypothalamic-pituitary-thyroid axes. Alterations in the sleep-wake cycle associated with depression and recent findings of possible effects of temperature regulation on mood have resulted in investigations of circadian rhythm disturbances as possible etiologic factors in depression.[12] Some consistent abnormalities in sleep EEGs (polysomnograms) among depressed patients include shortened rapid eye movement (REM) latency and increased REM duration and density (i.e., number of rapid eye movements per REM period).

Although bipolar disorder has generally been viewed as a state of excess of neurotransmitters such as norepinephrine and dopamine, Post (1992) proposed that bipolar disorder represents a kindling phenomenon. Kindling (also known as sensitization) is a phenomenon that occurs in laboratory animals when continuous stimulation is applied to their brains to cause seizures. With repeated stimulation, the animal will eventually have seizures without the need of the external stimulation. Post has suggested that the course in bipolar disorder reflects a kindling effect.[13] The kindling phenomenon may explain the finding by several research groups that the incidence of previous episodes is one of the best predictors of future relapses in bipolar disorders.[14–16] The model may also explain why medications with antikindling effects, such as divalproex and carbamazepine, are beneficial in the treatment of bipolar disorder. Furthermore, it may explain some of the findings regarding the cause and effect association between life events and relapse in bipolar disorder. At the onset of the illness, the occurrence of life events is associated with the development of illness; as the frequency of episodes increases, the patient may have relapses even in the absence of life events.[17]

Investigations of neurotransmitters as well as studies of second-messenger systems, neuroimaging, and neuroendocrine functioning support the view that mood disorders involve a profound alteration in multiple body systems, including many hypothalamic functions such as the regulation of sleep, wakefulness, appetite, eating, and neuroendocrine control of peripheral endocrine organs, particularly the adrenal glands, thyroid, and gonads. Unfortunately, conventional diagnostic techniques, including X-rays, magnetic resonance imaging (MRI) scanning, and blood laboratory tests, are not useful at this time in the clinical setting. However, significant abnormalities on biological testing are seen in mood disorder patients that are being pursued in the research setting. The focus of research into the pathophysiology of mood disorders indicates that these biological changes are profound and that most of the systems, although not all, returned to normal when the patient experienced symptomatic remission.[18,19]

Panic Disorder and Obsessive-Compulsive Disorder   Although no biological test is available for practical diagnostic use for panic disorder and obsessive-compulsive disorder (OCD), both have strong biologic underpinnings that derive from a variety of sources, including biochemical and neuroimaging studies. This area has been reviewed in detail by Popp and colleagues.[20] The most convincing evidence demonstrating the biologic nature of panic disorder derives from studies in which panic attacks are produced in susceptible individuals under controlled laboratory conditions using biochemical probes. Intravenous infusion of DL-lactate solution,[21] inhalation of air enriched with carbon dioxide, and oral administration of caffeine or yohimbine are well-studied means of inducing panic symptoms.[22] PET scans of panic disorder patients' brains during lactate-induced attacks or anticipatory states suggest specific dysfunctional areas of the limbic system.[23,24] Animal studies also suggest the importance of noradrenergic activity in the locus caeruleus in panic disorder.[25] Neuropsychiatric investigations of OCD have focused on the importance of serotonergic transmission. The strongest evidence in support of a serotonergic mechanism is the consistent observation of positive clinical effects produced by serotonergic antidepressants.[26–28]

Therapeutic Interventions in Conjunction with Drug Therapy

Mood Disorders   Patients will present to advanced practice nurses with symptoms of depression ranging from mild to severe. In mild forms of depression, the client may have symptoms lasting over two weeks and express some difficulty performing daily tasks. Individuals with mild forms of depression are best helped with short-term brief psychotherapy or crisis intervention if the symptoms are associated with a specific stressful event.

People with moderate depression have more symptoms with greater severity than people with mild depression. People with moderate forms of depression may not have had previous episodes of depression or have co-morbid conditions that can exacerbate depressive symptoms, such as substance abuse, debilitating medical conditions, or symptoms of anxiety, panic, and euphoria. Studies suggest that 50 percent of individuals suffering from mild to moderate depression will have symptom remission in the acute phase (which typically lasts from 6 to 12 weeks) following treatment with psychotherapy alone.[2] In situations where the advanced practice nurse is not a psychiatric clinical specialist, clients diagnosed with mild to moderate forms of depression may be referred to a specialist in psychotherapy.

At this time, there is insufficient empirical evidence to warrant the continuation of psychotherapy alone in mild to moderate forms of depression after the acute phase.[2] If there is no symptom improvement after 6 weeks of treatment with psychotherapy, or if clients express insufficient relief from depressive symptoms after 12 weeks, advanced practice nurses should consider strongly treatment with antidepressant medication.[2]

Interpersonal and supportive psychotherapy are used as adjuncts to pharmacologic treatment of patients with severe depression who have had recurrences or situational crises involving family or work and who have co-morbid personality disorder. Family or marital therapy is strongly indicated for clients with major mental illness to educate family members about the disease, negotiate conflicts, and formulate effective intervention strategies to manage behaviors counterproductive to recovery.

Group therapy is appropriate for patients with a wide range of mental disorders. Hypomanic patients who are verbally abusive are not appropriate for group psychotherapy. Groups assist patients in developing interpersonal skill and insight into their illness. Psychotherapeutic groups are an integral part of partial or day programs in most psychiatric facilities. Self-help or support groups organized by patients in recovery or their families are discussed under compliance.

Anxiety Disorders   Cognitive-behavioral therapy (CBT) is the first line of psychotherapy used in the treatment of anxiety disorders. The basic precept of CBT is that all behavior is learned. If behavioral responses are learned, then theoretically, behavior can be reversed or extinguished provided there are the right incentives and reinforcement. Recent studies report that half of patients with anxiety disorders show improvement with a combination of CBT and medication.[29] Despite the clear clinical efficacy of combined treatment, one study found that although 75 percent of the children were referred for behavioral therapy, only a third actually initiated treatment.[30] Parents' reasons for not following through with the treatment recommendations included cost and lack of qualified behavioral therapists.[30]

Desensitization and exposure theory are two CBT approaches used to treat panic disorder and agoraphobia. In desensitization, patients face the feared object or situation repeatedly, for increasing periods of time. For example, if a child was school phobic, the child would have a schedule of gradually increasing time in the classroom, first perhaps with a parent and then without. Desensitization is effective in treating between 60 and 90 percent of patients diagnosed with panic attacks or phobias.[29]

Whether the patient is in individual, family, or group psychotherapy, the goal of the therapist remains the same—to prevent relapse. Studies have demonstrated that patients who have formed a therapeutic alliance with their primary care provider are more compliant, less likely to relapse, and need lower doses of medication.[31] Advanced practice nurses need to be both prudent and creative about ways they can provide patients with access to a finite number of reimbursed therapy sessions.

Group therapy and day programs are more likely to be reimbursed than individual psychotherapy, and crisis, brief, or cognitive-behavioral therapies are more likely to be approved than interpersonal psychotherapy. During follow-up visits for medication maintenance a brief, solution-focused approach can be used to address immediate issues that may contribute to relapse. The most therapeutic and cost-effective treatment plans are those that knit together services offered by mental health professionals and community or volunteer organizations.

Self-help groups are an effective treatment for preventing relapse, especially for individuals with substance abuse disorders. Alcoholics Anonymous, founded in 1935, is perhaps the oldest and most well-established patient self-help organization. Other self-help organizations offering education, support, and advocacy services to patients and their families include: The National Depressive and Manic Depressive Association (NDMDA), 730 North Franklin St., Suite 501, Chicago, IL 60610; The Phobia Society of America, 133 Rollins Ave., Suite 4B, Rockville, MD 20852; The Obsessive-Compulsive (OC)

Foundation, P.O. Box 9573, New Haven, CT 06535; and The National Alliance for the Mentally Ill, 200 N. Glebe Road, Suite 1015, Arlington, VA 22203-3754.

Patient Variables
Demographic Factors

Age Mood and anxiety disorders can occur at any age. The average age of onset for anxiety disorders is in the early 20s, and the late 20s for mood disorders. Findings from the latest Epidemiologic Catchment Area (ECA) study suggest that the age of onset for major mental illness is steadily declining.[32] There is debate about which, or how, social-cultural factors have interacted to put the baby-boomer generation at greater risk for depression than their predecessors. Although the answer to why there appears to be a cohort effect may never be fully understood, there does appear to be a greater risk for major depression among younger cohorts.

Although the incidence of depression may be increasing among younger cohorts, the risk of suicide is twice as great in the elderly than the general population.[33] The high mortality for depression among the aged underscores the importance of conducting a careful medical history and mental status examination to properly distinguish between the signs and symptoms of depression and dementia (see Table 16-4). The elderly should be routinely asked if they have thoughts of ending their life or a plan for committing suicide. Expired or stockpiled medications should be collected and properly disposed of by visiting nurses or family members. The elderly who are isolated should be referred to community-based day programs and religious or outreach agencies. For the aged diagnosed with major depression, the most effective treatment is a combination of brief psychotherapy with antidepressant medication.[33]

The overall incidence of depression in children is estimated to be between 1 and 9 percent for primary school children and 4 to 7 percent for adolescents.[35] A recent meta-analy-

TABLE 16-4

Clinical Features Distinguishing Depression from Dementia

Depression	Dementia
Short duration	Long duration
Expresses frustration during cognitive testing	Confabulates during cognitive testing
Little effort to perform simple tasks	Difficulty performing simple tasks
Pervasive changes in mood	Affect labile
Symptoms worse in morning	Symptoms worse in evening
Family and personal history of depression	Family history of dementia
Patient frequently complains of deficit	Patient often unaware of deficit

SOURCE: Adapted from Gitlin.[34]

sis of the treatment of children with TCAs found that TCAs were not superior to placebo and half of the subjects on placebo experienced a significant improvement in depressive symptoms.[35] This finding suggests that the *process of care* is at least as efficacious as the psychoactive effects of medication for youngsters experiencing depression. When formulating a treatment plan for children and adolescents with major mental illness, it is important to remember that removing children from abusive environments and initiating family, group, and individual psychotherapy may be just as beneficial as prescribing a medication.

Children under the age of 16 exhibiting severe or unremitting symptoms of depression, suicidal ideation, psychosis, or self-mutilation should be referred to a child psychiatric nurse clinical specialist or a child psychiatrist. Children suffering from the more severe forms of mental illness are likely to have a chronic course and are best treated with multimodal therapy. As an adjunct to psychopharmacology, multimodal therapy may include family therapy, individual psychodynamic psychotherapy, or cognitive-behavioral therapy.

Gender   Women are twice as likely to be diagnosed with mood or anxiety disorders than men. Epidemiological studies have concluded that the higher prevalence of mood and anxiety disorders among women is not a function of diagnostic bias or health-seeking behavior.[7] The increased susceptibility of women to major mental illness appears to be associated with physiological and developmental gender differences.

Race, Ethnicity, and Social Class   Rates of mood disorders are similar across racial and ethnic groups. Although the rates are similar, some ethnic groups may present with more somatic complaints or are more descriptive about their symptoms than others. Anxiety disorders and dual diagnosis (major mental illness concomitant with substance abuse) are more common among African-Americans and Hispanics than the general population. For obsessive-compulsive disorder, the gender difference is smaller, and there is a higher incidence among whites than African-Americans.

Differences in prevalence across social class have been found in bipolar disorder with the lowest incidence occurring among lower socioeconomic classes and the highest incidence occurring among the middle to upper classes.[36] Data from the ECA study found that schizophrenia was diagnosed more frequently among African-Americans than whites; however, when controlling for social class, these differences disappeared.[37] The overwhelming majority of individuals diagnosed with an eating disorder are white women in the middle to upper social classes. Recent evidence suggests that as developing cultures and ethnic groups are assimilated to Western culture, the incidence of eating disorders begins to rise.[38]

Diagnostic Factors

Grief Reaction   People suffering from a normal grief reaction exhibit many of the same symptoms as individuals suffering from mild forms of depression. The clinical features that distinguish a grief reaction from mild depression include: (1) A grief reaction is time-limited to two to six months; (2) generally, individuals experiencing a grief reaction are able to carry out normal daily activities; and (3) symptoms in a grief reaction steadily remit without treatment over the course of several weeks. Bereavement groups, short-term solution-focused psychotherapy, or crisis therapy is an appropriate therapeutic intervention for patients experiencing a grief reaction.

Major Depression   The diagnosis of a depressive illness is made by the intensity, pervasiveness, and persistence of the mood symptoms as well as by the interference of the depressed mood with the person's usual social and physiological functioning. Several features distinguish clinically ill patients from those with normal mood. In addition to the disturbances of mood, patients suffering from a depressive illness will exhibit a combination of the following features: (1) changes in neurovegetative signs, indicated by disturbances in sleep, appetite, and sexual interest; (2) reduced desire and ability to perform the usual, expected social roles; (3) suicidal thoughts or acts; and (4) disturbances in reality testing, manifested by confusion, profound sense of worthlessness, or ruminations. Suicidal ideation and evidence of a thought disorder usually indicate a need for immediate psychiatric consultation and may lead to hospitalization.

In the more severe forms of depression, the patient is incapacitated by the symptoms of depression. Patients with severe forms of depression are more likely to have had previous episodes of depression, have a family history of depression, and express suicidal ideation. The DSM-IV criteria for major depression requires evidence of 5 out of the 8 symptoms listed in Table 16-5 for at least two weeks.[39] Other symptoms which are common in major depression are tearfulness (94 percent), diurnal variation (64 percent), and hopelessness (51 percent).[32]

TABLE 16-5

DSM-IV Diagnostic Criteria for Major Depressive Episode

Five (or more) of the following symptoms are present for most of the day, nearly every day for at least two weeks. The symptoms cause significant impairment in psychosocial functioning and are not due to a general medical condition or the physiological effects of illicit substances or medication. The percentage of patients presenting with these symptoms is indicated in parentheses.

1. Depressed mood (100%) (in children and adolescents, can be irritable mood).
2. Marked diminished interest or pleasure in activities.
3. Unintended weight gain or loss (66%) of more than 5% of body weight in a month (in children and adolescents failure to make expected weight gains).
4. Changes in sleep pattern including insomnia (100%) or early morning wakening (in children and adolescents may see hypersomnia).
5. Psychomotor agitation or retardation (76%).
6. Fatigue (76%).
7. Feelings of worthlessness; excessive or inappropriate guilt.
8. Difficulty concentrating or indecisiveness (91%).
9. Recurrent thoughts of death; recurrent suicidal ideation (82%) or suicide attempt (15%).

SOURCE: Reprinted with permission from the *Diagnostic and Statistical Manual of Mental Disorders,* 4th ed. Copyright 1994 American Psychiatric Association.[32]

Psychotic (Delusional) Depression   Psychotic depression has many of the same features of major depression and in addition the patient shows evidence of a thought disorder. Individuals with psychotic depression, which includes postpartum depression, typically have many somatic delusions or exhibit paranoid ideation. Individuals suffering from the more severe forms of psychotic depression may be so regressed that they are incontinent and unable to perform basic self-care activities.

Schatzberg and Rothschild[40] have argued that there are sufficient data and clinical reasons to designate major depression with psychotic features as a distinct depressive syndrome. Generally, the content of the delusions or hallucinations is consistent with the depressive themes. Such mood-congruent psychotic features include delusions of guilt, delusions of deserved punishment, nihilistic delusions, or somatic delusions. Less commonly, the content of the hallucinations or delusions has no apparent relationship to depressive themes. Such mood-incongruent psychotic features include persecutory delusions, delusions of thought insertion, delusions of thought broadcasting, and delusions of control. Some studies have suggested that psychotically depressed patients have residual social and occupational impairment but not depression and psychosis at 1 year[18] and 5 years[41] after the initial index episode. Patients with psychotic depression have a poor prognosis and greater short-term morbidity and mortality than do nonpsychotic depressed patients.

It is important to make the distinction between psychotic and nonpsychotic depression because patients with psychotic depression respond better to a combination of a TCA and a neuroleptic than to TCA monotherapy or neuroleptic monotherapy.[40] SSRIs in combination with neuroleptics are less well studied but may be effective as well.[42] New atypical antipsychotic medications such as clozapine, risperidone, and olanzapine (which currently have the indication for the treatment of schizophrenia in the United States) may also have a role in the treatment of patients with psychotic depression (Reference 43 and Rothschild, et al., unpublished data).

Postpartum Depression   In general, the symptoms that characterize postpartum depression do not differ from symptoms in a nonpostpartum episode. Typically, symptom onset occurs within four weeks postpartum. Symptoms may include psychotic features such as delusions that the newborn is possessed by the devil or will be doomed to a terrible fate.[39] Psychotic features appear from 1 in 500 to 1 in 1000 deliveries and typically are more common in primiparous women.[44] In both the psychotic and nonpsychotic presentations, there may be associated suicidal ideation, obsessional thoughts regarding violence to the child, insomnia (i.e., early morning awakening), spontaneous crying long after the usual duration of "baby blues" (i.e., three to seven days postpartum), panic attacks, and disinterest in the infant.[39]

Since the number of women choosing to breastfeed is increasing,[45] the clinician may be faced with the question as to whether antidepressant medication can be prescribed to women who are breastfeeding. To date, breast milk excretion studies have demonstrated that antidepressants are present in breast milk, with a milk/serum ratio that is typically greater than or equal to 1.0,[46] but the clinical significance of this is unclear. Adjusting both the schedule of dosing of the antidepressant and the infant's feeding schedule may considerably reduce the concentration of the drug to which the infant is exposed. It is highly recommended that the clinician discuss the medication and potential interactions with the infant's pediatrician. The delay in hepatic maturity may affect the metabolism of psychotropic agents and potentially alter the serum levels of other medications prescribed for the infant. In those complicated cases of women on psychotropic medications who are breast-feeding, it is also often advisable to obtain a consultation from a psychiatric specialist.

Bipolar Disorders A small number of patients (less than 2 percent of the general population) may present initially with major depression and later exhibit symptoms of mania or bipolar illness. The DSM-IV criteria for hypomania, which is a milder or briefer form of mania, are listed in Table 16-6. Manic episodes are characterized by all the same symptoms as hypomania as well as delusions or hallucinations. The symptoms in mania are so severe as to markedly impair normal daily functioning or require immediate hospitalization.

Ninety percent of patients diagnosed with bipolar disorder will experience another episode of illness with the second episode occurring, on average, in 4 years. Noncompliance with medication, marital discord, and divorce are prominent treatment problems in patients diagnosed with bipolar disorder. To minimize the debilitating psychosocial effects of recurrence, the American Psychiatric Association practice guidelines for the treatment of bipolar disorder stress the need for a long-term, supportive psychotherapeutic relationship.[47] Advanced practice nurses who diagnose a first episode of bipolar disorder should always consider referring the patient to a psychiatric clinical specialist for long-term supportive psychotherapy and medication.

Thought Disorders

Patients presenting to the advanced practice nurse with florid psychotic symptoms should have a careful neurological exam to rule out psychosis due to neurologic impair-

TABLE 16-6

DSM-IV Diagnostic Criteria for Hypomanic Episode

The presence of three or more of the following symptoms for at least 4 days:

1. Inflated self-esteem or grandiosity (86%)*
2. Need for sleep decreases significantly from usual sleep pattern (i.e., feels rested after 3 hours of sleep when normally sleeps 7 hours) (90%)
3. Pressured speech or very talkative (99%)
4. Flight of ideas or racing thoughts (93%)
5. Distractibility (100%)
6. Hyperactivity
7. Increase in risk-taking behavior (i.e., gambling, promiscuity (11%), speeding, physical or verbal altercations)

*Percentage of patients presenting with symptoms.

SOURCE: Reprinted with permission from the *Diagnostic and Statistical Manual of Mental Disorders*, 4th ed. Copyright 1994 American Psychiatric Association.[32]

ment and a toxic screen to rule out substance-induced psychosis and/or withdrawal. On interview if the patient exhibits symptoms characteristic of severe or chronic mental illness (such as schizophrenia or bipolar disorder), has been nonresponsive to psychotropic medication in the past, or has multiple psychosocial issues (such as questions of child neglect and abuse), the patient should be referred to a psychiatric clinical specialist for evaluation and follow-up (see Table 16-7). Suicidal or homicidal threats are

TABLE 16-7

Clinical Features of Mental Illness Warranting Referral

Psychiatric Symptoms	Examples
Psychotic Behavior	
Hallucinations	Hearing voices
Delusions	Believes that he/she has unusual powers
Bizarre behavior	Engages in ritualistic behavior which has special meaning
Racy and tangential thinking	Jumps quickly from one topic to another
Marked risk-taking behavior	Speeding in car, gambling excessively
Marked increase in libido	Making inappropriate sexual remarks
Depersonalization	Feeling like an outside observer of one's mental or bodily functions
Suicide Risk	
History of recent trauma or loss	Death of significant other, loss of job, loss of possessions due to natural disaster
History of past suicide attempts	Has taken an overdose of medication
Has a suicide plan	Even vague references—"I feel like jumping in front of a car"—should be taken seriously
Has the means	Owns a gun, has lethal amount of medication
Refuses to contract for safety	Is unable to state that he/she will not follow through with suicide plan
Poor coping skills	Feels hopeless
Has few social supports	"I have no one to live for"
History of substance abuse	Alcoholic or history of impulsive behavior when under the influence of illicit drugs
Neurovegetative Signs	
Marked change in weight	Weighing 70% of ideal body weight
Marked change in sleep	Sleeping 3 to 4 hours less than usual
History of Severe Mental Illness	
Past personal history or family history of schizophrenia, manic-depressive illness, chronic or severe eating disorders, and depression	
Family history of suicide or suicide attempts	

symptoms that warrant immediate referral to psychiatric specialists and may require hospitalization.

Eating Disorders   Anorexia nervosa and bulimia typically present in adolescence or young adulthood. Populations at risk include athletes (especially runners or gymnasts), models, and dancers.[38] Both disorders have physical sequelae which may precipitate referral to the advanced practice nurse for a medical evaluation. Although anorexic patients may wear bulky clothes to hide their emaciated appearance, the physical signs of anorexia are easily assessed. Physical signs and symptoms of anorexia nervosa include amenorrhea, constipation, abdominal pain, cold intolerance, fatigue, hypotension, hypothermia, dry skin, lanugo, bradycardia, and edema. Laboratory abnormalities include elevated growth hormone levels, increased plasma cortisol, and reduced gonadotropin levels.

The physical signs of bulimia tend to be more subtle. The bulimic patient may present with a weight that is appropriate for his or her height and stature. Significant weight fluctuations of 10 to 20 lbs should alert the advanced practice nurse to the possibility that the patient may be bulimic. There are several physical signs characteristic of bulimia including calluses on the knuckles, an enlargement of the parotid glands, erosion of dental enamel, and in extreme cases, esophageal tears. Laboratory abnormalities are common in bulimia and may include elevated serum cholesterol, hypocalcemia, or hypokalemic alkalosis.

Electrolyte and nutritional imbalances in both anorexia nervosa and bulimia can cause weakness, stress fractures, or in extreme cases, cardiac arrhythmia and death. One in ten patients dies from the complications of an eating disorder.[38] Any patient who presents at 60 percent of his or her ideal body weight, has marked electrolyte imbalances, or is suicidal should be evaluated for immediate hospitalization. Intravenous fluids or nasogastric feedings should be initiated for dehydrated patients whose medical condition is clearly compromised.

An interdisciplinary team approach is generally used in the management of eating disorders. Advanced practice nurses or internists may treat the medical symptoms, nutritionists advise on proper diet regimens, and psychiatric clinical specialists provide cognitive-behavioral, family, or group psychotherapy.[38] Patients seen at the first episode who are not medically compromised and do not exhibit co-morbid psychiatric symptoms should be referred for CBT or short-term psychotherapy.[48]

Pharmacologic treatment is often used in combination with psychotherapeutic approaches. A meta-analysis of the efficacy of antidepressants in the treatment of bulimia found that on average, binge episodes decreased 67 percent.[49] Although these findings are encouraging, it is also important to note that only a small number of patients completely abstained from bingeing or purging behavior and medication had mixed effects on symptoms of anxiety or depression.

In contrast to studies supporting the efficacy of pharmacologic treatment for bulimia, controlled trials of antidepressants in the treatment of anorexia are inconclusive.[48] The course and prognosis of anorexia nervosa is similar to treatment-resistant depression. Frequent checks of plasma blood levels may help determine if the dose is inadequate or if there are problems with treatment compliance. However, even with adequate plasma levels the client may remain unresponsive to medication treatment. Given the chronic and sometimes intractable course of anorexia nervosa, advanced practice nurses are advised to consult colleagues or the literature for the most up-to-date information on medication treatment strategies.

Anxiety Disorders   Anxiety is a subjective emotional and physiological state experienced by everyone at some point in their lives. Anxiety warrants therapeutic intervention when individuals are incapable of controlling their apprehension and are so preoccupied with worrisome thoughts that it interferes with their sleep, ability to rest, and concentration for at least six months. Generalized anxiety disorder is the most prevalent of all psychiatric conditions with an estimated lifetime prevalence rate of 15 percent. Nearly a quarter of medical inpatients have anxiety symptoms severe enough to warrant pharmacologic intervention.[50]

Cognitive-behavioral therapies, such as progressive relaxation and sensory imagery, are very effective for mild forms of anxiety. The choice of medication in the treatment of generalized anxiety disorder varies depending upon the frequency and duration of symptoms. Benzodiazepines and buspirone are the most common pharmacologic treatments. Meditation, massage therapy, acupuncture, and hydrotherapy are alternative approaches that are not well studied, but may offer patients symptomatic relief.

Approximately 1.5 percent of the general population meet the criteria for panic disorder with the highest incidence (13 percent) being among alcoholics. Panic attacks occur suddenly and have prominent physical symptoms that may resemble an acute myocardial infarction. Cardiac signs and symptoms characteristic of panic disorder include sweating, shortness of breath, palpitations, tachycardia, chest pain, dizziness, paresthesia, chills, hot flashes, nausea, or abdominal distress. The presence of psychological symptoms characteristic of panic disorder assists in making a differential diagnosis; these symptoms include derealization, detachment, fear of losing control, and fear of death. Medications or other medical conditions that present with anxiety or panic-like symptoms include excessive caffeine ingestion, diet pills, decongestants, benzodiazepine withdrawal, hypoglycemia, and hyperthyroidism.

Once a proper differential diagnosis has been made, the treatment of panic disorders should include both medication and cognitive-behavioral therapy. Pharmacologic treatments for panic disorder include the SSRIs, TCAs, MAOIs, and benzodiazepines. Progressive relaxation and desensitization techniques are effective in the vast majority of patients with the diagnosis of panic disorder.

Obsessive-compulsive disorders (OCDs) have approximately the same incidence among the general population (2 percent) as anxiety disorders. In OCD, medication effects on target symptoms may take longer and require higher doses of antidepressants. The severity of symptoms after five weeks of optimal pharmacologic treatment is the best predictor for long-term outcome in patients with OCD.[30]

The most effective medications for the treatment of OCD are potent inhibitors of 5-HT reuptake such as clomipramine, fluvoxamine, fluoxetine, paroxetine, and sertraline.[51] Forty to sixty percent of OCD patients are unresponsive even when given adequate trials of these medications. For patients who do experience some symptom relief, the relapse rate following discontinuation of pharmacotherapy is extremely high (90 percent).

Because of the chronicity and high relapse rate among patients diagnosed with OCD, regular follow-up visits and periodic telephone screening for medication compliance are essential for proper long-term management. There are mixed reports on the efficacy of CBT in the treatment of OCD. Nevertheless, patients whose symptoms are not responsive to pharmacologic treatment should be referred to a psychiatric clinical specialist for a trial of cognitive-behavioral psychotherapy.

Posttraumatic Stress Disorder   To be diagnosed with posttraumatic stress disorder (PTSD) an individual must have experienced a traumatic event that is outside the range of normal human experience. The National Comorbidity Study estimates that the lifetime prevalence of PTSD is 7.8 percent. Although men are exposed to more traumatic events than women, women are twice as likely to develop symptoms of PTSD. In general, the earlier and more frequent the trauma, the poorer the long-term prognosis.[52] For example, 80 percent of young children who are severely burned exhibit symptoms of PTSD one to two years later, compared to 30 percent of adults.[32] Symptoms may begin hours or years after the traumatic event and include flashbacks, insomnia, outbursts of anger, hypervigilance, and an exaggerated startle response.

In an acute episode, patients with PTSD experience vivid flashbacks of the trauma, accompanied by symptoms of hyperarousal such as tachycardia, tremors, and sweating. In extreme cases, clients may appear to dissociate or even hallucinate. Cognitive therapies, such as grounding techniques, are useful to reorient the patient and mobilize healthy defenses. The volatility of the patient's affect and rage can make management of patients with PTSD challenging for advanced practice nurses.

It is advisable to use a multidisciplinary approach with the psychotherapist as the principal person who works through the emotionally laden material with the patient. Primary care providers who are peripheral to the psychotherapy are discouraged from probing into the patient's past for details and descriptions about the traumatic event. The major short-term goal of providers, other than the psychotherapist, should be to diffuse the overwhelming affect and minimize psychotic episodes—not to "uncover" repressed recollections, "confront" the perpetrator, or "get the patient in touch with his or her feelings."

Medication is used as an adjunct to psychotherapy to moderate the acute exacerbations of PTSD symptoms. Because the symptom profiles can be so diffuse and variable over time, advanced practice nurses should continually reassess the medication regimen, adjusting dosages or initiating new trials of medications from different classes in response to any significant change in mental status.

Patients with PTSD generally present with a predominance of affective and hyperarousal symptoms. Investigations have shown the efficacy of TCAs, MAOIs, and SSRIs. Mood stabilizers such as lithium, carbamazepine, and valproate may be used to manage mood lability and outbursts of rage. As psychotherapy progresses, recounting traumatic material may trigger psychotic-like behavior. Antipsychotics can be added as a PRN or daily dose depending on the frequency and severity of symptoms. Beta blockers are often prescribed to manage persistent arousal symptoms assuming there are no medical contraindications.[53] Benzodiazepines should be used cautiously in patients with PTSD because of their potential for abuse and disinhibiting effects.[54]

Premenstrual Dysphoric Disorder   Many women experience physical changes occurring around the time of their menses such as fatigue, bloating, breast tenderness, headaches, and edema. In addition to these physical signs, women diagnosed with premenstrual dysphoric disorder (PDD) also experience abrupt changes in mood that can have a marked impact on their social functioning. Psychological symptoms include irritability, mood lability, and depression. To definitively make the diagnosis of PDD, patients should rate their mood daily for at least 2 months. Changes in mood or other affective symptoms should be circumscribed around the time of menses and have a measurable, deleterious effect on the patient's ability to function.

There are a wide range of pharmacologic and alternative treatments that have been proposed for PDD. One of the complicating factors in evaluating the efficacy of these proposed treatments is that in the few published controlled trials, there has been a very high placebo response rate (40 percent).[34] Because the symptoms cluster around the time of menses, the first line of treatment is usually hormonal therapies. The most effective hormonal treatments are Gn-RH agonists and danazol followed by estrogen. The efficacy of oral contraceptives and progesterone is unclear. Antidepressants, in particular the SSRIs, appear to be as effective as the hormonal therapies. Limiting the use of antidepressants to the time of menses has been suggested, but remains controversial. Alprazolam and buspirone also have been reported to be useful in the treatment of PDD.

Substance Abuse   Approximately one-third of patients diagnosed with major mental illness abuse alcohol or other substances.[55] Studies report co-morbidity rates which range from 15 to 65 percent for major depression and schizophrenia, and about half of all patients diagnosed with bipolar disorder.[56] In general, when prescribing medication to patients with a history of substance abuse, advanced practice nurses must balance the pharmacologic risks, (which include psychoactive potential, reinforcement potential, tolerance, and withdrawal) against the risks of undertreating a psychiatric disorder. Alcohol and illicit substances alter the P-450 cytochrome system, hepatic metabolism, as well as the levels of neurotransmitters.[56] When, for how long, and if a client must be abstinent or in recovery prior to prescribing psychotropic medication is controversial. Advanced practice nurses should refer to the Treatment Improvement Protocols (TIPS) published by the U.S. Department of Health and Human Services for detailed recommendations on the pharmacologic management of patients with dual diagnoses.[55]

Compliance and Management of Side Effects

Changes in neurovegetative signs such as sleep, appetite, or psychomotor activity are relatively straightforward to quantify and record over time. Monitoring the effectiveness of psychopharmacologic medication on subjective emotional states is a far more complicated process. Several measurement instruments have been devised to more objectively evaluate the efficacy of medications on target symptoms and side effects. These instruments are listed in Table 16-8.

Target symptoms can be identified through interviews and the use of rating scales. Advanced practice nurses should actively engage the patient in an open dialogue about which symptoms are the most problematic or which symptoms he or she would like to see relieved by the use of medication. Once the target symptoms have been identified, the next step is to try to determine how much change the patient wishes to see in these symptoms. For example, the patient may ordinarily sleep only six hours a night, but now is sleeping just three hours. Other patients may not feel rested unless they have nine hours of sleep. Clarifying expectations about the effects of medications—positive and

TABLE 16-8

Commonly Used Rating Scales for Psychiatric Disorders

Scale	Condition	Copyright
MMSE (Mini Mental Status)	Generic for all psychiatric disorders	Pergamon Press
GAS (Global Assessment Scale)	Generic for all psychiatric disorders	AMA
BPRS (Brief Psychiatric Rating Scale)	Generic for all psychiatric disorders	Overall, J.E.
SANS (Scale for Assessing Negative Symptoms)	Thought disorders	Andreasen, N.C.
SAPS (Scale for Assessing Positive Symptoms)	Thought disorders	Andreasen, N.C.
AIMS (Abnormal Involuntary Movement Scale)	Tardive dyskinesia	Guy, W.
Hamilton Depression Scale	Mood disorders	Hamilton, M.
Hamilton Anxiety Scale	Anxiety disorders	Hamilton, M.
Yale-Brown OCD Scale	Obsessive-compulsive disorders	Goodman, W.K.

negative—helps to dispel any false expectations or understanding of how the medication may affect behavior. When evaluating the response of patients to antidepressants, it is important to remember that the symptoms of depression resolve gradually (usually over several weeks). The dysphoric mood state is typically the last state of depression to improve. In the initial stage of treatment the patient may report improvement in energy level, sleep disturbance, or somatic complaints. The clinician may also observe that the patient smiles for the first time or has improved cognitive processes. However, the patient may report that he or she still feels depressed or that "the medication is not working." If the clinician observes signs of improvement in depression (or the patient's family reports improvement), it is important to continue the antidepressant currently prescribed because the early signs of improvement may predict a full response.

Reasonable ranges should be given to the client for when the therapeutic effects should become evident. Advanced practice nurses should be candid with the patients that side effects are likely to be experienced first and therapeutic effects some time later. Some advanced practice nurses prefer to give patients a handout on all the potential side effects of medication, while others prefer to review orally the most common side effects and limit written material to those side effects that are serious and warrant immediate medical attention. The method of educating the patient is secondary to the process of eliciting information throughout the medication trial about the existence of side effects. The key is to develop a therapeutic alliance, identify bothersome side effects early, and intervene so the patient remains compliant.

In addition to written material, education about the medication may include more formal didactic presentations (i.e., medication education groups). Consumer advocacy groups (such as the National Alliance for the Mentally Ill) sponsor local patient and family support groups, as well as educational sessions about the therapeutic benefits of psychopharmacologic therapies. Pharmaceutical companies also have written or video materials about the use of medication to treat mental illness that can be useful for patient and family education.

Relapse or rehospitalization of patients with major mental illness is most often precipitated by a failure to comply with the medication treatment regimen. It is estimated that half of all patients who have been prescribed psychopharmacologic medications for the treatment of major mental illness are noncompliant. Noncompliance can be due to either primary or secondary factors. Primary noncompliance may be a function of cost, proximity to a pharmacy, or a conscious decision by the patient to refuse the medication. The rate of primary noncompliance is estimated to be about 20 percent.[31]

Advanced practice nurses should be able to anticipate during an interview many of the factors contributing to primary noncompliance. It is important not to make assumptions about ability to pay for medication. Patients should be asked directly if cost will be a problem. Use of generic brands is one strategy for minimizing cost. Dispensing medication samples in accordance with state rules and regulations is another option for limiting out-of-pocket expense. Advanced practice nurses should also familiarize themselves with private and state indigent care funds that may be used toward the purchase of medication.

Patients who make a conscious decision to stop taking their medication generally fall into two groups: those who believe they are no longer in need of medication and those who can no longer tolerate objectionable side effects. Bipolar patients are at high risk for primary noncompliance because they find the euphoric hypomanic state preferable to their baseline mental status. Patients who insist that they are no longer in need of medication should be tapered gradually during a period of time when there is less stress in their lives. Frequent telephone contacts to monitor changes in mental status are useful so that the medication regimen can be quickly reinstituted if necessary.

Secondary noncompliance occurs when patients miss a dose, forget their medication, run out of medication and forget to get an order for a refill, or take the wrong dose at the wrong time. The estimated incidence of secondary noncompliance ranges between 15 to 90 percent.[31] Secondary noncompliance may be due to cognitive difficulties, misunderstanding the daily schedule, abuse, tolerance, or diversion by others in the household. Patients at highest risk for secondary noncompliance are those with dementia or substance abuse.

Depending upon the cause, nurses can intervene with education strategies and drug-dispensing devices (weekly pill boxes) or by engaging family members to assist in proper adherence to the medication schedule. For children and adolescents, or patients with chronic schizophrenia, simple behavioral reinforcement programs are often helpful. Depot antipsychotic medication is also an option for the chronic mentally ill who have difficulty adhering to an oral medication regimen. On a cautionary note, a recent study associated the high incidence of tardive dyskinesia in African-Americans with high doses of depot medication.[37]

The simplest way to avoid side effects is to never prescribe more than one medication in the same class (the patient just gets double the chance of experiencing side effects, not double the therapeutic effect) and to be conservative with increasing the dose. The higher the dose, the more likely the patient will experience side effects. Many psychotropic medications take weeks before patients may experience a therapeutic effect. "Start low and go slow" should be the motto for all advanced practice nurses.

If the patient is complaining about problematic side effects, first determine if the side effect is related to the dose or when the medication is ingested. For example, if the patient complains of sedation, find out if the patient is taking the medication in the morning. If the patient is and it is a once a day dose, then recommend taking it in the evening. If the patient complains of nausea, find out if the patient is taking the medication on an empty or full stomach and then suggest he or she do the opposite. If the medication is taken once a day, then try administering the medication in divided doses.

If the side effects are dose-related, consideration should be given to lowering the dose. In panic disorders, it is not uncommon for patients to experience hyperarousal with a dose increase in SSRIs or TCAs. If patients complain after a dose increase, then go back to the original dose; wait a day or two (depending upon the half-life), and then increase the dose half again as much. If the side effects are so troublesome that the patient may stop the medication entirely, consideration should be given to switching to another drug within that class if the patient has received some therapeutic benefit. If the patient has received no therapeutic benefit, it is advisable to switch to another class of medication. Tapering medication is always recommended to avoid withdrawal or rebound effects. Washout periods are discussed later in this chapter but obviously are an important consideration when switching to different classes of medication.

Clients with eating disorders present a unique set of challenges for medication compliance. Anorexic clients may refuse or severely restrict anything by mouth including medication. Psychoeducation or behavioral programs may improve compliance, but for some clients who are severely regressed and need supplemental nasogastric feedings, it may be necessary to obtain legal guardianship. With bulimic patients, absorption may be compromised by the use of laxatives or by vomiting. Clients with bulimia should be directed to take their medications during periods of the day when they are least likely to engage in bingeing and purging activity.

Prescription of Medications
Depression
The goals of the initial treatment of depression are threefold: (1) to reduce and ultimately remove all the signs and symptoms of the depressive disorder, (2) to restore the patient's ability to function at his or her job or within his or her social setting, and (3) to reduce the likelihood of a relapse or the recurrence of the depression. A consultation or referral to a psychiatrist should be considered if one is unsure of the diagnosis or, if there is co-morbid medical illness, a lack of response to the medication, or a severe functional impairment (see Table 16-7). Referral is always advisable if the patient shows signs of psychosis such as hallucinations or delusions. If one suspects bipolar disorder or if there is suicidal ideation or even distorted reasoning that may be psychotic in nature, referral is a sensible choice. Since there is a relationship between psychosocial problems and depression, if the patient has responded to medication but has residual psychosocial problems, a referral to a psychotherapist would be appropriate.

Over the past 45 years, remarkable advances have been made in the development of medications to treat depressive illness. In general, approximately 65 to 80 percent of depressed outpatients receiving an antidepressant will show marked improvement.[57,58] There is no evidence that any one antidepressant or class of antidepressants is more efficacious or works at a faster rate of speed than any other antidepressants. However, antidepressants differ in their mechanisms of action, side-effect profile, and toxicity in overdose. The past 10 years have seen a dramatic increase in the number of antidepressants available to treat depression with the advent of the selective serotonin reuptake inhibitors (SSRIs) and other new antidepressant agents. These newer medications have an improved side-effect profile over older classes of medications like the TCAs and MAOIs and were developed specifically to treat depression. The development of these antidepressants differs from the serendipitous "discovery" of the TCAs and MAOIs.

The medications commonly used to treat depression are summarized in Table 16-9. In general, a clinical trial of an antidepressant medication lasts 4 to 6 weeks. Patients and their families must be educated that the response rate is slow and subtle. Side effects of antidepressants, if they occur, are likely to occur early in the treatment before the positive beneficial effects of the medication begin. The prescription of an antidepressant is almost certainly appropriate in the case of a patient with moderate to severe depression, whether or not psychotherapy is also used. An antidepressant prescription is also indicated for a patient experiencing a recurrence of depression.

Medication Selection   Since clinical studies show that all antidepressants are equally efficacious, the practitioner could select any one of the medications listed in Table 16-9. Several key factors that should be considered when selecting an antidepressant medication for a patient include (1) the ease with which one will be able to achieve the therapeutic dose, (2) the global safety of the drug, (3) the patient's prior response if he or she has been prescribed the drug previously, (4) any co-morbidity that may be present, (5) the type and extent of the side effects, (6) the drug's half-life, and (7) the cost of the drug within the context of the cost of treating the entire disease.

Dosage Range   It is important to titrate the dose of an antidepressant medication based upon the clinical response. The usual therapeutic dose ranges of the antidepressants are shown in Table 16-9. In practice, most mental health and primary care practitioners often use an SSRI as their first-line antidepressant because of ease of prescription and benign side-effect profiles.

Dosing an SSRI   The SSRIs are a new and widely prescribed class of antidepressants. One of the reasons for the popularity of this class is the ease of prescribing. The majority of patients treated for depression respond to the starting dose or mid-range dose of SSRIs. Patients should be started on the 1-pill-per-day starting dose for each SSRI [fluoxetine 20 mg/day, paroxetine 20 mg/day (10 mg for the elderly), sertraline 50 mg/day]. After a 2 to 4 week trial, the dose may be raised by 50 mg/week to a maximum of 200 mg/day for sertraline, by 10 mg/week to a maximum of 50 mg/day for paroxetine, and to a maximum of 80 mg/day for fluoxetine. Before the dose of any antidepressant is titrated, the patient should be evaluated for early signs of response. Since the SSRIs

TABLE 16-9

Dose Ranges of Antidepressants

Generic Name	Brand Name	Usual Therapeutic Dose Range, mg/day*
SSRIs		
Fluoxetine	Prozac	20–80
Paroxetine	Paxil	20–50
Sertraline	Zoloft	50–200
Other		
Bupropion	Wellbutrin	200–450
Venlafaxine	Effexor	75–375
Nefazodone	Serzone	300–500
Mirtazapine	Remron	15–45
Heterocyclics		
Amoxapine	Asendin	150–450
Maprotiline	Ludiomil	150–200
Trazodone	Desyrel	150–300
Tricyclics		
Amitriptyline	Elavil, Endep	150–300
Desipramine	Norpramin, Pertofrane	150–300
Imipramine	Tofranil, Janimine, Sk-Pramine	150–300
Nortriptyline	Pamelor, Aventyl	50–150
MAOIs		
Phenelzine	Nardil	45–90
Tranylcypramine	Parnate	30–50

*Dosage ranges are approximate. Many patients will respond at relatively low dosages (even below ranges given above); others may require higher dosages.

have a flat dose response curve, the starting dose of the SSRI is usually the same as the ending dose. By contrast, the TCAs require titration. High doses of SSRIs (although often well tolerated by patients) are usually not required, although trials of standard doses for up to 6 to 8 weeks may be needed.[59,60]

Dosing a TCA   The prescription of TCAs requires gradual titration of the patient's dose until a therapeutic dose is achieved (see Table 16-9 for therapeutic ranges). For most TCAs the usual starting dose is 25 or 50 mg at bedtime with gradual increases by 25- or 50-mg increments to a dose range of approximately 150 to 300 mg/day (with the exception of nortriptyline, which is usually half these amounts). Most patients will not be able to tolerate the therapeutic dose without gradual titration.

Use of MAO Inhibitors   Before the advent of the SSRIs and other newer agents, the pharmacologic choices for the treatment of depression were limited to the TCAs, MAOIs, electroconvulsive therapy (ECT), and lithium. Prior to 1988, MAOIs were often the second-line agents after the TCAs. Currently, given the wide array of choices for pharmacologic treatment, MAOIs are rarely used in the primary care setting and are reserved more for treatment-resistant patients being treated by specialists. However, because some patients are being treated with MAOIs, the advanced practice nurse needs to be aware of several important drug-drug and food-drug interactions.

Patients prescribed MAOIs are susceptible to hypertensive crises from drug-drug or food-drug interactions. Patients taking MAOIs require special tyramine-free diets in which foods with high levels of tyramines are avoided. The MAOIs should not be given concomitantly with or in temporal proximity to SSRIs because the combinations can result in the potentially fatal serotonin syndrome. The symptoms of the serotonin syndrome include hyperthermia, muscle rigidity, and autonomic hyperactivity which can progress to coma and death.

When switching from an MAOI to any of the SSRIs, a washout period of 2 weeks is recommended. When switching from an SSRI to an MAOI, a washout period of 2 weeks is recommended for sertraline and paroxetine; a 5-week washout period is recommended when switching from fluoxetine to an MAOI.

Global Safety   Drug overdose is always an important consideration with depressed patients. Due to the greater toxicity associated with TCAs, an overdose of one of these agents may prove to be fatal. TCAs are the third most common cause of drug-related death (following alcohol-drug combinations and heroin).[61] TCAs also rank fourth in overdoses seen in emergency departments.[62] A total of 70 to 80 percent of patients who take TCA overdoses do not reach the hospital alive.[63] For these reasons, the newer agents offer an important advantage in their wider margin of safety in overdose.

It is important to note that higher blood levels of TCAs and their metabolites may cause serious cardiac conduction disturbances that can prove to be fatal. Monitoring TCA blood levels and regular electrocardiograms is especially recommended for the elderly, those with compromised medical health, those showing clinical symptoms of toxicity, those on higher-than-average doses, and those with certain preexisting cardiac conditions.

Half-life   The half-life of an antidepressant is important in case the patient experiences an adverse reaction and quick removal of the medication is indicated. Most TCAs have a half-life of about 24 h, while that of SSRIs is shorter, averaging approximately 20 h. The notable exception is fluoxetine, which has a half-life of two to three days; it has an active metabolite with a half-life of 7 to 9 days. The pharmacokinetic profiles of the serotonin reuptake inhibitors are shown in Table 16-10. Long washout periods also may be significant when the practitioner wants the medication to leave the patient's body quickly (e.g., when mania is induced or side effects become unbearable, when pregnancy is discovered, when concurrent medical problems develop, or when other medications must be added).

TABLE 16-10

Pharmacokinetic Profiles of the Serotonin Reuptake Inhibitors

	Fluoxetine	Paroxetine	Sertraline
Half-life	2–3 days	24 hours	26 hours
Metabolite activity	Equal	Essentially inactive	Substantially less
Half-life of metabolite	7–9 days	—	2–4 days
Washout period	35–45 days	7 days	7 days
Steady state	35–45 days	7 days	7 days

Cost   The typical cost of the commonly prescribed antidepressants is shown in Table 16-11. It is important to keep in mind that the cost of the medication is only a small part of the total cost of the treatment of depression. A study of economic outcomes in a health maintenance organization indicated that the mean annual cost per patient for therapy with a TCA was $960.00, while the mean annual cost per patient for therapy with an SSRI was $508.00.[64] Although the price per pill of an SSRI is frequently greater than the cost per pill of a TCA, the medications are only a small part of the total cost. Other costs such as visits to the outpatient clinic or hospitalization (should it occur) are much more costly. Since patients on TCAs often have more side effects and require titration of the medication, they need more frequent visits to the clinic, and the total depression-related direct cost for TCAs is greater than the total mean cost for treatment with an SSRI. Thus, if one takes a narrow view of depression-related treatment cost, one might come to the erroneous conclusion that TCAs are the least expensive. However, if one takes a broad view of the total depression-related treatment cost, SSRIs are actually more cost-effective. Thus, formularies or managed care plans which restrict access to SSRIs in preference for TCAs are not only exposing the patients to medications with more toxic side effects, but are also creating greater costs for themselves and the health care system as a whole.

Ease of Use in Achieving a Therapeutic Dose   Achieving the proper therapeutic dose is a serious problem with many antidepressants. A recent study observed that only 54 percent of patients studied had received adequate dose and duration of antidepressant treatment.[65] A review of the records of psychiatric patients enrolled in a large HMO over a 2-year period was conducted to determine whether drug category made a difference in the number of patients who received treatment of adequate dosage and/or duration.[65] In this study, patients treated with an SSRI were more likely to receive an adequate dose and duration of treatment than those treated with TCAs or other medications. It has also been found that in clinical practice, adequate dose and duration are achieved more often with SSRIs than with bupropion, secondary amine tricyclics, tertiary amine tricyclics, or trazodone.

TABLE 16-11

Approximate Average Wholesale Price of Medications

Medication		Cost per Tablet $	Medication		Cost per Tablet $
Antidepressants			Pamelor	10 mg	0.50
SSRIs				25 mg	1.00
Paxil	10 mg	1.98		50 mg	1.89
	20 mg	2.07		75 mg	2.88
	30 mg	2.13	* Desipramine	25 mg	0.27
	40 mg	2.25		50 mg	0.53
Prozac	10 mg	2.36		75 mg	0.62
	20 mg	2.42		100 mg	1.07
Zoloft	50 mg	2.16	* Nortriptyline	10 mg	0.38
	100 mg	2.22		25 mg	0.76
Luvox				50 mg	1.50
	50 mg	2.07		75 mg	2.13
	100 mg	2.13	* Imipramine	10 mg	0.05
				25 mg	0.06
Other				50 mg	0.09
Wellbutrin	75 mg	0.62	* Amitriptyline	25 mg	0.07
	100 mg	0.83		50 mg	0.11
Wellbutrin SR	100 mg	0.72		75 mg	0.15
	150 mg	0.74		100 mg	0.19
Effexor	25 mg	1.02			
	37.5 mg	1.05	**MAOIs**		
	50 mg	1.08	Nardil	15 mg	0.42
Serzone	100 mg	0.97	Parnate	10 mg	0.50
	150 mg	0.97	**Anxiolytics**		
	200 mg	0.97	Alprazolam	0.25 mg	0.54
Remeron	15 mg	1.98		0.50 mg	0.67
	30 mg	2.04		1.0 mg	0.89
	1.0 mg	0.91		2.0 mg	1.54
	2.0 mg	1.27	Klonopin	0.5 mg	0.80
			Buspar	5 mg	0.62
Heterocyclics				10 mg	1.08
*Trazodone			Xanax	0.25 mg	0.65
	50 mg	0.30		0.50 mg	0.81
	100 mg	0.48		1.0 mg	1.08
	150 mg	0.89		2.0 mg	1.84
Tricyclics					
Norpramin	25 mg	0.65			
	50 mg	1.22			
	75 mg	1.55			
	100 mg	2.04			

*Generic.

Prior Response   Another consideration when selecting an antidepressant medication is prior response. If the patient had been treated with a particular antidepressant in the past and the patient's experience with the drug was positive, a new prescription for the same medication would be appropriate. However, it is important to determine why the patient stopped taking the medication. For example, if side effects were a problem, a different medication may be advisable. In addition, probing to determine whether any new problems have developed, such as cardiovascular disease, may influence your selection of the antidepressant. Another possibility is that the patient is on new medications which may result in drug-drug interactions with the previously prescribed antidepressant (e.g., an anticholinergic medication and a TCA).

Side Effects The side effects from antidepressants occur because of activation or blockade of neuronal receptors. Examples include blockade of the alpha$_1$-adrenergic receptor, the histamine (H$_1$) receptor, and the muscarinic receptor. Examples of agonist effects would include increases in asynaptic serotonin levels affecting postsynaptic serotonin receptors.

Table 16-12 provides a summary of antidepressant side effects. Newer agents such as the SSRIs do not cause the side effects commonly seen with the TCAs and MAOIs; this is also a major reason for their wide acceptance and frequent use among psychiatric and nonpsychiatric practitioners.

Drug-Drug Interactions It is important for the practitioner to keep in mind potential drug-drug interactions between the antidepressant and other medications the patient may be taking. For example, anticholinergic side effects of the TCAs can be additive with anticholinergic side effects of other medications (e.g., an antispasmodic). Sedative antidepressants combined with other medications that have sedating properties may also be problematic. The use of most TCAs and SSRIs in combination with MAOIs is contraindicated. The SSRIs are metabolized extensively in the liver by the cytochrome P-450 microsomal enzyme system. Inhibition occurs at therapeutic doses of the SSRIs and consequently can produce drug interactions of clinical significance.[67] Fluoxetine, its equally potent metabolite norfluoxetine, and paroxetine are significantly more potent inhibitors of cytochrome P-450 II D6 than sertraline and its principal metabolite *N*-desmethylsertraline. These differences are evident in vitro[68,69] and in vivo.[70,71]

The cytochrome P-450 II D6 isoenzyme is important in the metabolism of many commonly prescribed medications including TCAs, antiarrhythmics (e.g., quinidine), haloperidol, some benzodiazepines, codeine, and dextromethorphan (the ingredient found in over-the-counter medications such as Dristan, Comtrex, Tylenol Cold and Flu, Robitussin DM, and Benylin DM). The inhibitory effects of SSRIs on the cytochrome P-450 isoenzymes may slow the metabolism or inhibit the clearance of affected drugs and thereby produce higher plasma concentrations. Thus, it may be necessary to lower the dosage of affected drugs if therapy of fluoxetine or paroxetine is initiated or start with a lower dose of the affected drug when it is added to an ongoing regimen of an SSRI. Likewise, when the SSRI is withdrawn from therapy, it may be necessary to increase the dose of the co-administered drug.

Other medications (e.g., nefazodone, SSRIs) may be potent inhibitors of the cytochrome P-4503A4 isoenzyme, and the practitioner needs to use caution in using medications that are metabolized by P-4503A4. For example, the antihistamines terfenadine and astemizole are contraindicated when a patient is taking nefazodone.[72] Alprazolam

TABLE 16-12

Side-Effect Profiles of Antidepressant Medications

Drug	Central Nervous System			Cardiovascular		Other	
	Anticholinergic*	Drowsiness	Insomnia/ agitation	Orthostatic hypotension	Cardiac arrhythmia	Gastrointestinal distress	Weight gain (>6 kg)
SSRIs							
Fluoxetine	0	0	2+	0	0	3+	0
Paroxetine	0	0	2+	0	0	3+	0
Sertraline	0	0	2+	0	0	3+	0
Other							
Bupropion	0	0	2+	0	1+	1+	0
Nerazadone	0	2+	0	1+	0	1+	0
Venlafaxine	0	1+	1+	0	0	3+	0
Mirtazapine	1+	4+	0	2+	0	0	4+
Heterocyclics							
Amoxapine	2+	2+	2+	2+	3+	0	1+
Maprotiline	2+	4+	0	0	1+	0	2+
Trazodone	0	4+	0	1+	1+	1+	1+
Tricyclics							
Amitriptyline	4+†	4+	0	4+	3+	0	4+
Desipramine	1+	1+	1+	2+	2+	0	1+
Doxepin	3+	4+	0	2+	2+	0	3+
Imipramine	3+	3+	1+	4+	3+	1+	3+
Nortriptyline	1+	1+	0	2+	2+	0	1+
Protriptyline	2+	1+	1+	2+	2+	0	0
Trimipramine	1+	4+	0	2+	2+	0	3+
MAOIs	1+	1+	2+	2+	0	1+	2+

*Dry mouth, blurred vision, urinary hesitancy, constipation.

†0 absent or rare; 1+ to 2+, in between; 3+ to 4+, relatively common; MAOIs, monoamine oxidase inhibitors.

SOURCE: Adapted from Rothschild AJ.[66]

and triazolam are also metabolized by cytochrome P-4503A4, so a dosage reduction of the benzodiazepine is recommended.[72]

Patients who are on concomitant medications and in whom drug-drug interactions may be an issue may warrant a consultation and/or referral to a psychiatrist.

Treating Symptoms versus Syndrome It is critical to remember that when one is treating patients suffering from depression that the goal is alleviation of the entire syndrome and not just one or two symptoms of the depressive disorder (e.g., anxiety, insomnia). SSRIs and other antidepressants effectively treat not only the depression but also the anxiety or insomnia associated with depression. Prescribing an antidepressant that is very sedating, such as amitriptyline or trazodone, for a depressed patient with insomnia will result initially in that patient sleeping better. However, insomnia is only one of many symptoms of depression, and a 50-mg starting dose of amitriptyline will do very little for the total syndrome of major depression and its accompanying symptoms of hopelessness, poor energy, anhedonia, and suicidal ideation. Therapeutic doses of sedating antidepressants (150 to 300 mg/day) are necessary to treat the total syndrome, but they may result in daytime sedation. If a sleep disturbance develops during SSRI treatment, the addition of a sedating antidepressant (e.g., trazodone) at a low dose as a sleeping medication is often effective.[73]

Anxiety is also commonly observed in patients with major depression.[74] If anxiety is one of the symptoms of a major depressive episode, an antidepressant will alleviate anxiety. In contrast, if only an antianxiety agent (e.g., buspirone or benzodiazepine) is prescribed for a patient with depression, only the anxiety symptoms will be alleviated and the syndrome of major depression will not be treated adequately. Although the patient may be more distressed by the anxiety symptoms, the clinician should evaluate the patient for other symptoms of depression. Unlike anxiety, major depression may be characterized by anhedonia (loss of interest or pleasure in usual activities), fatigue, weight/appearance changes, sad affect, and excessive guilt. In addition, patients with major depression will have early morning awakening (awakening at 3 or 4 A.M.) without being able to fall back asleep, whereas those with an anxiety disorder often have trouble falling asleep but usually do not have early morning awakening once they are asleep.

Scheduling Follow-up Visits Follow-up on the patient with depression should begin within the first seven days after the initial contact. After the first week of treatment, follow-up should occur a week or two after the start of medication, depending on the severity of symptoms and a need for dosage titration. If the patient has severe symptoms, a referral may be in order; otherwise, a visit every two to three weeks should be adequate. Giving the patient ongoing support is essential in order to enable the clinician to determine clinical response and the need for dosage adjustments. Although it is possible for patients to experience significant improvement in the symptoms of major depression within the first week, this is not common. In fact, if the patient contacts the advanced practice nurse immediately after the antidepressant is prescribed and profusely thanks him or her for starting the antidepressant, two things should be considered: (1) The patient is bipolar and has switched into hypomania or mania (and a referral to a mental health practitioner should be made) or (2) it is a placebo effect.

Although the occurrence of mania with antidepressant therapy is not always predictable, a thorough patient and family history for bipolar disorder before starting medications may reveal risk factors for bipolar disorder. If a placebo effect is suspected, the patient should be encouraged to continue to take the medications, but the clinician should not be surprised if in 7 to 10 days the patient reports that the medication "has stopped working."

Anxiety Disorders

Generalized Anxiety Disorder   Many studies have demonstrated the efficacy of benzodiazepines (BZDs) in the acute treatment of anxiety and generalized anxiety disorder. The anxiolytics work quickly to reduce symptoms in many patients, with most improvement occurring in the first week of treatment. BZDs should be used with the lowest possible dose for the shortest possible time.

Benzodiazepines should be used cautiously in patients with a substance abuse history because of the potential to develop psychological and physical dependence. Twenty-five to 45 percent of patients treated with benzodiazepines develop dependency after 2 years of treatment.[50] Other studies have found that the efficacy of benzodiazepines diminishes significantly after 3 to 4 months of treatment.[53]

In light of the clear evidence suggesting diminished efficacy and a high propensity for dependence, the use of benzodiazepines should be vigilantly monitored and time-limited. Patients whose symptoms persist throughout the day respond better to long-acting benzodiazepines such as clonazepam. If the anxiety episodes are more circumscribed, use of shorter-acting benzodiazepines such as alprazolam or lorazepam should be considered. Examples of benzodiazepines used to treat anxiety include diazepam (15 to 40 mg/day), clonazepam (1 to 4 mg/day), and alprazolam (2 to 6 mg/day).

Buspirone, an azaspirone anxiolytic, does not interact with brain BZD receptors but has been shown to be as effective as BZDs for generalized anxiety disorder. Buspirone, in contrast to the BZDs, does not cause sedation, memory, or psychomotor impairment. Buspirone also does not interact with alcohol and has no potential for abuse. Buspirone has a slower onset of anxiolytic action (1 to 2 weeks) than the BZDs. Patients who have been treated with benzodiazepines in the past may become impatient with the delay in therapeutic effect. The dose range of buspirone is from 15 to 60 mg/day.

Panic Disorder   The pharmacotherapy of panic disorder includes high-potency benzodiazepines (alprazolam or clonazepam) and/or antidepressants. Patients who present with extreme or intolerable distress can be treated initially with a high-potency benzodiazepine. Alprazolam therapy can be initiated at a dosage of 0.5 mg twice a day and titrated gradually to within the 2 to 6 mg/day range. It is useful to prescribe the medication in divided dosages (3 to 4 times a day) to avoid interdose rebound anxiety. Since clonazepam is slower to reach a steady-date serum level, the clinician should be careful to avoid titrating the dose up too quickly. The dose range for clonazepam of 1 to 4 mg/day is adequate for the majority of patients. Given clonazepam's longer half-life, bid dosing is usually adequate to maintain a steady anxiolytic effect.

Antidepressants take longer to be effective in panic disorder but are effective antipanic agents, with the exception of bupropion and trazodone. Patients with panic disorder are particularly sensitive to the activating side effects of antidepressant medication and so it is advisable to use small doses and titrate slowly. Imipramine is the most widely studied tricyclic for the treatment of panic disorder and agoraphobia and is generally considered an effective antipanic agent. Imipramine should be started at doses of 25 to 50 mg and gradually increased. Most patients achieve a therapeutic benefit at 150 to 250 mg/day, although it can be increased to 300 mg/day.

Theoretically despiramine should work as well as imipramine because it is the main metabolite of imipramine. However, imipramine may be more serotonergic than desipramine, which may give it greater efficacy, assuming that the serotonin system is important in panic disorder. MAOIs are also effective antipanic and antiphobic agents. Phenelzine has been shown to be a very effective agent for panic disorder. Although adverse effects tend to be less troublesome than with TCAs, dietary restrictions may limit the usefulness of MAOIs in some patients. In treatment-refractory OCD patients, some clinicians have found it helpful to combine an SSRI with clomipramine.[26] However, caution should be used when using this combination because of the danger of producing a toxic clomipramine level through induction of the P-450 enzyme system by the SSRI. Treatment of those patients suffering from treatment-resistant OCD may be more appropriately managed by a psychiatrist.

Recent studies have suggested the efficacy of SSRIs in panic disorder. The following dosages are recommended: sertraline at 25 mg/day, paroxetine at 10 mg/day, fluoxetine at 5 to 10 mg/day, and fluvoxamine at 50 mg/day. When restlessness and akathisia are prominent reactions or when greater acute relief of anxiety is needed, the temporary use of adjunctive high-potency BZDs can help a patient tolerate the initial weeks of antidepressant treatment. In general, as with the TCAs, the final treatment SSRI dose is most commonly at the low end of the dose range although some patients may require dosages at the higher levels.

Obsessive-Compulsive Disorder The pharmacotherapy of obsessive-compulsive disorder (OCD) is based primarily on the use of serotonergic antidepressants. Due to their potent selective reuptake properties and benign side-effect profile, the SSRIs (fluoxetine, sertraline, fluvoxamine, paroxetine) are often the initial choice of treatment. When treatment with an SSRI is not effective, a switch to the serotonergic TCA clomipramine may be helpful. Although most clinicians believe that the dosages of the SSRIs needed in the treatment of OCD patients are more toward the higher end of the dose range, a study using sertraline found that 50 mg/day was as effective as higher dosages in the treatment of OCD patients.[28] For patients who fail to respond to SSRI monotherapy, the addition of the 5-HT agonist buspirone, at a dosage of 10 mg three times a day, has been reported to be helpful.[75]

In contrast to patients suffering from depression, patients with OCD respond more slowly to the medication and thus trials of the medication should be longer (e.g., 10 to 12 weeks). Although the medications are extremely effective in alleviating symptoms in OCD patients, they may not be completely effective in eradicating all symptoms. For example, a patient who may be exhibiting compulsive checking behaviors several times an hour may on the medication have a decrease in symptoms to where he or she is only exhibiting these behaviors 3 or 4 times a day. Nonpharmacologic therapies (e.g., cognitive-behavioral therapy) may be effective in alleviating residual symptomatology. In treatment-refractory OCD patients, some clinicians have found it helpful to combine an SSRI with clomipramine.[26] However, caution should be used when using this combination because of the danger of producing a toxic clomipramine level through induction of the P-450 enzyme system by the SSRI. Treatment of those patients suffering from treatment-resistant OCD may be more appropriately managed by a psychiatrist.

Use of Medication with Special Populations

Pregnancy   The U.S. Food and Drug Administration (FDA) classifies the teratogenic effects of prescription medications in five categories ranging from category A (controlled studies show no risk) to X (studies have demonstrated clear fetal risk which outweighs any possible benefits to the mother) (see Chapter 6). Most psycho-pharmacologic medications are classified by the FDA in category C (risk cannot be ruled out). Some psychoactive medications, especially the barbiturates and benzodiazepines, are category D (positive evidence of risk to the human fetus). Three psychoactive medications—benzphetamine, temazepam, and triazolam—have been associated with fetal abnormalities and are explicitly contraindicated in pregnancy.

The paucity of research on the use of psychotropic medication in pregnancy makes weighing the potential risks to the fetus against the therapeutic benefits for the mother extremely difficult. There is also the additional problem that abruptly discontinuing medications, such as the benzodiazepines, could cause withdrawal symptoms that place the mother and developing fetus at an even greater risk. It is prudent for advanced practice nurses to consult with an obstetrician and a psychiatrist prior to prescribing or discontinuing psychopharmacologic medications to pregnant women. A general guide for the choice of medication during pregnancy can be seen in Table 16-13.

Adolescents   There are no studies on the long-term effects of psychopharmacologic medications on brain function, cognitive development, behavior, or physical health in children and adolescents.[77] As a general rule, psychopharmacologic medication should be prescribed only when there is consistent evidence from a variety of sources (parents, teachers, primary care providers) of an urgent clinical need, and there have been reasonable trials of other nonpharmacologic interventions. Prior to prescribing psychopharmacologic medication, advanced practice nurses should request permission from the patient (or from parents or guardians if the patient is a minor) to speak to other adults who have frequent contact with the patient outside the home (such as teachers, coaches, pediatric primary care providers, or social service personnel). Only by conferring with other adults who observe the adolescent in a variety of settings can there be a complete evaluation of how the problematic behavior is impacting normal development.

An interdisciplinary treatment plan should always include an explicit rationale delineating the potential benefits of prescribing a medication against any known or unknown long-term risks. The medical record should also reflect that such information has been communicated in person or in writing to the patient, or if the patient is a minor, to their parents or guardians. Adolescents should be active participants in the informed consent process and be given age-appropriate material describing the uses and side effects of medication.

TABLE 16-13

A Guide for the Use of Psychopharmacologic Medications During Pregnancy

Choice of Medication
Greatest documentation of prior use
Lower FDA risk category (B>C>D)
Few or no metabolites
Shorter half-life of elimination
Fewer side effects
Dose of Medication
Minimal effective dose
No medication in first trimester if possible
Adjust dose as body fluid volume changes
Reduce or taper dose 2 weeks prior to delivery
Adjust breastfeeding to dose schedule to minimize infant exposure
Communication
Obtain written informed consent
Document discussion of risk and benefit with client in the medical record
Consult with an obstetrician and psychiatrist specializing in the care of pregnant women prior to prescribing or discontinuing medication
Communicate medication regimen to client's pediatrician or pediatric nurse practitioner and update on any changes in dosages prior to delivery

SOURCE: Reprinted with permission from the *American Psychiatric Press Textbook of Psychopharmacology.* Copyright 1995 American Psychiatric Press.[7]

After puberty, adolescents are prescribed doses that are equivalent to those for adults. There are more studies evaluating the risks and benefits of TCAs than the newer SSRIs in the treatment of children and adolescents. In clinical practice, because the side-effect profile of SSRIs is so superior to that of TCAs, the SSRIs are generally accepted as the first line of medication treatment. Other prescribing considerations include (1) using multiple daily dosing rather than once-a-day dosing to minimize side effects, (2) tapering TCAs over 10 days to avoid cholinergic rebound, and (3) a longer period (8 to 10 weeks) to see a therapeutic effect on target symptoms.[35]

The Elderly Chapter 7 on drug therapy in the elderly reviews the appropriate use of antipsychotic medication for the aged. Physiological changes such as a decrease in total body water, slower liver metabolism, and slower renal clearance prolong excretion and increase blood levels of medication in the elderly.[78] Delays in excretion, in combination with multiple or complicated medication regimes, put the elderly at greater risk for drug-drug interactions and toxic side effects. Advanced practice nurses should always consider whether disruptive, incoherent behavior exhibited by the elderly may be associated with the toxic or additive effects of multiple medications. If toxic effects are suspected and medication is discontinued, the washout period will take considerably longer than for healthy adults.

SUMMARY

The responsibility for advanced practice nurses to diagnose and treat anxiety disorders and major depression has, and will continue, to grow. This trend is in part due to the newer medications, which are simpler to prescribe and have fewer side effects, as well as the economically driven constraints on specialist referrals. Although psychotropic medication may alleviate many of the symptoms that initially bring a patient to seek treatment from APNs, a pill cannot be wholly effective in managing the syndrome of major mental illness or in helping patients cope with social and psychological consequences of their illness.

In recognition of this shift in treatment responsibility to the primary care setting, throughout this chapter, indications for referral or consultation to a psychiatric clinical specialist or psychiatrist have been highlighted. Advanced practice nurses may find that these recommendations for specialist referral and treatment are fiercely resisted by managed care providers or other insurers. In the face of such resistance, advanced practice nurses must act as strong, unwavering advocates on behalf of their patients to receive health care benefits that are likely to prevent recurrence or hasten recovery.

There is extensive empirical evidence that psychotropic medication can markedly improve the course and sequelae of major mental illness. Although the scientific evidence proving the efficacy of psychotherapy is less compelling, that should not dissuade advanced practice nurses from using psychotherapy as an adjunct to pharmacologic treatment, especially for patients with other co-morbid conditions. There are several studies that have demonstrated that psychopharmacology in conjunction with psychotherapy offers patients the best chance for sustaining mental health. Psychotropics may make a miraculous difference in people's lives, but they are not and should not be viewed as a miracle cure.

REFERENCES

1. U.S. Senate. *Deinstitutionalization, mental illness and medications.* Committee on Finance (May 10, 1994). Washington, DC: U.S. Government Printing Office, 1995.
2. *Depression in Primary Care. Vol. 1 (Diagnosis and Detection); vol. 2 (Treatment of Major Depression).* Rockville, MD: Agency for Health Policy Research, 1993.
3. National Institute of Mental Health: *Decade of the Brain—Medications.* Washington, DC: National Institutes of Health, 1995, Pub. no. 95-3929.
4. Laraia MT, Beeber LS, Callwood GB, et al: Psychiatric Mental Health Nursing Psychopharmacology Project. Washington, DC: American Nurses' Association, 1994.
5. Spitzer RL, Williams JBW, Kroenke K, et al: Utility of a new procedure for diagnosing mental disorders in primary care: The PRIME-MD 1000 study. *JAMA* 272:1749–1756, 1994.

6. Ellison JM, Gold I: *Practical Implementation and Risk Management Aspects of the Nurse Clinical Specialist/Supervising Physician Relationship*. Wellesley, MA: Massachusetts Psychiatric Society, 1996.

7. Grady TA, Sederer LI, Rothschild AJ: Depression, in Sederer LI, Rothschild AJ (eds). *Acute Care Psychiatry: Diagnosis and Treatment*. Baltimore: Williams & Wilkins, 1997, pp 83–121.

8. Bunney WE, Davis JM: Norepinephrine in depressive reactions. *Arch Gen Psychiatry* 13:483–494, 1965.

9. Schildkraut JT. The catecholamine hypothesis of affective disorders: A review of supporting evidence. *Am J Psychiatry* 122:509–522, 1965.

10. Maas JW: Biogenic amines and depression. Biochemical and pharmacological separations of two types of depression. *Arch Gen Psychiatry* 32:1357–1361, 1975.

11. Baldessarini RJ: The basis for amine hypotheses in affective disorders: A critical evaluation. *Arch Gen Psychiatry* 32:1087–1093, 1975.

12. Schwartz PJ, Brown C, Wehr TA, et al: Winter seasonal affective disorder: A follow-up study of the first 59 patients of the National Institute of Mental Health seasonal studies program. *Am J Psychiatry* 153:1028–1036, 1996.

13. Post PM: Transduction of psychosocial stress into the neurobiology of treatment of affective disorders. *Am J Psychiatry* 149:999–1010, 1992.

14. Tohen M, Waternaux CM, Tsuang MT, et al: Four-year follow-up of 24 first-episode manic patients. *J Affect Disord* 19:79–86, 1990.

15. Keller MB, Shapiro RW, Lavori PW, et al: Relapse in major depressive disorder: Analysis with the life table. *Arch Gen Psychiatry* 39:911–915, 1982.

16. Harrow M, Goldberg JF, Grossman LS, et al: Outcome in manic disorders: A naturalistic follow-up study. *Arch Gen Psychiatry* 47:665–671, 1990.

17. Goodwin FK, Jamison KR: *Manic-Depressive Illness*. New York: Oxford University Press, 1990.

18. Rothschild AJ, Samson JA, Bond TC, et al: Hypothalamic-pituitary-adrenal axis activity and one-year outcome in depression. *Biol Psychiatry* 34:392–400, 1993.

19. Ribeiro SCM, Tandon R, Grunhaus L, Greden JF: The DST as a predictor of outcome in depression: A meta-analysis. *Am J Psychiatry* 150:1618–1629, 1993.

20. Popp S, Ellison JM, Reeves P: Neuropsychiatry of the anxiety disorders, in Ellison JM, Weinstein CS, Hodel-Malinofsky T (eds): *The Psychotherapist's Guide to Neuropsychiatry: Diagnostic and Treatment Issues*. Washington, DC: American Psychiatric Press, 1994.

21. Cowley DS, Arana GW: The diagnostic utility of lactate sensitivity in panic disorder. *Arch Gen Psychiatry* 47:277–284, 1990.

22. Nutt D, Lawson C: Panic attacks: A neurochemical overview of models and mechanisms. *Br J Psychiatry* 160:165–178, 1992.

23. Reiman EM, Fusselman MJ, Fox PT, et al: Neuroanatomical correlates of anticipatory anxiety. *Science* 243:1071–1074, 1989.

24. Reiman EM, Raichle ME, Robins E, et al: Neuroanatomical correlates of a lactate-induced anxiety attack. *Arch Gen Psychiatry* 46:493–500, 1989.

25. Charney DS, Woods SW, Nagy LM, et al: Noradrenergic function in panic disorder. *J Clin Psychiatry* 51(Suppl):5–11, 1970.

26. Zetin M, Kramer MA: Obsessive-compulsive disorder. *Hosp Community Psychiatry* 43:689–699, 1992.

27. Goodman WK, McDougle CJ, Price LH: Pharmacotherapy of obsessive compulsive disorder. *J Clin Psychiatry* 53(Suppl):29–37, 1992.

28. Greist J, Chouinard G, DuBoff E, et al: Double-blind parallel comparison of three dosages of sertraline and placebo in outpatients with obsessive-compulsive disorder. *Arch Gen Psychiatry* 52:289–295, 1995.

29. Sperry L: *Psychopharmacology and Psychotherapy Strategies for Maximizing Treatment Outcomes.* New York: Brunner/Mazel, 1995.

30. Leonard HL, Swedo SE, Lenane MC, et al: A 2- to 7-year follow-up study of 54 obsessive-compulsive children and adolescents. *Arch Gen Psychiatry* 30:429–439, 1993.

31. Bond AJ, Lader MH: *Understanding Drug Treatment in Mental Health Care.* New York: Wiley, 1996.

32. Andreasen NC, Black DW: *Introductory Textbook of Psychiatry,* 2d ed. Washington, DC: American Psychiatric Press, 1995.

33. Gomez GE, Gomez EA: Depression in the elderly. *J Psychosoc Nurs Ment Health Serv* 31(5):28–33, 1993.

34. Gitlin MJ: *The Psychotherapist's Guide to Psychopharmacology,* 2d ed. New York: The Free Press, 1996.

35. Laraia MT: Current approaches to the psychopharmacologic treatment of depression in children and adolescents. *JCAPN* 9(1):15–26, 1996.

36. Tohen M: Mania, in Sederer LI, Rothschild AJ (eds): *Acute Care Psychiatry: Diagnosis and Treatment.* Baltimore: Williams & Wilkins, 1997, pp 141–165.

37. Glazer WM, Morgenstern H, Doucette J: Race and tardive dyskinesia among outpatients at a CMHC. *Hosp Community Psychiatry* 45(1):38–42, 1994.

38. Wilfley DE, Grilo CM: Eating disorders: A women's health problem in primary care. *Nurse Pract Forum* 5(1):34–45, 1994.

39. American Psychological Association: *Diagnostic and Statistical Manual of Mental Disorders,* 4th ed. Washington, DC: American Psychiatric Press, 1994.

40. Schatzberg AF, Rothschild AJ: Psychotic (delusional) major depression: Should it be included as a distinct syndrome in DSM-IV? *Am J Psychiatry* 149:733–745, 1992.

41. Coryell W, Keller M, Lavori P, Endicott J: Affective syndromes, psychotic features and prognosis. I: Depression. *Arch Gen Psychiatry* 47:651–657, 1990.

42. Rothschild AJ, Samson JA, Bessette MP, Carter-Campbell J: Efficacy of the combination of fluoxetine and perphenazine in the treatment of psychotic depression. *J Clin Psychiatry* 54:338–342, 1993.

43. Rothschild AJ: Management of psychotic treatment-resistant depression. *Psych Clin North Am* 19:237–252, 1996.

44. Kendell RE, Charlmers JC, Platz C: Epidemiology of puerperal psychoses. *Br J Psychiatry* 150:662–673, 1987.

45. Briggs GG, Freeman RK, Yaffe SJ, in Mitchell CW (ed): *Drugs in Pregnancy and Lactation,* 4th ed. Baltimore: Williams & Wilkins, 1994, pp 1–8.

46. Buist A, Norman TR, Dennerstein L: Breastfeeding and the use of psychotropic medication: A review. *J Affect Disord* 19:197–206, 1990.

47. American Psychological Association: Practice guidelines for the treatment of patients with bipolar disorder. *Am J Psychiatry* 151:1–31, 1994.

48. Jimerson DC, Wolfe BE, Brotman AW, Metzger ED: Medications in the treatment of eating disorders. *Psychiatr Clin North Am* 19(4):739–754, 1996.

49. Wolfe BE: Dimensions of response to antidepressant agents in bulimia nervosa: A review. *Arch Psychiatr Nurs* 9(3):111–121, 1995.

50. Blair DT, Ramones VA: Psychopharmacologic treatment of anxiety. *J Psychosoc Nurs* 32(7):49–53, 1994.

51. McDougle CJ, Goodman WK, Leckman JF, Price LH: The psychopharmacology of obsessive compulsive disorder. *Psychiatr Clin North Am* 16(4):749–765, 1993.

52. Chu JA: Trauma and dissociative disorders, in Sederer LI, Rothschild AJ (eds): *Acute Care Psychiatry: Diagnosis and Treatment.* Baltimore: Williams & Wilkins, 1997, pp 195–219.

53. Taylor CB: Treatment of anxiety disorders, in Schatzberg AF, Nemeroff CB (eds): *The APA Textbook of Psychopharmacology.* Washington, DC: American Psychiatric Press, 1995, pp 641–655.

54. Baily K, Glod CA: Post-traumatic stress disorder: A role for psychopharmacology? *J Psychosoc Nurs* 29(9):42–43, 1991.

55. Ries R: Assessment and treatment of patients with coexisting mental illness and alcohol and other drug abuse. Rockville, MD: Department of Health and Human Services (Pub. No. 94–2078), 1994.

56. Decker KP, Ries RK: Differential diagnosis and psychopharmacology of dual disorders. *Psychiatr Clin North Am* 1(4):703–717, 1993.

57. Chan CH, Janicak PG, Davis JM, et al: Response of psychotic and nonpsychotic depressed patients to tricyclic antidepressants. *J Clin Psychiatry* 48:197–200, 1987.

58. Baldessarini RJ: Current status of antidepressants: Clinical pharmacology and therapy. *J Clin Psychiatry* 50:117–126, 1989.

59. Stoll AL, Pope HG, McElroy SI: High dose fluoxetine: Safety and efficacy in 27 cases. *J Clin Psychopharmacol* 11:225–226, 1991.

60. Schweitzer E, Rickels K, Amsterdam JD: What constitutes an adequate antidepressant trial for fluoxetine? *J Clin Psychiatry* 51:8–11, 1990.

61. Beaumont G: The toxicity of antidepressants. *Br J Psychiatry* 154:454–458, 1989.

62. Callaham M, Kassel D: Epidemiology of fatal tricyclic antidepressant ingestion: Implications for management. *Ann Emerg Med* 14:1–9, 1985.

63. Kulig K: Management of poisoning associated with "newer" antidepressant agents. *Ann Emerg Med* 15:1039–1045, 1986.

64. Sclar DA, Robison LM, Skaer TL, et al: Antidepressant pharmacotherapy: Economic outcomes in a health maintenance organization. *Clin Therapeutics* 16:715–730, 1994.

65. Katzelnick DJ, Kobak KA, Jefferson JW, Griest JH: Prescribing patterns of antidepressant medications for depression in a health care organization. Dean Foundations for Health, Research and Education. Poster session. Orlando, FL: New Clinical Drug Evaluation Unit, June 2, 1995.

66. Rothschild AJ: Adherence to antidepressant therapy. *Fed Pract* April 13(Suppl):16, 1996.

67. Ciraulo OA, Shader RI: Fluoxetine drug-drug interactions. I: Antidepressants and antipsychotics. *J Clin Psychopharmacol* 10:48–50, 1990.

68. Preskorn S: Recent pharmacologic advances in antidepressant therapy for the elderly. *Am J Med* 94(suppl 5A):2–12, 1993.

69. Crewe HK, Lennard MS, Tucker GT, et al: The effect of selective serotonin re-uptake inhibitors on cytochrome P4502D6 (CYP2D6) activity in human liver microsomes. *Br J Clin Pharmacol* 34:262–265, 1992.

70. Brosen K, Hansen JG, Nielsen KK, et al: Inhibition by paroxetine of desipramine metabolism in extensive but not in poor metabolizers of sparteine. *Eur J Clin Pharmacol* 44:349–355, 1993.

71. Preskorn SH, Alderman J, Chung M, et al: Pharmacokinetics of desipramine coadministered with sertraline or fluoxetine. *J Clin Psychopharmacol* 14:90–98, 1994.

72. Manufacturer's prescribing information, 1994, in *Physician's Desk Reference,* 49th ed. Oradell, NJ: Medical Economics Company, 1995.

73. Nierenberg AA, Alder LA, Peselow E, et al: Trazodone for antidepressant-associated insomnia. *Am J Psychiatry* 151:1069–1072, 1994.

74. Coryell W: Anxiety secondary to depression. *Psychiatr Clin North Am* 13:685–698, 1990.

75. Markovitz PJ, Stagno SJ, Calabrese JR: Buspirone augmentation of fluoxetine in obsessive-compulsive disorder. *Am J Psychiatry* 147:798–800, 1990.

76. Schatzberg AF, Nemeroff CB (eds): *The American Psychiatric Press Textbook of Psychopharmacology.* Washington, DC: American Psychiatric Press, 1995.

77. Schatzberg AF, Cole JO: *Manual of Clinical Psychopharmacology,* 2d ed. Washington, DC: American Psychiatric Press, 1991.

78. Strome T, Howell T: How antipsychotics affect the elderly. *Am J Nurs* 5:46–50, 1991.

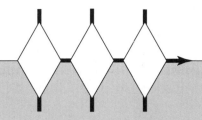

Chapter 17

MANAGEMENT OF CHEMOTHERAPY SIDE EFFECTS

Gail Wilkes

INTRODUCTION

The use of chemicals to treat malignancy dates back to at least the 1500s when heavy metals were used.[1] It was not until the 1940s, however, that chemotherapy was used scientifically. Following an accident involving nitrogen mustard gas stored for possible wartime use, it became apparent that exposure to this substance caused bone marrow aplasia, or destruction of bone marrow elements. Subsequently, nitrogen mustard was used in the treatment of lung cancer and lymphoma. Also in this decade, it was demonstrated that methotrexate could be used effectively in the management of childhood leukemia. Since then, major classes of antineoplastic agents have been introduced, as well as new technology to deliver drugs such as liposomes. However, the administration of effective doses of chemotherapy with manageable toxicity still challenges provider and patient.

For many nurses, the term *antineoplastic agents*, sometimes referred to as *cancer chemotherapy*, means the administration of drugs to the point of known toxicity, which may be life-threatening. This is in direct contrast to the prescription and administration of most other drugs, which are prescribed using doses that do not result in toxicity. In fact, provider and patient education focuses on assessment of possible drug side effects so that the drug dose or drug may be changed before the patient experiences severe toxicity. This paradigm shift in the use of antineoplastic agents is understandable as the drug action is intended to kill malignant cells with drugs that to date are unable to distinguish between normal and malignant cells. New technology, such as the encapsulation of cancer chemotherapy agents in liposomes to deliver the drug directly to the tumor site, is promising and is available for two drugs: doxorubicin (Doxil) and daunorubicin (Daunaxome). Following an overview of chemotherapy, this chapter will focus on symptom management to minimize drug toxicity in patients receiving cancer chemotherapy.

BRIEF OVERVIEW OF CHEMOTHERAPY AND TOXICITY

Cancer chemotherapy may be recommended as *curative* first-line therapy for certain malignancies, such as acute leukemia. In the treatment of solid tumors, it may be given as *adjuvant* therapy, as in breast cancer, to eliminate micrometastasis following surgical resection of the tumor. In addition, cancer chemotherapy may be given as *neoadjuvant* therapy to reduce tumor size so that surgical resection is possible, as with certain head and neck or esophageal cancers. In the management of more advanced tumors, *sensitizing* chemotherapy may be prescribed in combination with radiation so that the chemotherapy enhances the cellular effects of the radiation therapy and improves tumor response. High, potentially lethal doses of active agents may be given in an effort to cure malignancies with a poor prognosis or solid tumors that have recurred, followed by *stem cell rescue* or *bone marrow transplantation*. Finally, cancer chemotherapy may be recommended for *palliation* of solid malignancies that are advanced and unresectable or which recur following primary therapy, as well as advanced hematologic malignancies. Chemotherapy may offer significant advantages in improving quality of life, but the potential benefit must be carefully weighed against expected and potential toxicities.

Most cancer chemotherapy agents are either *cytostatic* (preventing cell division) or *cytocidal* (causing cell death) and affect cell DNA and/or RNA so that cell replication is prevented or the cell dies. The mechanism of action can be *cell cycle–specific*, where the injury to the cell occurs during a specific phase or phases of the cell cycle, or *cell cycle–nonspecific*, where injury occurs during all phases of the cell cycle. Cell cycle–specific agents are generally more effective against tumors that divide frequently, such as leukemia, while cell cycle–nonspecific agents are effective in the treatment of cancers that not only have dividing cells, but also cells in the resting phase that would normally escape chemotherapy. As tumors enlarge, they grow more slowly due to restricted nutrition (blood supply) so that cells in the center of the tumor are not actively dividing and are in the resting phase. See Fig. 17-1 for classification of agents and activity in relationship to the cell cycle.

Generally, in an effort to minimize toxicity, chemotherapeutic agents are used in combination to maximize cell kill. Drugs used together should (1) be active against the tumor when used alone, and together should be synergistic or additive; (2) have different mechanisms of action; (3) produce toxicities in different organ systems so maximal doses can be used without severe morbidity; and (4) have toxicities that occur at different times.[2]

As new drugs are considered for their antitumor activity, clinical trials are used to determine the maximum tolerated dose of a drug (phase I), drug activity in specific tumor types (phase II), and comparison of the new agent as compared to standard drug(s) (phase III). During these trials, the recommended drug dose is determined. For most agents these doses are calculated based on body surface area as determined by a nomogram considering height and weight. More precise, patient-individualized dosing can be determined by calculation of the drug concentration (area under the curve) for

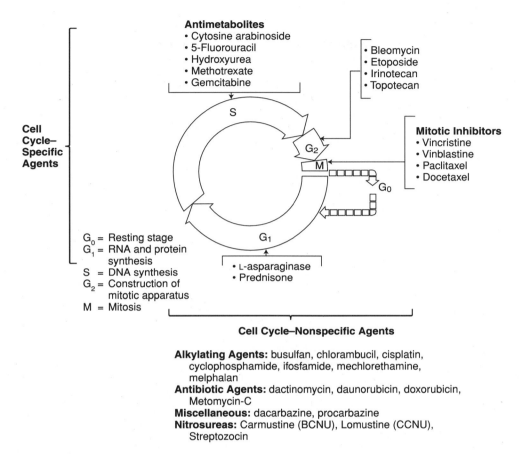

Antimetabolites
• Cytosine arabinoside
• 5-Fluorouracil
• Hydroxyurea
• Methotrexate
• Gemcitabine

• Bleomycin
• Etoposide
• Irinotecan
• Topotecan

Cell Cycle–Specific Agents

Mitotic Inhibitors
• Vincristine
• Vinblastine
• Paclitaxel
• Docetaxel

G_0 = Resting stage
G_1 = RNA and protein synthesis
S = DNA synthesis
G_2 = Construction of mitotic apparatus
M = Mitosis

• L-asparaginase
• Prednisone

Cell Cycle–Nonspecific Agents

Alkylating Agents: busulfan, chlorambucil, cisplatin, cyclophosphamide, ifosfamide, mechlorethamine, melphalan
Antibiotic Agents: dactinomycin, daunorubicin, doxorubicin, Metomycin-C
Miscellaneous: dacarbazine, procarbazine
Nitrosureas: Carmustine (BCNU), Lomustine (CCNU), Streptozocin

Figure 17-1 Cell-cycle specificity.

certain drugs, e.g., carboplatin (Paraplatin), so that the therapeutic margins can be determined. Carboplatin is an analogue of cisplatin, and as drug excretion is renal, clinical testing demonstrated that the plasma concentration of the drug over time was determined by the patient's pretreatment renal function; as expected, the degree of hematologic toxicity, e.g., thrombocytopenia, could also be predicted by the patient's pretreatment renal function.[3] Scientifically, the therapeutic index (therapeutic range) for this drug can be determined by deducting the dose associated with the undesired toxicity (thrombocytopenia) from the drug dose (plasma concentration) associated with the highest efficacy (tumor response).[4] Since the pharmacokinetics of carboplatin are predictable, recommended drug dosages take into consideration the patient's ability to excrete the drug (glomerular filtration rate, or GFR) so that the amount of active drug available in the plasma is more precise (area under the concentration-versus-time curve, or AUC). Calvert[3] has determined a formula used to calculate appropriate drug doses in milligrams by multiplying the area under the curve (AUC) by the sum of the GFR plus 25, and a special dose-determining calculator is available from the drug manufacturer (Bristol Myers Squibb).

In patients with advanced malignancy, often the tumor directly or indirectly affects organs involved in drug metabolism. It is very important for the prescribing provider, as well as for the nurse who administers the drug, to be very familiar with the drug's metabolism and excretion routes, as well as the patient's laboratory values of function. Clearly increased drug serum levels will occur if the drug is not excreted completely (due to impaired renal and/or hepatic metabolism), if the drug is sequestered in a body sanctuary (e.g., methotrexate in pleural effusion or ascites), or if the drug is given with drugs having similar metabolic pathways (e.g., 6-mercaptopurine and allopurinol; allopurinol inhibits xanthine oxidase, which normally metabolizes 6-mercaptopurine into an inactive metabolite). If the drug is excreted renally or hepatically and a patient has impaired renal and/or hepatic function, the drug dose should be reduced as directed by the manufacturer.

The advanced practice nurse plays a critical role in ensuring that the variables affecting toxicity that can be controlled are controlled. Patient assessment of psychosocial and physiological parameters form the foundation of care. Often patients are anxious about their diagnosis and its connotation of life-threatening illness, and this is compounded by fear and possible misunderstanding caused by myths about cancer chemotherapy. Initially, it is important to determine the patient's understanding of the malignancy, goals of treatment including those of chemotherapy, and beliefs about cancer chemotherapy. Informed consent is required for patients undergoing clinical trials, and because of the potential for severe toxicity, most clinicians also recommend this for standard therapy to ensure that patients have received appropriate education and the opportunity to ask questions prior to beginning therapy. Careful patient/family education and anxiety reduction can improve patient tolerance, compliance with recommended therapy, and quality of life. Other parameters to assess include the patient's ability to learn and perform self-assessment and care, financial ability to purchase antiemetics and a thermometer, and whether the patient has access to a telephone to call the provider if complications arise.

As most agents interfere with normal cell populations that have frequently dividing cells, physiologic parameters most often include baseline assessment of complete blood count and differential, renal or hepatic function tests depending upon route of drug excretion, oral mucosa, presence of head hair and significance of hair loss to the patient, reproductive function and goals, and organ function as directed by the specific drug(s) being administered. For example, renal function must be assessed for cisplatin, a heavy metal which can lead to renal failure if precautions are not followed. Ifosfamide can cause severe bladder hemorrhage so the urine must be assessed for presence of red blood cells. The anthracycline agents doxorubicin and daunorubicin may cause cardiotoxicity with higher cumulative dosing so baseline ejection fractions must be determined and monitored periodically during therapy. Certain drugs may be toxic to the lung parenchyma, such as bleomycin or with high cumulative dosing, the nitrosureas (carmustine), so baseline pulmonary function testing must be performed and monitored during and after therapy.

MINIMIZING TOXICITY AND OPTIMIZING PATIENT RESPONSE

Toxicities can arise at predictable times following chemotherapy administration, depending upon the drug. Table 17-1 shows selected examples of common toxicities. Symptoms arise from damage to frequently dividing cell populations such as bone marrow, the mucosa of the gastrointestinal tract (nausea/vomiting, stomatitis, diarrhea), gonads, and hair follicles and from injury to organ systems such as the heart, lungs, and kidneys. The following sections examine each of these systems, indicating specific patient risk assessment, management strategies, and points of emphasis for patient/family education for self-care.

Bone Marrow Suppression: Neutropenia

The bone marrow is constantly active, with the pleuripotent stem cell producing early precursor cells, which mature into the early or formed blood cell elements that are released into the circulation (neutrophils and lymphocytes to protect against infection, platelets to prevent bleeding, and red blood cells to provide oxygen and remove carbon dioxide from the tissues).

Chemotherapy *may* interfere with stem cell division, but commonly interferes with the frequently dividing cell precursors in the bone marrow. See Fig. 17-2 for the cascade of development of the formed cell blood elements. Since the formed blood cell elements are mature, they do not divide and are thus unaffected by chemotherapy. The *nadir* (or lowest blood count reached following chemotherapy) occurs when the mature cells die at a predictable time after chemotherapy administration and are not replaced. For neutrophils, this time is usually 7 to 10 days after drug administration. While the neutrophil lives 6 to 12 hours, additional neutrophils adhere to the blood vessel margins and are then released into the circulation through demargination. Platelets live 10 days; red blood cells, 120 days. Chemotherapy prevents the bone marrow from producing replacements temporarily. The bone marrow recovers with production of normal white blood cell, neutrophil, and platelet counts within 21 to 28 days so that chemotherapy can be administered again at that time. However, some agents do produce a delayed nadir (e.g., mitomycin C, melphalan, carmustine) occurring 27 to 32 days following drug administration with recovery of normal cell counts 6 to 8 weeks following administration. Table 17-2 shows the expected nadirs of common chemotherapy agents. It is important to remember that some agents do not affect the bone marrow, namely, bleomycin, vincristine, and L-asparaginase.

Risk Factors

Factors that influence the degree of bone marrow depression following myelosuppressive chemotherapy are advancing age (reduced functional bone marrow), high drug

TABLE 17-1

Temporal Occurrence of Common Toxicities

Timing of Occurrence	Common Toxicities
Immediate onset: hours to days after drug administration	General: nausea/vomiting; phlebitis; hyperuricemia; renal failure; anaphylaxis; skin rash; teratogenicity; diarrhea
	Specific agents: hemorrhagic cystitis: cyclophosphamide; radiation recall: Actinomycin-D; fever, chills: bleomycin; hypertension: procarbazine; hypotension: etoposide; renal failure: cisplatin
Early onset: days to weeks	General: leukopenia (neutropenia), thrombocytopenia, alopecia, stomatitis, diarrhea, megaloblastosis
	Specific agents: paralytic ileus: vincristine; hypercalcemia: estrogens, antiestrogens; hypomagnesemia: cisplatin; pancreatitis: L-asparaginase; fluid retention: estrogen, steroids; pulmonary infiltrates: methotrexate, bleomycin; ototoxicity: cisplatin
Delayed onset: weeks to months	General: anemia, aspermia, hepatocellular damage, hyperpigmentation, pulmonary fibrosis
	Specific agents: peripheral neuropathy: vincristine, cisplatin, paclitaxel; cardiac necrosis, cardiomyopathy: doxorubicin, cyclophosphamide; SIADH: cyclophosphamide, vincristine; hemolytic uremic syndrome: mitomycin C
Late onset: months to years	General: sterility, hypogonadism, premature menopause, second malignancy
	Specific agents: hepatic fibrosis/cirrhosis: methotrexate; encephalopathy: methotrexate + cranial XRT; cancer of the bladder: cyclophosphamide

SOURCE: Modified from Perry and Yarbro.[5]

doses, protein-calorie malnutrition, reduced bone marrow reserve (due to factors such as alcoholic fatty marrow or infiltration of the bone marrow by a tumor called myelophthisis), decreased drug metabolism, prior radiotherapy to sites of bone marrow production (long bones, skull, sternum, ribs, limb girdles, vertebrae, sacrum), and drug sequestration in a physiologic sanctuary with slow continued drug release.

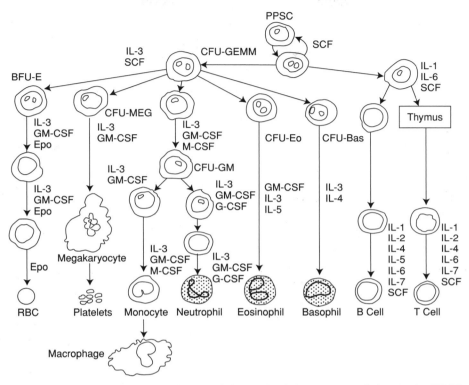

Figure 17-2 Bone marrow cascade with growth factor stimulation. Hematopoietic cascade. (PPSC = pluripotent stem cells; BFU = burst-forming unit; CFU = colony-forming units; CSF = colony-stimulating factor; GM = granulocyte-macrophage; GEMM = granulocyte, erythrocyte, macrophage, megakaryocyte; Epo = erythropoietin; IL = interleukin; SCF = stem cell factor.) (Reprinted with permission from Wujick.[6])

Since the neutrophil is the first line of protection against bacterial invasion, neutropenia predicts the incidence of infection. Neutropenia is defined as an absolute neutrophil count (ANC) of less than 2500 cells/mm³ The ANC is calculated as follows:

$$ANC = WBC \times \frac{Neutrophils + Bands}{100}$$

Minimal risk for infection exists when the absolute neutrophil count is 1000 to 1500/mm³, but risk increases to moderate as the ANC falls to 500 to 1000/mm³ and is severe when the ANC is less than 500 cells/mm³. Not only the degree of neutropenia but also the duration of neutropenia determine infection risk. Studies have shown for patients with an ANC of less than 100/mm³ for three weeks, the infection risk is 100 percent.[8]

Initial bacterial infection in the neutropenic patient develops quickly, and in at least 85 percent of patients it arises from the patient's own endogenous flora that colonize skin and pulmonary, GU, and GI tracts.[9] Fever is the most common first sign of infection, and as there are few neutrophils, classic signs such as pus formation or consolidation on a chest X-ray are absent. Fever of 101°F (38.3° C) in a neutropenic patient that

TABLE 17-2

Expected Nadir Occurrence of Common Agents

Drug Class	Nadir (days after drug administration)	Recovery (days after drug administration)
Alkylating Agents		
mechlorethamine (nitrogen mustard)	7–15	28
melphalan (Alkeran)	14–21	42–50
busulfan (Myleran)	11–30	24–54
chlorambucil (Leukeran)	14–28	28–42
cyclophosphamide (Cytoxan)	8–14	18–25
ifosfamide (Ifex)	Mild	14–21
cisplatin (Platinol)	14	21
carboplatin (Paraplatin)	14–21	28–35, but may take 4–6 weeks
dacarbazine (DTIC)	21–28	28–35
nitrosureas		
carmustine (BCNU)	26–30	35–49
lomustine (CCNU)	40–50	60
streptozocin (Zanosar)	Nonmyelosuppressive	
Antimetabolites		
cytosine arabinoside (ARA-C)	12–14	22–24
fluorouracil (5FU)	7–14	16–24
methotrexate (MTX)	7–14	14–21
mercaptopurine (6MP)	7–14	14–21
hydroxyurea (Hydrea)	18–30	21–35
Plant Alkaloids		
vincristine (VCR)	Relatively nonmyelosuppressive	
vinblastine (VLB)	5–9	14–21
vinorelbine (Navelbine)	7–8	15–17
paclitaxel (Taxol)	8–11	21
docetaxel (Taxotere)	9	15–21
Topoisomerase Inhibitors		
topotecan (Hycamtin)	8–15	11–20
irinotecan (Camptosar)	21–29	27–34
Podophyllotoxins		
etoposide (Vepsid)	9–14	20–22
Antitumor Antibiotics		
bleomycin (Blenoxane)	Nonmyelosuppressive	
daunorubicin (Daunomycin)	10–14	21
doxorubicin (Adriamycin)	10–14	21–24
dactinomycin (Actinomycin)	14–21	22–25
mitomycin C (Mutamycin)	28–42	42–56
Miscellaneous		
mitoxantrone (Novantrone)	8–10	14+
procarbazine (Matulane)	25–36	36–50

SOURCE: Modified from Dorr and Fritz,[7] pp. 103–104, and Barton-Burke et al.,[2] p. 101.

is untreated can result in death within 48 hours in up to 50 percent of patients, as sepsis develops rapidly.[10] Gram-negative bacteria, such as *Enterobacteriaceae* or *Pseudomonas aeruginosa*, are associated with the most severe infections. In the last decade, gram-positive infections such as *Streptococcus*, often associated with indwelling intravenous catheters or the use of prophylactic antibiotics, have become more common.[11] Secondary infections may occur as well, caused by members of the herpesvirus family, either as an initial infection or as reactivation of a latent virus or fungi, such as *Candida albicans*.

Management

Neutropenic fever can often be prevented by the prophylactic administration of granulocyte [G-CSF, such as filgrastim (Neupogen)] or granulocyte-macrophage [GM-CSF, such as sargramostim (Leukine, Prokine)] colony-stimulating growth factors. These agents stimulate the production and maturation of specific cell lineages, especially the neutrophils. Not only is neutrophil recovery accelerated, but the functions of phagocytosis and antibody-dependent cytotoxicity are enhanced so that the neutrophils are more effective in attacking invading microorganisms. Assessment of the patient's or family's ability to learn to administer the drug subcutaneously is critical, along with careful instruction in technique and timing of drug administration. The drug is well tolerated, and the patient and family should learn to anticipate bone pain and to use strategies of self-management such as the administration of NSAIDs such as Motrin.

Patient and family teaching about self-care to prevent infection and self-assessment to alert providers of any changes are critical. Often, the patient is at home when he or she becomes neutropenic, and if the patient becomes infected, early intervention can minimize morbidity and mortality. Prevention strategies include systematic oral care and assessment, avoiding sources of infection, avoiding trauma to skin and mucous membranes, maintaining optimal pulmonary and urinary function, and good perineal hygiene. Self-assessment strategies include taking a temperature, assessing skin and mucous membranes for changes, and reporting changes, including pain and fever higher than 100.4° F.

Assessment of patients includes risk factors, physical parameters, and diagnostic evaluation. Risk factors are (1) degree and duration of neutropenia, (2) lack of evidence of bone marrow recovery, (3) breaks in skin or mucosal barriers (e.g., mucositis, diarrhea), (4) clinical instability, and (5) underlying co-morbidity such as any other organ dysfunction.[12]

Anatomic sites where infection commonly occurs are perirectal mucosa, oral mucosa, lung, skin, and sinuses. Because the classic signs of inflammation are absent, physical assessment focuses on the presence of fever, pain or tenderness, and complete inspection and palpation as appropriate of skin, mucous membranes (mouth and rectum), lungs, sinuses, and IV or implanted catheter sites and subcutaneous tunnel. Any suspicious sites should be cultured. Further diagnostic testing is performed appropriate to signs, symptoms, and past medical history. Cultures performed at the first sign of fever include blood cultures, both peripherally and through indwelling central catheters.

Initially, if cultures of suspicious sites do not reveal a source, broad-spectrum antibiotics are administered, and if the patient remains febrile after 5 to 7 days of treatment, a secondary infection is assumed.[13] Common antibiotics used in the management of neutropenic fever are the ß-lactams such as the penicillins (e.g., carbenicillin), cephalosporins (e.g., ceftazidime), carbapenems (imipenem-cilastin), and monobactams (e.g., aztreonam); aminoglycosides (e.g., gentamycin); fluoroquinolones (e.g., norfloxacin); glycopeptides (e.g., vancomycin); antivirals such as acyclovir; and antifungals such as amphotericin B and ketoconazole.

Bone Marrow Suppression: Thrombocytopenia

Circulating platelets have a life-span of about 10 days, after which they are normally replaced by platelets released from the maturing megakaryocytes in the bone marrow. Platelet production in the bone marrow is suppressed by most chemotherapy agents, and in addition, platelet destruction is accelerated. As the bone marrow recovers, platelets reattain a normal range following the recovery of the neutrophils. Risk for bleeding increases as the platelet count falls below 100,000 cells/mm^3, reaching moderate risk at 50,000 cells/mm^3 and severe risk under 20,000 cells/mm^3.

Risk Factors

Factors which compound the risk of bleeding are combination radiotherapy and/or myelosuppressive chemotherapy, decreased marrow reserve related to bone marrow infiltration by tumor (myelophthisis), concurrent administration of platelet-damaging drugs (e.g., antidepressants, NSAID, ASA), presence of disseminated intravascular coagulation (DIC), and fever during platelet replacement transfusion, resulting in platelet destruction.

Currently, no available platelet growth factor is commercially available to prevent thrombocytopenia, but research is underway in interleukin-2 and -3, thrombopoietin, and PIXY-321.

Management

Patient assessment includes platelet count and other clotting studies as appropriate, medication profile for any interacting drugs or platelet-damaging drugs (e.g., ASA, NSAIDs), and assessment of evidence of bleeding (petechiae, bruising, bleeding from the GI or GU systems, or if thrombocytopenia is severe, increased incidence of visual floaters), changes in vital signs such as hypotension and tachycardia, and neurological signs that might suggest intracranial bleeding if thrombocytopenia is severe (e.g., headache, somnolence, confusion).

Management goals are the prevention of bleeding or stabilization if bleeding occurs. Strategies include patient and family teaching to (1) prevent bleeding or injury (no aspirin-containing drugs, no NSAIDS, use of electric razor, avoid flossing teeth) and (2) to report any signs and/or symptoms of bleeding. Important nursing actions are (1) avoidance of clinical procedures that may damage mucosal barriers (rectal suppositories, enemas), (2) application of pressure for 5 to 10 minutes to venipuncture sites, (3) avoidance of IM injections, and (4) replacement of platelets as indicated, with use of premedication to prevent febrile reaction and increase platelet survival as appropriate.

Bone Marrow Suppression: Anemia

Although bone marrow suppression caused by chemotherapy temporarily decreases the production of erythrocyte precursors, the long life of 120 days of the red blood cell, and the fact that red blood cells can be transfused, help make anemia, if it occurs, easily managed. Another cause of anemia related to chemotherapy is direct kidney damage by the drug cisplatin, causing decreased production of erythropoietin with a consequent decrease in red blood cell production. There may be an increase in the size of erthyrocytes (peripheral macrocytosis) due to folic acid depletion and megaloblastic changes in the bone marrow when methotrexate is given.[14]

Risk Factors

Risk factors are related to (1) specific drug, cumulative amount administered, and dose of drug; (2) decreased bone marrow reserve related to myelophthisis; (3) presence of anemia of chronic disease; (4) prior or concurrent radiotherapy to bone marrow sites with resulting bone marrow fibrosis; and (5) active bleeding.

Management

Patient assessment factors include (1) degree and duration of anemia, (2) signs and symptoms of anemia as shown in Table 17-3, (3) nutrition status and iron intake, and (4) activity level. Management may include administration of recombinant epoetin alfa [r-Hu erythropoietin (Procrit)] to use endogenous body resources to make red cells. Alternatively, red blood cells can be transfused. Prior to transfusion, the red blood cells should be irradiated to remove lymphocytes and then transfused using a leukocyte-removal filter, thus preventing sensitization. Other measures include patient teaching to alternate rest and activity, conservation of energy, diet high in iron (e.g., green leafy vegetables, liver), and iron supplements as appropriate.

Nausea and Vomiting

Nausea and vomiting related to chemotherapy can be *acute*, occurring within 24 h of drug administration; *delayed*, occurring after 24 h and continuing for as long as 5 to 7 days, related to the delayed excretion of active drug metabolites; and *anticipatory*, occurring as a conditioned response to sights, sounds, or other sensations associated with the experience of chemotherapy administration.

Cancer chemotherapy–induced nausea and/or vomiting is mediated by at least three pathways. Classically, direct stimulation of the true vomiting center in the medulla causes the physiologic responses of retching, vomiting, and nausea. Bloodborne cancer chemotherapy stimulates the chemoreceptor trigger zone (CTZ) in the area postrema of the floor of the fourth ventricle in the brain, which then stimulates the true vomiting center. This is mediated by a number of neurotransmitters, especially dopamine and serotonin. In the past, the principal antiemetic drugs were the phenothiazines, such as

TABLE 17-3

Anemia: Degree and Symptomatology

Degree of Anemia	Hemoglobin (mg/dL); Hematocrit (%)	Associated Signs and Symptoms
Normal	Males: 14–18; 42–52 Females: 12–16; 37–47	None
Mild	8–12; 31–37	Pallor, fatigue, sweating on exertion; tachycardia, palpitations, dyspnea with exertion
Severe	<8; <25	Headache, dizziness, irritability, pallor, sensitivity to cold, anorexia, symptomatic fatigue, exercise intolerance; dyspnea, tachycardia, palpitations at rest; systolic ejection murmur, S_3; difficulty concentrating; difficulty sleeping; menstrual irregularities, male impotence

SOURCE: Modified from Barton-Burke et al.[2] and Rieger and Haeuber.[15]

prochlorperazine (Compazine) or perphenazine (Trilafon), which are dopamine antagonists, or high-dose metoclopramide (Reglan), which at high doses possess both dopamine- and serotonin-antagonistic qualities. In addition, there may be a degree of delayed gastric emptying and gastroparesis, caused by agents such as cisplatin. Drugs such as metoclopramide probably not only provide dopamine antagonism, but also enhanced gastric emptying. It is now believed that delayed nausea and/or vomiting are largely mediated by dopamine. Thus, dopamine antagonists are the drugs of choice to prevent delayed nausea and vomiting.

In addition, classical conditioning can occur most often in younger adult patients who experience severe nausea and vomiting after chemotherapy. Subsequent severe nausea and vomiting are stimulated by the sights or sounds associated with the chemotherapy experience, such as the smell of alcohol swabs, the sight of the nurse who administered the drug, or the sight of the color of the chemotherapy agent. This is mediated by descending pathways from the cortex and can be reduced or prevented by the administration of amnesiac and anxiolytic drugs such as the benzodiazepines [lorazepam (Ativan)] prior to chemotherapy. In addition, behavioral techniques to decondition the patient may be very helpful.

More recently, it has become clear that the major emetogenic pathway for acute nausea and vomiting is actually related to injury to the enterochromaffin cells in the proximal gut wall, which then release serotonin. A secondary feedback loop is also engaged so that the release of serotonin stimulates the release of additional serotonin. This neurotransmitter then stimulates the vagal afferent fibers, stimulating the vomiting center directly and the CTZ indirectly. Serotonin inhibitors such as granisetron (Kytril) and ondansetron (Zofran) are effective in preventing nausea and vomiting caused by severely emetogenic agents such as cisplatin. Further, the addition of dexamethasone (Decadron) enhances protection from emesis. Clinical research continues, and new agents will be forthcoming, along with further elucidation of the complex phenomenon of chemotherapy-related nausea and vomiting.

Risk Factors

Patient factors that increase risk for the development of nausea and vomiting are age (younger > older), gender (female > male), increased anxiety, and a history of past experiences of nausea and vomiting (e.g., with pregnancy). A past history of moderate alcohol use appears to be protective. The antiemetic potential of the drug and the dose of the drug are also important predictors of risk. Clearly, as the dose increases, so does the risk. Table 17-4 lists the relative emetogenic potential of commonly used antineoplastic agents.

TABLE 17-4

Emetogenicity of Antineoplastic Agents

Emetic Potential	Agent/Dose (mg/m^2)	Onset (Latency: hours)	Reported Duration (hours)
Very High: >90%	cisplatin ≥ 75 mg	1–6	48–72+
	nitrogen mustard	0.5–2	6–24
	streptozotocin	1–6	12–24
	dacarbazine ≥ 500mg	0.5–6	6–24
	cyclophosphamide > 1g	4–12	12–24+
	cytarabine >500–1000 mg	1–4	12–24
	carmustine ≥ 200 mg	2–6	4–24
	melphalan, high dose	0.3–6	6–12
	lomustine ≥ 60 mg	4–6	12–24
High: 60–90%	cisplatin < 75 mg	1–6	48–72
	dacarbazine < 500 mg	1–6	6–24
	cyclophosphamide < 1 g	4–12	12–24+
	cytarabine 250–500 mg	2–4	12–24
	carmustine < 200 mg	2–6	4–24
	lomustine < 60 mg	4–6	12–24
	doxorubicin ≥ 75 mg	4–6	6–24+
	methotrexate ≥ 200 mg	4–12	3–24+ days
	procarbazine	24–72	variable
	etoposide, high dose	4–6	12–24
	ifosfamide	—	—
	carboplatin	4–9	12–48

(continued)

TABLE 17-4

Emetogenicity of Antineoplastic Agents (continued)

Emetic Potential	Agent/ Dose (mg/m^2)	Onset (Latency: hours)	Reported Duration (hours)
Moderate: 30–60%	cyclophosphamide < 750 mg	4–12	12–24+
	fluorouracil ≥ 1000 mg	3–6	24+
	doxorubicin	4–6	6–24+
	daunorubicin	2–6	24
	asparaginase	—	—
	cytarabine 20–200 mg	2–4	12–24
	methotrexate > 100 mg	4–6	6+
	mitoxantrone	1–4	48–72
	mitomycin	1–6	2–12
	teniposide	—	—
Moderately low: 10–30%	fluorouracil < 1000 mg	—	—
	doxorubicin ≤ 20 mg	—	—
	cytarabine ≤ 20 mg	3–12	—
	etoposide	3–8	6–12
	melphalan	6–12	—
	vinblastine	4–8	—
	hydroxyurea	—	—
	bleomycin	3–6	—
	melphalan	6–12	—
	mercaptopurine	4–8	—
	methotrexate < 100 mg	4–12	3–12
	paclitaxel	—	—
Low: <10%	vincristine	4–8	—
	busulfan	—	—
	chlorambucil	4–12	—
	thioguanine	—	—
	cyclophosphamide (oral)	—	—
	thiotepa	—	—
	hormones	—	—
	steroids	—	—

SOURCE: Reproduced with permission from Wickham,[16] p. 220.

Management

Prechemotherapy assessment should include anxiety level, risk of developing nausea and vomiting, tolerance of past chemotherapy and effectiveness of antiemetics used, and self-care ability. If the patient experiences nausea and vomiting, assessment of fluid balance and electrolyte balance and a plan for repletion are necessary. Skin turgor, evidence of rapid weight loss, changes in orthostatic vital signs, and cardiac function should be closely assessed as well. Subsequent cycles of chemotherapy should be preceded by more aggressive antiemetics. Antiemetic agents provide the cornerstone of management and offer high degrees of protection. The goal is to prevent nausea and vomiting so that anticipatory symptoms do not arise. Since it is clear that multiple pathways are involved, it is important to use aggressive, combination antiemetics to prevent nausea and vomiting when highly emetic agents are administered. In addition, the antiemesis should be continued for the period of drug excretion so that the patient does not experience breakthrough nausea and vomiting. This is preferable to using mild antiemetics and waiting to see if the patient develops nausea and/or vomiting. Further it is important to continually assess the efficacy of the antiemetic(s) and the incidence of drug side effects. Table 17-5 presents the common classes of antiemetic agents, side effects, and recommended doses.

For highly emetogenic agents, combination antiemetic therapy might include the following:

- Granisetron 1 mg IV (or 2 mg PO) plus dexamethasone 20 mg IV 15 min prior to the administration of chemotherapy; alternatively, ondansetron 32 mg IV plus dexamethasone 20 mg IV. If the patient is anxious, then lorazepam 1 to 2 mg PO, or 0.5 to 1.0 mg IV should be added.
- Metoclopramide 3mg/kg plus dexamethasone plus a benzodiazepine provides equivalent potency to granisetron.[24]
- Moderately emetogenic chemotherapy requires antiemesis with a phenothiazine plus a corticosteroid, a single agent serotonin antagonist (IV or oral), or a lower dose of ondansetron (Zofran).[17]
- Chemotherapy agents with low to moderate emetic potential require a phenothiazine as a single agent, or low-dose metoclopramide. Oral dopamine antagonists are appropriate for initial antiemesis for agents with low to mild risk.

Patient education is extremely important to help clarify misconceptions, as many patients may have heard or known of patients who experienced severe nausea and vomiting "that was worse than the cancer." Major advancements in the form of the serotonin antagonists have revolutionized the prevention of chemotherapy-induced nausea and vomiting. In addition, it is important that patients be instructed to self-administer prescribed oral antiemetics to prevent delayed nausea and vomiting, such as perphenazine or prochlorperazine plus low-dose metoclopramide after cisplatin chemotherapy. If nausea is experienced, patients should be instructed to drink fluids such as ginger ale or flat soda; avoid fatty, fried, or spicy foods; eat foods at room temperature or that are cool; and to call the provider for persistent nausea or vomiting unresponsive to prescribed antiemetics (e.g., vomiting lasting more than 1 to 2 days or vomiting more than 2 times a day for 1 to 2 days), if the patient is unable to keep down food or fluids, or if any blood is seen in the vomitus.

Today, in an era of cost containment and managed care, the availability of effective antiemetics may still be elusive. The cost of a single prechemotherapy dose of serotonin antagonist may cost $160 (Zofran, 32-mg vial, 1996). The advanced practice nurse

(text continues on page 393)

TABLE 17-5

Commonly Used Antiemetics in Cancer Chemotherapy

Drug Class Drug Name	Recommended Dosage	Indications	Side Effects
Serotonin Antagonists			
Granisetron (Kytril)	IV: 10 µg/kg IV over 5 min PO: 1 mg bid or 2 mg single dose beginning 30–60 min prior to chemotherapy	Highly emetogenic chemotherapy	Mild constipation, diarrhea, headache
Ondansetron (Zofran)	IV: 32 mg IV over 15–30 min or 0.15 mg/kg q 4 hours × 3 beginning 30 min prior to chemo; studies have shown titration of dose based on emetogenic potential of chemo[17] PO: 8 mg po tid; first dose 30 minutes prior to chemo, then at 4 and 8 h after first dose, then tid	Full IV dose indicated for highly emetogenic chemotherapy. Oral doses indicated for moderately emetogenic chemotherapy	Mild constipation, diarrhea, headache; rarely with rapid infusion of drug: orthostatic hypotension, dizziness, transient blindness, resolving in minutes to hours
Phenothiazines			
Prochlorperazine (Compazine)	PO: 5, 10, 25 mg q 4–6 h Slow release: PO: 10, 15, 30 mg q 12 h. PR: 25 mg q 4-6 h. IM/IV: 5–40 mg q 3–4 h (mix in 50 mL 5% dextrose or NS and infuse over 20–30 min)[18]	Standard doses: low to moderately emetogenic chemotherapy High doses: moderately emetogenic chemotherapy	Sedation, hypotension, extrapyramidal side effects (e.g., dystonia)
Perphenazine (Trilafon)	PO: 4 mg q 4–6 h (max. 30 mg in 24 h) IV: 5 mg IVB q 4–6 h[19]	Moderately emetogenic chemotherapy	Sedation, hypotension, extrapyramidal side effects (e.g., dystonia)
Butyrophenones			
Droperidol (Inapsine)	IM/IV: 0.5–2.5 mg q 4–6 h or drip[20]	Moderately emetogenic chemotherapy	Sedation, restlessness, extrapyramidal side effects (less severe than with phenothiazines), tardive dyskinesia; can induce respiratory depression when used with narcotic analgesics

	Dose	Indication	Adverse Effects/Comments
Substituted Benzamides			
Metoclopramide HCl (Reglan)	IV: 1–3 mg/kg IV 30 min before chemotherapy administration then repeat q 2 h for 2–4 doses PO: for delayed nausea/vomiting: 20–40 mg q 4 h × 24, or 0.5 mg/kg qid × 4 days beginning 24 h after cisplatin together with dexamethasone 8 mg bid days 1–2, and 4 mg days 3–4[21]	Highly emetogenic chemotherapy Delayed nausea and vomiting following cisplatin	Sedation, akathesia (restlessness), and other extrapyramidal side effects; diarrhea
Benzodiazepines			
Lorazepam (Ativan)	IV: 0.5–1.5 mg/m² (max 2 mg) IVP or IVB, 30 min prior to chemotherapy PO: 1–3 mg 30 min prior to chemotherapy; q 4–6 h postchemotherapy[22]	Anxiety, anticipatory nausea/vomiting Used in combination with primary antiemetic +/– dexamethasone	Arousable sedation, but may be profound; prolonged amnesia, hypotension, perceptual disturbances, urinary incontinence. Risk for respiratory depression. Dose must be reduced in the following: elderly, debilitated patient, patient with severe hepatic dysfunction
Glucocorticoids			
Dexamethasone (Decadron)	IV: 10–20 mg 30 min prior to chemo, then q 4–6 h as needed PO: 4 mg q 4 h × 4 doses, beginning 1–8 h prior to chemotherapy[23]	In combination with primary antiemetic; will increase complete protection from nausea/vomiting by 15%	IVP administration: perineal burning; lethargy, weakness, mood changes, hyperglycemia (use with caution in diabetics), leukocytosis, insomnia, agitation following therapy. Avoid in patients with psychosis

(continued)

TABLE 17-5

Commonly Used Antiemetics in Cancer Chemotherapy (continued)

Drug Class Drug Name	Recommended Dosage	Indications	Side Effects
Cannabinoids Dronabinol (Marinol)	PO: 5–7.5 mg/m² 1–3 h before chemotherapy, then 2–4 h post for 4–6 doses per day	Patients who have failed standard antiemetics; more effective than placebo, may be as effective as prochlorperazine; not effective against cisplatin	Mood changes, disorientation, drowsiness, muddled thinking, dizziness; brief impairment of perception, coordination, sensory functions. Rarely, dry mouth, increased appetite, general increase in central sympathomimetic activity (increased HR, postural hypotension); increased CNS toxicity in elderly
Antihistamines Diphenhydramine (Benadryl)	IV: 25–50 mg prior to chemotherapy or 25 mg q 4 h × 4 during metoclopramide antiemesis PO: 25–50 mg q 4 h IM: 25–50 mg q 4 h	Slight antiemetic activity; used together with a phenothiazine or high-dose metoclopramide to prevent extrapyramidal side effects	Drowsiness, dry mouth, dizziness

must be cognizant of the patient risk profile and be articulate about the cost-benefit ratio to advocate for the appropriate medication. Clearly, the cost of a inpatient hospitalization for uncontrolled nausea and vomiting is more expensive than a single dose of antiemetic, and if the antineoplastic agent is highly emetogenic, this is an important dimension of the discussion. Patients with advanced malignancy under hospice care may experience financial constraints as well in the selection of appropriate antiemetics, and the advanced practice nurse must draw from knowledge of effective agents or combinations of agents to provide effective control of nausea. As most managed care groups and hospices have developed standards of pharmacologic management of nausea and vomiting, it is imperative that advanced practice nurses are present on the committees making decisions about available and recommended agents.

Stomatitis

While mucositis refers to inflammation of the mucosal lining of the gastrointestinal tract, stomatitis refers specifically to the mucosa lining the mouth. Chemotherapy directly and indirectly causes this inflammation, which can progress to desquamation and ultimately to ulceration. The stem cells of the oral mucosa lie in the deep squamous epithelium above the basement membrane. These cells have a life span of 3 to 5 days, and the outer epithelial layer is replaced entirely every 7 to 14 days. As the mature mucosal cells are sloughed off due to the normal wear and tear of digestion, the frequently dividing stem cells are injured *directly* by the chemotherapy and are unable to replace the sloughed cells. This results in thinning of the oral mucosa. *Indirectly*, as bone marrow stem cells are also depressed following chemotherapy, the subsequent neutropenia contributes to infection and increased stomatotoxicity.

Normally, the oral mucosa is pink, moist, and intact without debris. Beginning 5 to 7 days after chemotherapy, the oral mucosa may appear pale and dry, with dry tongue and raised papillae and ridging of the buccal mucosa, and the patient may experience a burning sensation. This may progress during days 8 to 10 to a red, dry, and wrinkled mucosa. The tongue may appear swollen with a protective white coating; isolated mucosal ulcerations may appear, and the patient may complain of pain and altered taste perception. The mucosa and tongue may appear intensely inflamed 11 to 14 days after chemotherapy with dry and cracked lips; large areas of painful ulceration may be present, along with infection or bleeding. The patient may not be able to eat or drink. In severe cases, the patient may require parenteral narcotics for pain control and nutrition to promote healing until the patient is able to take oral nutrition. As the bone marrow recovers, so does the oral mucosa, with resolving inflammation, and granulation of the ulcerated areas occurring after day 14.[25] A grading system is shown in Table 17-6.

Antimetabolite chemotherapy agents most commonly cause stomatitis (cytosine arabinoside, 5-fluorouracil, 6-mercaptopurine, methotrexate, 6-thioguanine), but other agents that may have this toxicity to a lesser degree are the antibiotics (actinomycin, doxorubicin, bleomycin sulfate, daunomycin, mitomycin C, mitoxantrone), plant alkaloids (vinblastine sulfate), and the taxanes (paclitaxel and docetaxel).

TABLE 17-6

Stomatitis Grading System

Grade	Characteristics
Grade I	Generalized erythema
Grade II	Increased erythema, isolated small ulceration or infection
Grade III	Confluent ulcerations with infection >25% of mucosa, or unable to drink liquids
Grade IV	Hemorrhagic ulcerations and/or unable to drink liquids or eat solid food

Research on granulocyte and granulocyte-macrophage colony-stimulating factors has shown that administration of these agents to prevent febrile neutropenia in fact reduces the incidence of stomatitis in patients receiving stomatotoxic chemotherapy.[26] The use of oral cryotherapy has been shown to reduce the incidence of 5-fluorouracil-induced stomatitis and involves having the patient suck ice chips for five minutes prior to the bolus administration of the drug and again 25 minutes afterwards.[27]

Risk Factors

Patient risk factors that enhance the development of stomatitis when receiving stomatotoxic chemotherapy are exposure to alcohol and tobacco, poor oral hygiene, poor nutritional status, ill-fitting dentures, and receiving steroids that promote superinfection.

Management

Prechemotherapy assessment should include an assessment of the teeth and oral mucosa. If dental work needs to be performed, it should be done prior to beginning treatment to reduce the incidence of infection. Patients should be taught systemic oral cleansing involving brushing, rinsing, flossing, and lip moisturizing. Although hydrogen peroxide solutions are generally avoided because they damage early granulation tissue and hinder healing, 0.25% strength hydrogen peroxide may be appropriate for patients with thick secretions or oral tumors, who need to use a mucolytic cleanser. Alternatively, sodium bicarbonate solutions may be used. If the patient is at risk for severe neutropenia and the risk of an oral infection becoming systemic is of concern, prescribing oral rinses with chlorhexidine has been shown to reduce the incidence of infections.[28] Flossing should be avoided if it is painful, if the platelets are less than 50,000/mm³, of if the leukocyte count is less than 1500/mm³.[29] A moisturizer should be applied to the lips to prevent cracking, and the patient should be encouraged to drink 3 L of fluid daily.

If the patient has xerostomia, pilocarpine may be prescribed to increase secretions. Sucking sugarless candy may also stimulate secretions. The patient should be taught to assess for changes in the oral mucosa and for signs and symptoms of infection or bleeding. *Candida albicans* is a common superinfection, especially if the patient is taking steroids. However, infections can be fungal, bacterial, or viral, and suspicious sites should be cultured. Patients who are seropositive for the herpes simplex virus who are receiving immunosuppressive therapy should receive prophylaxis with an antiviral agent such as acyclovir.[30]

Diarrhea

Diarrhea can be defined as the passage of 2 or 3 stools in excess of normal elimination pattern pretreatment, and it is graded as Grade I toxicity. More severe toxicity is shown in Table 17-7. The intestinal mucosal epithelial cells (villi and microvilli) are characterized by rapid cell division (high mitotic rate) and a cell generation time of 24 hours. Normally 20 to 50 million epithelial cells are shed every hour, and rapid cell division is necessary to replace these cells. Chemotherapy, especially the antimetabolite drugs and the topoisomerase inhibitor irinotecan (Camptosar), interferes with cell division, preventing replacement of the sloughed cells. Mucosal cells atrophy and become inflamed; the villi and microvilli shorten and become denuded; and the inflamed mucosa produces large amounts of mucus, which stimulates peristalsis. Rapid transit time of intestinal contents, plus the damaged mucosal epithelium, prevents absorption of nutrients, water, and electrolytes.[31] In addition, there may be other mechanisms, such as the cholinergic-mediated acute diarrhea associated with irinotecan. Diarrhea may be an indication to stop or hold further therapy, as continued therapy may cause intestinal perforation and severe morbidity (e.g., 5-fluouracil, irinotecan, methotrexate); a complete symptom analysis must be obtained prior to drug administration.

Risk Factors

Patient risk factors include (1) administration of antimetabolite- or topoisomerase-inhibiting drugs (2) use of cathartics, (3) ingestion of high-fiber foods, and (4) baseline elimination pattern of loose stools.

TABLE 17-7

Grading of Severity of Diarrhea Based on the National Cancer Institute Common Toxicity Grading Criteria

Grade I	Grade II	Grade III	Grade IV
Increase of 2–3 stools/day over pretreatment pattern	Increase of 4–6 stools/day, nocturnal stools, or moderate cramping	Increase of 7–9 stools/day or severe cramping	Increase of ≥ 10 stools/day; grossly bloody diarrhea; need for parenteral support

Management

Patient assessment factors include (1) patient baseline elimination pattern, (2) dietary and medication profile, and (3) self-care ability. Management strategies are directed toward control of diarrhea, prevention of dehydration and electrolyte imbalance, and maintenance of nutritional status. Interventions include administration of antidiarrheal medications (e.g., loperamide), hydration, and electrolyte repletion as needed. Patient and family teaching includes (1) elimination of the use of cathartics, (2) dietary teaching about elimination of foods that stimulate peristalsis, e.g., high-fiber foods, fruits, and raw vegetables; (3) dietary teaching about inclusion of high-calorie, and high-protein, low-residue foods, as well as small, frequent meals (e.g., cottage cheese, cream cheese, yogurt, custard); (4) intake of 3 L of fluid each day; (5) perianal skin care; and (6) reporting of persistent diarrhea or presence of blood in the stool.

Gonadal Dysfunction

Chemotherapy, depending upon the drug and dose being administered, may threaten sexual and reproductive health on many levels. First, the reproductive tissues are composed of frequently dividing gonadal cells in men, while women receive their full complement of ovarian follicles at birth. For women, alkylating agents are the most damaging, causing a loss of ova and an increase in the mutation rate. Women aged 35 and over are most apt to develop ovarian fibrosis and failure. Amenorrhea experienced by young women is usually reversible but often becomes irreversible after age 30. Women with ovarian failure experience symptoms of early menopause (hot flashes, amenorrhea, vaginal dryness, dyspareunia). In addition, many drugs are mutagenic and teratogenic so that the need for birth control measures is an important consideration prior to therapy in women of childbearing age. In some areas and situations, women may be able to bank oocytes or cryopreserve embryos.

For men, temporary or permanent sterility may result. There is damage and destruction of testicular germ cells and epithelium of the seminiferous tubules. Oligospermia or azoospermia may develop 90 to 120 days after treatment begins, and normal sperm levels may take several years to return after therapy is completed. However, testosterone levels are not altered. For men who wish to father a child, sperm banking is an option. However, depending upon the type of malignancy, the viability of sperm may be uncertain (e.g., in lymphoma or testicular cancer).

It is important to remember that not all drugs may cause reproductive injury, and even with known drugs, results may be unpredictable. In addition, many men and women who have received chemotherapy have gone on to have healthy children. The most significant variables are the age of the patient and the specific drug(s), dose(s), and duration of therapy.

Sexual dysfunction that may occur includes decreased libido, dyspareunia (females), and erectile dysfunction (males).

Risk Factors

Patient risk factors include drug and dosage, duration of therapy, age (women), prior surgical procedures, prior radiation therapy to the pelvis, concurrent medications (e.g., narcotics, antihypertensives), presence of depression and/or fatigue, and type of malignancy.

Management

Patient management strategies include prechemotherapy assessment of sexual health and reproductive goals, teaching and counseling concerning options as appropriate (e.g., sperm banking), and birth control measures. During and after chemotherapy, it is important to help patients and their partners discuss coping strategies, and if necessary, refer them for specialized counseling. Testosterone replacement therapy, if not contraindicated, may help men with decreased libido. Patient teaching concerning self-care measures must be individualized, and, for instance, may include the use of water-based lubricants to decrease vaginal dryness for women with symptoms of early menopause.

Alopecia

The hair follicles comprise the fourth major cell population that is frequently dividing and thus is vulnerable to the effects of chemotherapy. These cells have a high mitotic rate, and usually 90 percent of the hair follicles are in the growth phase (anagen).[2] In fact, hair growth measures about 0.35 mm every 24 h.[32] Although there is little physical damage or morbidity associated with hair loss, there is an enormous psychological impact, and in some cases, the fear of hair loss may prevent an individual from accepting even lifesaving chemotherapy.

Alopecia is reversible and can occur by two mechanisms. First, atrophy or necrosis of the hair shaft bulb causes constriction and bisection of the hair shaft so that it breaks off, usually at the hairline, resulting in *patchy, thin hair*. A second mechanism is root damage resulting in *complete alopecia*. Strands of hair fall out spontaneously or with brushing.

Many drugs cause varying degrees of hair loss that often are dose-dependent. In addition, drugs with long half-lives of active metabolites, such as doxorubicin, the nitrosureas, and cyclophosphamide, produce severe hair loss.[7] Table 17-8 shows drugs commonly associated with alopecia. Usually, hair loss begins about two weeks after initial chemotherapy. Degrees of hair loss are (1) minimal (less than 25 percent of hair lost, and noticeable only to the patient) (2) moderate (25 to 50 percent of hair is lost with obvious thinning), and (3) severe (greater than 50 percent loss). Hair grows back about 3 to 5 months after the completion of chemotherapy (anagen or growth phase of hair follicle is 3 months), but may be a different texture or color.

Risk Factors

Risk factors for alopecia are (1) specific drug, dose, schedule, and whether given in combination with other alopecia-producing drugs; (2) concurrent radiotherapy to the scalp that causes alopecia; (3) usual hair care practices and use of hair-damaging substances; (4) other medical conditions such as hypothyroidism; and (5) concurrent use of medications such as prednisone.

TABLE 17-8

Drugs Causing Significant Alopecia

bleomycin	irinotecan
cyclophosphamide	methotrexate
dactinomycin	mitomycin C
daunorubicin	mitoxantrone
doxorubicin	melphalan
5-fluorouracil	paclitaxel
ifosfamide	vincristine

Management

Prechemotherapy assessment and teaching includes anticipated impact of hair loss and strategies to minimize loss. If complete alopecia is expected, assisting the patient in obtaining a wig prior to hair loss is a helpful strategy. In addition, for patients receiving adjuvant chemotherapy, hair loss may symbolize the malignancy and be the only visible sign of cancer. Other important strategies are gentle hair care and avoidance of harsh hair-coloring solutions, or perms and curling irons; use of a scarf or cap at night in cold climates to minimize heat loss; and assessment and bolstering of effective coping strategies. Although hair preservation techniques such as the use of a scalp tourniquet with or without local scalp icing have been used in the past, use today is avoided largely due to concern over creation of a sanctuary and site for scalp metastasis.

The next section addresses direct injury to specific organs, and drugs causing toxicity to the heart, lungs, and kidneys, along with preventative measures, will be discussed.

Cardiotoxicity

A number of chemotherapeutic agents can cause acute and long-term changes in cardiac function. Within 24 hours of drug administration, *acute* electrocardiogram changes (e.g., sinus tachycardia, arrhythmias) may occur rarely with some drugs, such as doxorubicin, which are self-limiting and require no intervention, or paclitaxel, which requires drug cessation and a modification in drug administration. Other drugs, such as 5-florouracil or cisplatin, rarely may cause angina with ST-segment changes that require drug discontinuation.[33] *Subacute* changes may occur rarely within four to five weeks after drug administration and are related to pericarditis, which is usually reversible. *Chronic* changes involve the anthracycline agents (doxorubicin, daunorubicin) that intercalate the DNA base pairs in the cell nucleus and cause direct injury to the myofibrils with resultant loss of contractility. Over time, with cumulative doses greater than 550 mg/m^2 for doxorubicin, this leads to decreased left ventricular contractility, increased myocardial workload and hypertrophy, and congestive failure. However, with careful monitoring of baseline and periodic cardiac ejection fractions by nuclear medicine studies, early damage can be identified and congestive heart failure prevented. The risk of injury is heightened when doxorubicin is given in combination with cyclophosphamide or if radiotherapy has been given to the thorax; in these cases the maximum cumulative dose is 350 mg/m^2.

With high-dose chemotherapy for bone marrow transplantation or stem cell rescue, some standard drugs may now cause cardiac damage.

Efforts to minimize cardiotoxicity of the anthracycline agents, which have excellent activity against many tumor types, have included drug delivery systems using liposomes (Doxil, Daunaxome), and the development of drugs such as dexrazoxane (Zinecard), which is approved for use in women with breast cancer responsive to doxorubicin who have received more than 300 mg/m^2 cumulative dose. However, this drug also causes myelosuppression. Investigationally, the drug amifostine has also shown cardioprotection by its action as a scavenger of free radicals.[34]

Risk Factors

Patient risk factors include (1) drug(s) and dose(s) being administered (see Table 17-9 for a list of cardiotoxic drugs), (2) administration schedule (a low dose given more frequently or a dose given as a continuous infusion has less cardiotoxicity than a high dose given over a shorter time), (3) age (young children and adults over age 50), (4) pre-existing cardiovascular disease (e.g., hypertension, CAD) and (5) smoking history.

Management

Management strategies are based on prevention of cardiotoxicity, and if prevention is not possible, early identification of the dysfunction. Key patient assessment areas include patient risk factor profile; past administration of cardiotoxic drugs, cumulative dose received, and history of past radiotherapy to the chest; baseline cardiac studies (e.g., radionuclide cardiac scan, MUGA) if this is an initial dose, and comparison of periodic monitoring to the baseline study if this is a subsequent dose; cardiac systems review (history and PE including heart sounds, rate, rhythm, regularity, blood pressure, breath sounds, percussion of liver, and inspection for peripheral edema); serum electrolytes including potassium and calcium; and end organ function to assess drug excretion.

Interventions may rarely include drug cessation if ejection fraction falls below 55 percent and discussion with the physician about changing to another active but noncardiotoxic drug, teaching the patient to avoid tobacco use, and symptom management as needed.

Pulmonary Toxicity

Drugs most commonly associated with pulmonary toxicity are bleomycin (which is distributed preferentially to the skin and lungs), the nitrosureas (carmustine, busulfan), and less commonly methotrexate. The lung parenchyma, especially the alveoli and capillary endothelium, may be injured by two mechanisms. First *hypersensitivity pneumonitis* may rarely occur 7 to 10 days following bleomycin administration and requires drug cessation and management with corticosteroids and ventilatory support. Signs and symptoms include severe dyspnea, characteristic fever, diffuse infiltrates on

(text continues on page 403)

TABLE 17-9

Drugs with Potential to Cause Cardiotoxicity

Drug	Dosage	Cardiotoxicity	Occurrence	Comments
aminoglutethimide	250 mg PO qid	Hypotension, tachycardia	10%	Can occur at any time during treatment.
amsacrine (AMSA)	100 mg/m^2 IV qd × 3 or 75–150 mg/m^2 IV qd × 5	Ventricular fibrillation Cardiomyopathy	5%	Risk is increased by cumulative dose of greater than 900 mg/m^2 or greater than 200 mg/m^2 of AMSA in 48 h. Increased incidence with previous anthracycline exposure. Cardiac toxicity is enhanced by preexisting hypokalemia.
cisplatin	Unknown	Cardiac ischemia	Rare	Reports of myocardial infarction (MI), cerebrovascular accident (CVA) after treatment with cisplatin, velban, bleomycin, etoposide.
cisplatin-based combination therapy	Unknown	Arterial occlusion events, MI, CVA	Rare	
cyclophosphamide	120–270 mg/m^2 × 1–4 days	Hemorrhagic myocardial necrosis	Rare	Occurs with induced myelosuppression for bone marrow transplantation. Potentiates anthracycline-induced cardiomyopathy.
dactinomycin	0.25 mg/m^2 × 5 days	Cardiomyopathy	Rare	Seen with previous anthracycline exposure.
daunorubicin	400–550 mg/m^2 (lifetime dose)	Transient EKG changes Cardiomyopathy	0–41% 1.5%	Increased risk with concomitant cyclophosphamide or previous chest irradiation. Young children and the elderly are most susceptible.

Drug	Dose	Cardiac toxicity	Frequency	Comments
diethylstilbestrol (DES)	5 mg qd	Thromboembolic CVA, myocardial infarction	Frequent	Risk decreased by decreasing dose to 1 mg qd.
doxorubicin	450–550 mg/m² (lifetime dose)	Transient EKG changes Cardiomyopathy	2.2% 1–5%	Same as for daunorubicin.
doxydoxorubicin (DXDX; synthetic anthracycline)	25–30 mg/m²	CHF (cumulative dose-related cardiotoxicity with 250 mg/m²)	Rare	Radionuclide ejected fraction performed after patient receives 150 mg/m² cumulative dose. Repeat at each dose of 250 mg/m².
4′-epidoxorubicin (anthracycline analogue)	75 mg/m² q 3 weeks; 1100 mg/m² lifetime dose	Transient EKG changes, ventricular extrasystole CHF	1%	Spectrum of activity is similar to doxorubicin. Incidence of CHF is 1% when doses to 1100 mg/m² are given.
estramustine	600 mg/m² PO in 3 divided doses	Hypertension, angina, myocardial infarction, arrhythmias, pulmonary emboli	10–15%	Increased risk with history of cardiovascular disease.
estrogens	5 mg qd	CHF with ischemic heart disease, thromboembolic CVA	39%	Increased risk with history of cardiovascular disease.
etoposide (VP-16)	Unknown	Myocardial infarction	Rare	May be worsened with prior mediastinal XRT and preexisting coronary artery disease.
fluorouracil	12–15 mg/kg q week	Angina 3–18 hrs after drug administered	Rare	May occur in patients without preexisting cardiovascular disease. Can recur with subsequent doses. Cardiac enzymes are normal.

(continued)

TABLE 17-9

Drugs with Potential to Cause Cardiotoxicity (continued)

Drug	Dosage	Cardiotoxicity	Occurrence	Comments
mithramycin	25–50 mg/kg IV qod × 3–8 days	Cardiomyopathy	Rare	Exacerbates subclinical anthracycline-induced cardiotoxicity.
mitomycin	15 mg/m^2 q 6–8 weeks	Cardiomyopathy	Rare	Increased risk with previous chest irradiation or anthracycline exposure. Synergistic with anthracyclines.
mitoxantrone (Novantrone)	a. 12–14 mg/m^2 q 3 weeks b. 100 mg/m^2 lifetime dose with prior exposure to anthracyclines c. 160 mg/m^2 lifetime dose without prior exposure to anthracyclines	a. Transient EKG changes b. Decreased ejection fraction c. CHF	a. 28% b. 44% c. 2.1–12.5%	Increased risk of cardiomyopathy with previous anthracycline exposure, chest irradiation, or cardiovascular disease. CHF has occurred in patients who have not received prior anthracycline therapy.
paclitaxel (Taxol)	135 mg/m^2 or higher	Asymptomatic bradycardia; rarely may progress to heart block Rarely, chest pain, brief ventricular tachycardia or supraventricular tachycardia	29%	Asymptomatic bradycardia may occur during or up to 8 hrs after paclitaxel infusion; one fatal myocardial infarction has been reported.
vincristine and vinblastine	Unknown	Myocardial infarction	Rare	Phenomena not well described.

SOURCE: Barton-Burke et al.[2], pp. 156–157. Reproduced with permission of the publisher.

chest X-ray, and eosinophilia. Second, *pulmonary fibrosis and pneumonitis* may occur and are associated with higher cumulative doses of drugs (e.g., bleomycin, carmustine). Early signs and symptoms are dry, hacking cough, fine bibasilar rales with exertional dyspnea, and decreased diffusing capacity (DLCO) on pulmonary function studies. The chest X-ray may only show minimal changes, but fine reticular bibasilar infiltrates may appear. Later, dyspnea occurs at rest, along with tachypnea, fever, coarse rales, changes on chest X-ray (e.g., consolidation), significant decrease in DLCO, and hypoxemia. Risk is increased with prior or concurrent chest radiotherapy, high cumulative doses, or the inspiration of pure oxygen (bleomycin). Incidence of bleomycin toxicity is 5 to 11 percent, while that of carmustine is 20 to 30 percent with a mortality of 24 to 80 percent.[35]

Risk Factors

Patient factors that increase the risk of pulmonary toxicity are (1) elevated serum levels of pulmonary toxic drugs due to delayed drug metabolism or excretion (e.g., renal dysfunction resulting in impaired bleomycin drug excretion), (2) prior or concurrent chemotherapy with pulmonary toxic drugs and/or radiotherapy to the chest (bleomycin, carmustine, cyclophosphamide, doxorubicin), (3) age greater than 70 years, (4) pre-existing pulmonary disease (e.g., COPD, asthma), (5) smoking history, (6) exposure to industrial pulmonary irritants, (7) exposure to high oxygen concentrations following bleomycin administration, and (8) high cumulative drug doses (bleomycin: dose greater than 500 IU, but may occur at lower doses; carmustine: dose greater than 1000 mg/m^2).

Management

Patient management strategies are to prevent pulmonary toxicity by identifying patients at risk and acting on early pulmonary changes. The pulmonary system review should include a detailed history and physical assessment. If abnormalities are found, pulse oximetry, arterial blood gases, and a chest X-ray should be performed. Pulmonary function tests should be performed baseline and periodically during treatment if the patient is receiving bleomycin or carmustine. The drug should be discontinued if pulmonary function worsens. Patient education should include avoidance of smoking and reporting of changes in breathing patterns, especially the development of dyspnea on exertion.

Renal Toxicity

Toxicity to the kidneys can occur *directly*, through damage to the nephron, glomerulus, and renal blood vessels by the drug (e.g., cisplatin may cause proximal and distal renal tubular necrosis; high-dose methotrexate may precipitate in the tubules and collecting ducts in an acid urine causing obstructive nephropathy), or *indirectly* by the accumulation of metabolic end products after administration of chemotherapy to a patient with a sensitive, high tumor burden (tumor lysis syndrome, hyperuremic nephropathy). Fortunately, renal damage is largely preventable by ensuring adequate hydration and urinary output prior to and following drug administration, alkalinization of the urine to enhance drug or uric acid excretion, and use of allopurinol as appropriate to decrease the production of uric acid. Specific protocols must be followed for the administration of cisplatin, high-dose methotrexate, and during initial therapy of patients with high tumor burdens of a sensitive tumor (e.g., acute leukemia, small cell lung cancer, and lymphoma). Recently, amifostine (Ethyol) has been shown to protect normal tissues from cisplatin damage and has been approved to reduce the cumulative renal toxicity associated with repeated courses of cisplatin in patients with advanced ovarian or non–small cell lung cancer.[36] However, although amifostine does not appear to alter the efficacy of the anticancer agent, it is not approved for use in patients with potentially curable cancers.

Risk Factors

Patient factors that increase the risk of renal toxicity include (1) drug, dose, and administration schedule (cisplatin is a heavy metal and thus nephrotoxic; if the drug is given IV over 1 to 3 h in 3% normal saline, it is less nephrotoxic); (2) preexisting renal impairment; (3) concurrent administration of other renally toxic drugs (e.g., NSAIDs, aminoglycoside antibiotics, amphotericin B); (4) increased age; and (5) hypovolemia (possibly related to severe nausea and vomiting).

Management

Management goals are to prevent renal toxicity. Pretreatment assessment must include baseline BUN and serum creatinine, 24-h creatinine clearance (actual or estimated), patient hydration status (as evidenced by skin turgor, mucous membranes, weight compared to baseline), and self-care ability after chemotherapy administration. The drug should not be administered if the BUN and serum creatinine are abnormal or if the creatinine clearance is less than 60 mL/min, unless otherwise directed in the clinical protocol. The advanced practice nurse should discuss with the physician the benefit of further hydration to normalize renal function or selection of an alternative chemotherapeutic agent. In addition, serum electrolytes and magnesium should be determined. During and following chemotherapy administration, these studies should be monitored, along with BUN and serum creatinine. Other tests are determined by the drug(s) administered, such as urine pH (alkaline to enhance methotrexate and uric acid excretion) and urine osmolality (indicating tubular damage) and/or protein (proteinuria suggests damage to the renal glomerulus and tubules). Patients receiving cisplatin require IV repletion of magnesium and potassium, as acceptable; reversible damage to the kidneys prevents reabsorption of these substances in the distal renal tubule.

Patients should be instructed to drink 3 to 4 L of fluid a day for 1 day before and 3 days following chemotherapy administration. If not contraindicated, some of the fluid should contain salt (e.g., Gatorade). Patients should report nausea and vomiting so that a more effective antiemetic regime may be instituted, as this may predispose a patient to hypovolemia and renal dysfunction. Patients should avoid concurrent administration of NSAIDs and aspirin when receiving high doses of methotrexate, as these drugs are also protein bound, and higher serum levels of methotrexate may result with increased toxicity. Finally, patients should be compliant with their follow-up appointments so that renal function can be monitored closely.

SUMMARY

Cancer chemotherapy is an important modality for the systematic treatment of cancer. However, despite major advances, drug toxicity to normal tissues still presents a major challenge to patients and providers alike. Most toxicity can be anticipated and, if not prevented, at least identified early to minimize toxicity and long-term morbidity. The advanced practice nurse plays an important role in identifying patients at risk, developing management plans to minimize toxicity, and in empowering patients through self-care education. This chapter has reviewed cancer chemotherapy and discussed toxicity and management strategies in frequently dividing organ systems (bone marrow, gastrointestinal mucosa, gonads, hair follicles) and the specific organs of the heart, lungs, and kidneys.

REFERENCES

1. Burchenal JH: The historical development of cancer chemotherapy. *Semin Oncol* 4:135-148, 1977.
2. Barton-Burke MB, Wilkes GM, Ingwersen K: *Cancer Chemotherapy: A Nursing Process Approach*, 2d ed. Sudbury, MA: Jones and Bartlett, 1996.
3. Calvert AH, Newell DR, Gumbrell LA, et al: Carboplatin dosage: Prospective evaluation of a simple formula based on renal function. *J Clin Oncol* 7:1748–1756, 1989.
4. Tannock IF: Experimental chemotherapy, Tannock IF, Hill RP (eds): *The Basic Science of Oncology*, 2d ed. New York: McGraw-Hill, 1992, pp 338–359.
5. Perry MC, Yarbro JW: *Toxicity of Chemotherapy*. New York: Grune and Stratton, 1984.
6. Wujick D: Infection control in oncology patients. *Nurs Clin North Am* 28(3): 639–650, 1993.
7. Dorr RT, Fritz WL: *Cancer Chemotherapy Handbook*. New York: Elsevier, 1980.
8. Bodey GP, Buckley M, Sathe YS, et al: Quantitative relationship between circulating leukocytes and infections in patients with acute leukemia. *Am Intern Med* 64(2):328–340, 1966.
9. Pizzo PA, Robichaud KJ, Wesley R, et al: Fever in the pediatric and young adult patient with cancer: A prospective study of 1001 episodes. *Medicine* 61:153–165, 1982.
10. Carlson AC: Infection prophylaxis in the patient with cancer. *Oncol Nurs Forum* 12(3):60, 1985.
11. Rubin RH, Ferraro MJ: Understanding and diagnosing infectious complications in the immunocompromised host. *Hematol Oncol Clin North Am* 7:795–812, 1993.
12. Talcott JA, Siegel RD, Finberg R, et al: Risk assessment in cancer patients with fever and neutropenia: A prospective two-center validation of a prediction rule. *J Clin Oncol* 10:316–322, 1992.
13. Wujick D: Infection, in Groenwald SL, Frogge MH, Goodman M, Yarbro CH (eds). *Cancer Symptom Management*. Boston: Jones and Bartlett, 1996, pp 289–302.
14. Hoagland HC: Hematologic complications of cancer chemotherapy, in Perry MC (ed): *The Chemotherapy Source Book*. Baltimore: Williams & Wilkins, 1992, pp 498–507.
15. Rieger PT, Haeuber D. A new approach to managing chemotherapy-related anemia: Nursing implications of epoetin alfa. *Oncol Nurs Forum* 22:73, 1995.
16. Wickham R: Nausea and vomiting, in Groenwald SL, Frogge MH, Goodman M, Yarbro CH (eds): *Cancer Symptom Management*. Boston: Jones and Bartlett, 1996, pp 218–251.
17. Hesketh PJ, Beck TM, Uhlenhoop M, et al: Adjusting the dose of IV ondansetron plus dexamethasone to the emetogenic potential of the chemotherapy regimen. *Proc Am Soc Clin Oncologists* 13:433, 1994.

18. Carr B, Blayney D, Leong L, et al: A prospective, double-blind dose-response study of prochlorperazine therapy for cisplatin-induced emesis. *Proc Am Soc Clin Oncologist* 4:268, 1985.

19. Smaglia RA: Antiemetic effect of perphenazine versus prochlorperazine intravenously before cisplatin therapy. *Am J Hosp Pharmacol* 41 (March): 560, 1984.

20. Citron M, Johnson-Early A, Boyer M, et al: Droperidol: Optimal dose and time of initiation therapy. *Proc Am Soc Clin Oncologists*: 3:106, 1984.

21. Kris M, Gralla RJ: Antiemetic trials to control delayed vomiting following high-dose cisplatin. *Proc Am Soc Clin Oncologists* 5:1005, 1986.

22. Lazlo J, Clark RA, Harrison DC, et al: Lorazepam in cancer patients treated with cisplatin: A drug having antiemetic, amnesiac, and anxiolytic effects. *J Clin Oncol* 3:864–869, 1985.

23. Goodman M: Management of nausea and vomiting induced by outpatient cisplatin therapy. *Sem Oncol Nurs* 3(1) suppl 1:23–35, 1987.

24. Jones AL, Gee GL, Bosanquet N: The budgetary impact of 5-HT[3] receptor antagonists in the management of chemotherapy-induced emesis. *Eur J Cancer* 29A: 51–56, 1993.

25. Engleking C: Prechemotherapy nursing assessment in outpatient settings. *Outpatient Chemother* 3(1): 9–11, 1988.

26. Chi KH, Chen Sy, Chan WK, et al: Effect of granulocyte macrophage colony stimulating factor on oral mucositis in head and neck cancer patients with cisplatin, 5-FU and leukovorin therapy. *Proc Am Soc Clin Oncologists* 13:428, 1994.

27. Mahood DJ, Dose AM, Loprinzi CL, et al: Inhibition of fluourouracil-induced stomatitis by oral cryotherapy *J Clin Oncol* 9:449–452, 1991.

28. Ferretti GA, Ash RC, Brown C, et al: Control of oral mucositis and candidiasis in marrow transplantation: A prospective, double-blind trial of chlorhexidine digluconate oral rinse. *Bone Marrow Transplant* 3:483–493, 1988.

29. Beck SL, Yasko JM: *Guidelines for Oral Care*, 2d ed. Crystal Lake, IL: Sage, 1993.

30. Beck SL: Mucositis, In Groenwald SL, Frogge MH, Goodman M, Yarbro CH (eds): *Cancer Symptom Management*, Boston: Jones and Bartlett, 1996, pp 308–323.

31. Brager BL, Yasko JM *Care of the Client Receiving Chemotherapy*. Reston VA; Reston, 1984.

32. DeSpain JD: Dermatologic toxicity of chemotherapy. *Sem Oncol* 19:501–507, 1992.

33. Akhtar SS, Salim KP, Bano Z: Symptomatic cardiotoxicity with high-dose 5-fluorouracil infusion: A prospective study. *Oncology* 50: 441–444, 1993.

34. Dorr RT, Lasel KE: Anthracycline cardioprotection by amifostine (WR-2721) and its active metabolite (WR-1065). *Proc Am Soc Clin Oncologists* 13:435, 1994.

35. Wickham R: Pulmonary toxicity secondary to cancer treatment. *Oncol Nurs Forum* 13(5):69–76, 1986.

36. Kemp G, Roe P, Lurain J, et al: Amifostine pretreatment for protection against cyclophosphamide-induced and cisplatin-induced toxicities: Results of a randomized control trial in patients with advanced ovarian cancer. *Clin Oncol* 14(7): 2101–2112, 1996.

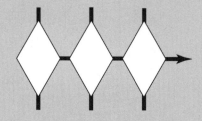

Part 3

CASE STUDY APPLICATIONS

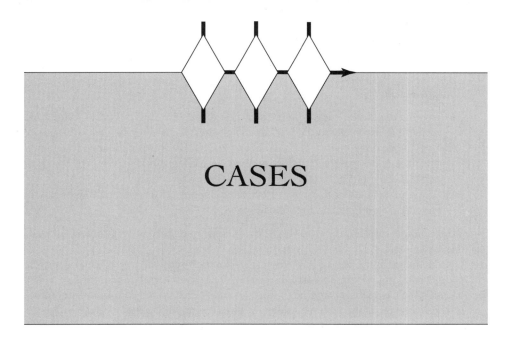

CASES

INTRODUCTION

This part of the book provides a variety of patient case write-ups that allow the reader to apply the various concepts and skills discussed in the earlier sections. Each case can be used to learn different concepts and thinking skills. The cases use varying formats and are presented purposefully in random order; i.e., they do not follow the sequence of topics in this book. Rather they challenge the student to integrate information from all chapters by presenting "real" patients with multiple medical and nursing problems.

The following exercises or questions can be used in almost every case:

1. Using the P-D-C approach:

P—Patient Analysis. Identify and explain the factors in assessment that relate to current and/or future drug therapy for this patient (see Case Analysis at end of Chap. 4):

> Evidence of drug effectiveness
> Variables that might affect pharmacokinetics and/or pharmacodynamics
> Indications of drug interactions (drug-drug, drug-food, or drug-lab test)
> Indications of possible adverse drug effects
> Factors affecting compliance

D—Drug Analysis. For each drug:

> Describe the drug's action and effects and why it is being used in this patient.
> Describe possible side effects and those that may be present in this patient.
> Describe the usual dosage and whether the drug dosage the patient is taking is within the recommended dosage and dosage schedule.
> Describe interactions with other drugs the patient is taking and with any foods, home remedies, and/or folk practices.
> Describe what the prescription should say (write an actual prescription).

C—Contextual Analysis

> Determine the cost of each drug (be sure to indicate whether the price is wholesale or retail and give the number of tablets or units of the drug the cost is based on.
>
> Identify other drugs that could have been prescribed for this patient and why they may not have been the choice of the prescribing clinician (or why the prescribed drug was chosen).
>
> Describe client factors that may affect compliance and what the clinician can do to increase compliance in this patient.

2. Write sample prescriptions for each drug, using the format or protocol in your agency or state.

3. Obtain the costs (retail and/or wholesale) for a 30-day supply of each drug the patient is taking. Compare costs for generic and brand name preparations.

4. Identify the assessments and laboratory tests that are needed to monitor the effectiveness as well as the adverse effects of drug therapy the patient is receiving.

CASE 1

Case A. D.

(Adapted from a case by Debra Swerda)

Age: 58; female

Allergies: penicillin, Percocet, codeine.

Reason for visit: "I am here for my physical exam. I have been doing okay. I just saw a podiatrist at the beginning of the month for the pain in my right foot and he gave me an injection which helped. I am going to see him again tomorrow."

Past illness/hospitalizations: Medical: asthma/COPD for several years; HTN for 10 years; angina for 5 years; anxiety and depression for several years; right foot pain for 4 months. Surgical: cholecystectomy 22 years ago; appendectomy 20 years ago; hysterectomy 16 years ago.

Current medications: Nasalcrom spray 4% prn; Theochrom 300 mg PO bid; Isordil 40 mg PO bid; imipramine 60 mg PO qhs; Naprosyn 500 mg PO bid; ASA 325 mg PO qd; Klonopin 0.05 mg PO 1 tab if needed; Nitrostat 0.3 mg PO 1 tab as needed; Ventolin inhaler in rotocap dispenser 2 puffs tid.

Problem: Routine physical health review.

Assessment

Health perception-health management: Client views her general health as "okay." "I take my medications as I'm supposed to." Has a >30-year history of smoking at least 2 packs of cigarettes/day, and has at times smoked up to 5 packs per day. States alcohol use includes "a few drinks during the week of wine or beer and sometimes more on weekends—usually grapefruit juice and vodka. Wears seat belts; does not do SBE.

Nutrition-metabolic pattern: Sample diet related: excess carbohydrates and fats; minimal high roughage (fruits and vegetables); does not take vitamins. Does not add salt to preparation of food. Has a good fluid intake, drinks several glasses of water/day and 2 cups of coffee or tea/day. States has a "very good appetite and has gained weight gradually over the past 20 years." Wears upper and lower dentures.

Elimination pattern: Daily bowel movement pattern with no c/o constipation; does not use laxatives. Has no problems with voiding or control in elimination.

Activity-exercise pattern: Does not participate in any form of physical exercise. Usual form of recreation consists of "going food shopping or out with friends." Client does experience SOB on exertion due to her asthma/COPD and this limits her physical activity and tolerance. Has hypertension and CAD. BP is well controlled at present; client is compliant with medications and does not require Nitrostat. Recently has had some right foot pain but feels that this did not interfere with her mobility.

Sleep-rest pattern: Average 6 to 8 h sleep/night; sleeps in own room. Uses two pillows to sleep with. Presleep activity is "usually watching TV." Perception of rest is good.

Cognitive-perceptual pattern: Sight corrected with glasses, changed 1 year ago; no change in hearing, taste, or smell. No perceived change in memory—"I'm all there." No change in sensory integrity; does not usually get headaches or have difficulty with sense of balance. Able to articulate well; does use an antidepressant.

Self perception–self concept pattern: Sees self as having to be there for her children. Client has a history of anxiety and sees a psychiatrist regularly for control and management of anxiety. "I'm doing real well with that—I haven't had any anxiety attacks in a long time and have never had to use my Klonopin."

Role-relationship pattern: Describes her children as "having a lot of problems. It has been really hard on me seeing them go through difficult times, but I'm there to help them in any way I can." Client is not employed and lives in a housing project with several of her children. She is divorced and presently is dating someone on a regular basis. Other social relationships confined to "a few close friends." She finds this sufficient.

Sexuality-reproductive pattern: Has 7 children, and has had 6 miscarriages. Had a hysterectomy 16 years ago. Perceived satisfaction with present sexual relationship.

Coping–stress tolerance pattern: Has had a lot of difficulty in the past with coping and stress. Has had a lot of family and social problems. States she "is doing very well now and managing pretty good."

Value-belief pattern: "I generally believe that if you try, things will work out for you. I'm not religious, but I have faith." States her children are important to her.

Review of Systems

General: Overall feels her state of health is "pretty good at present." Illnesses are controlled at present.

Integument: No eruptions, rashes; c/o dry skin on hands and feet; no disorders of hair or nails.

Head: No c/o of headaches; no history of trauma.

Eyes: Nearsighted and wears corrective glasses; last exam 1 year ago; no other visual disturbances.

Ears: Normal hearing; no tinnitus; no infections.

Nose: No epistaxis; no discharge.

Mouth, gums, and teeth: Wears upper and lower dentures; last saw dentist 1 year ago.

Throat and neck: No c/o sore throat, hoarseness, or neck pain or stiffness.

Breasts: No lumps, masses, discharge, or bleeding.

Resp: SOB with exertion; occasional productive cough; has frequent wheezing due to asthma/COPD.

CV: Has hypertension, well controlled with medication compliance. No c/o chest pain or palpitations.

GI: Appetite good; one BM every day; no melena; no jaundice or ulcers.

GU: No dysuria; hematuria; nocturia; no STD.

Musc: No muscle weakness; right foot pain controlled.

NP: No syncope, vertigo, dizziness; intelligent and well oriented × 3 spheres; sensorium intact; no paresthesias; affect appears good and mood appropriate.

Lymph-hemat: No abnormal bleeding; no adenopathy.

Endocrine: Prefers cold weather, has some difficulty tolerating heat; no excessive perspiration or polydipsia.

Physical Examination

VS: T 98.4 P 100 R 22 BP 120/80 HT 5 ft 4 in. WT 190 lb.

General: A. D. is an alert, pleasant, moderately obese 56-year-old white woman appearing about stated age who presents for a complete physical examination.

Skin: Pink; good turgor; warm; dryness on palms of hands and soles of feet; telangiectasis on right anterior chest.

Hair: Normal distribution and consistency.

Nails: No deformities; no clubbing; nail beds pink with good capillary refill.

Head: Symmetrical, normocephalic; normal hair distribution.

Face: No muscle weakness; appropriate facial expression.

Eyes: External eye structures symmetrical, without lesions; lashes and brows present; lacrimal apparatus nontender to palpitation, no excessive tearing; conjunctivae moist and clear; lens clear; sclera white; no defects of cornea or iris; PERRLA; can read newsprint 12 inches away; EOM normal; fundi not seen due to photosensitivity of client.

Ears: No masses, lesions of auricles or canals; tragus and auricle nontender to palpitation; canals have a small amount of soft yellow cerumen; noninflamed;

both TM pearly gray, no perforations; light reflex intact and landmarks discernible; able to identify whispered voice bilaterally; Weber test normal.

Nose: Nostrils patent bilaterally; no masses or tenderness; no septal deviation or perforations.

Mouth: Wears dentures; can clench teeth; mucosa pink; no lesions or masses; tongue protrudes in midline without tremor.

Pharynx: Mucosa pink, no lesions; tonsils present; gag reflex intact; uvula and soft palate rise in midline with phonation "ah."

Neck: Full ROM; no vein distention; carotid pulsations equal and of good quality; thyroid not palpable; trachea in midline; no lymphadenopathy.

Thorax: Chest movements symmetrical, good expansion bilaterally; AP diameter not increased; no tenderness; no axillary adenopathy.

Lungs: Fremitus equal bilaterally; wheezing heard in bronchi and lower lobes bilaterally.

Breasts: Symmetrical; no masses or tenderness; no retraction or nipple discharge.

Heart: No heaves, visible pulsations on anterior chest; no heaves, thrills, or rib retraction; PMI palpable at left 5th ICS; regular rhythm, rate 100/min; normal S1, S2, no extra heart sounds, murmurs, or gallops.

Abdomen: Abdomen obese; no visible masses, pulsations, or hernias; skin intact without lesions, well-healed transverse and vertical scars from previous surgeries.

Back: Normal curvature, no spinal tenderness, no CVA tenderness.

Extremities: No skin, hair, or nail abnormalities; no venous dilation; radial, brachial, femoral, popliteal, posterior tibial, and dorsalis pedis pulses all palpable and equal; no masses or tenderness; no right foot pain at present; no lymphadenopathy; fingers and toes dry and warm to touch; normal gait; full ROM; muscle strength intact; Romberg negative.

Genitalia: External: thinning pubic hair; no labial swelling or lesions, normal clitoris; no urethral redness, swelling or discharge; Skene's and Bartholin's glands not inflamed, perineum intact, and clean, no scars. Internal: Vagina: mucosa intact, atrophic, no bulging or masses. Uterus and cervix surgically absent. Adenexa: ovaries not palpated, no tenderness. Cul-de-sac: no palpable cystocele or retrocele; no bulging, tenderness, or masses. Discharge: no discharge; no odor. Pap: vaginal pool swab, gonorrhea, and chlamydia swabs and cultures sent to lab.

Rectal: Perineal skin and anus intact and clean; no external or internal hemorrhoids, no fissures or fistulae; sphincter tone slightly atrophic; no masses or tenderness; no visible stool or blood on glove, stool guaiac negative for occult blood.

Neurologic: Cerebral function: Alert and responsive, memory and orientation intact; appropriate behavior and speech. CN: ii-xii grossly intact. Cerebellar function: finger to nose, heel-toe walk coordination intact; gait normal; Romberg negative. Motor system: No weakness or tremor. Sensory system: Intact to light touch, pin prick; proprioception; vibration sensation.

Reflexes: Normal.

CASE 2

Case J. F.

(Adapted from a case by Elizabeth A. Casey)

Age: 26 years. Race: Caucasian. Nationality: German. Religion: Protestant. Marital status: single, lives with boyfriend and his 4-year-old son. Education: completed high school, one year of college, and secretarial school. Vocation: secretary in computer firm.

Family history: father (57) has 30-year history of depression; mother (54) has history of lupus; three sisters (30, 17, 13) alive and well.

Allergies: dust and pollen, penicillin and cephalosporins.

Past medical history: TMJ (ages 14-17), pelvic inflammatory disease (age 18), endometriosis, laparotomy × 2, laparoscopy × 5 (last three years ago); pneumonia (age 22); bronchitis (age 27); severe allergic reaction to Ceclor (six months ago), treated with three courses of prednisone over a three-month period; headaches.

Medical diagnoses: major depressive episode, seasonal allergic rhinitis.

Current medications: four years ago, J.F. was prescribed Zoloft 50 mg PO 1 tablet every morning for major depression and Seldane (terfenadine) 60 mg PO bid for relief of symptoms related to seasonal allergic rhinitis.

History of present illness: Spring 1990—developed allergies to dust and pollen (mild asthmatic symptoms, sneezing, rhinorrhea, lacrimation, and pruritus); treated with Seldane 60 mg PO bid and Azmacort 1 puff bid P.M. during the spring and summer months. May 1993—sought attention from primary care physician and social worker for clinical depression at the end of an eight-year love relationship (labile emotions, anxiety attacks, insomnia, anorexia with 30-lb weight loss, feelings of hopelessness, no suicidal ideation); treated with Zoloft 50 mg PO q A.M. and Xanax 0.1 mg PO tid. July 1993—BuSpar 10 mg PO tid added to counteract side effects of Zoloft (i.e., hot flashes, insomnia, decreased appetite, tremor); Xanax dosage changed to 0.05 to 0.1 mg PO at hs prn for insomnia.

Present medication regime: Seldane 60 mg PO bid, Zoloft 50 mg PO q A.M., BuSpar 10 mg PO tid, Azmacort 1 puff bid P.M. As doctor recommended, also takes vitamin E 800 mg PO daily, vitamin C 2000 mg PO daily, Stress Tabs 1 tab daily, multivitamin 1 tab daily; no other OTC drugs. Regular primary care visits every three months while on Zoloft and as needed for allergies. Sees social worker bimonthly.

Assessment

Health perception-health management pattern: Strictly adherent to medication regime. Never forgets to take medication. Stores medications in cool, dry place away from heat or direct sunlight and out of reach of children. Takes medications with water and no food. Has exercised in past but not presently due to busy schedule. Hopes to begin exercise program soon. Smokes a half pack of cigarettes per day. Aware of dangers but has no plan to stop anytime soon. Does not drink alcohol due to known precautions with Zoloft and BuSpar. Able to define illness and reasons for medications. Aware of side effects of drugs and reports immediately to physician. Aware of potential dangerous side effects of drugs and interactions and takes precautions. Does not take an OTC drug without consulting doctor.

Nutrition-metabolic pattern: Eats three meals daily with occasional snacks. Diet is high in dairy products (high fat). Eats red meat occasionally; otherwise, prefers chicken. Client is frequently thirsty and drinks 8 to 10 glasses of water per day; 1 cup of caffeinated coffee a day; no tea, and no carbonated beverages. Lost and gained 30 lb in past year. No height loss. Takes vitamins as recommended by physician. Appetite is fair. No food or eating discomfort; no swallowing discomfort. No stomach upset or pain; no nausea or vomiting. No skin lesions. Skin is normal with no excessive sweating. Normal hair distribution with no hair loss or thinning. Tends to bruise easily. Healing capacity is good.

Elimination pattern: Constipation prior to onset of menses (unchanged); otherwise, normal daily bowel elimination. Stool is brown and formed or semiformed. No discomfort with bowel elimination. No increase in flatulence. Does not use laxatives. No problems with micturation. No change in frequency. Urine is pale yellow and clear without odor.

Activity-exercise pattern: Sufficient energy throughout day for required activities. Becomes extremely tired between 8 and 10 P.M. Walks about 1.5 miles to and from work but does not engage in a formal exercise program. No episodes of dizziness or fainting. No complaints of increased sweating. Hobbies include sewing, needlepoint, cooking, decorating, and reading.

Sleep-rest pattern: No problem falling asleep between 10:30 and 11 P.M. but often wakes up in the middle of the night due to vivid dreams with inability to sleep for next two hours. Tries to get seven hours of sleep per night but usually gets only five or six. Infrequently takes Xanax 0.05 mg PO at hs if sleeping pattern poor for several nights. Does not feel tired during the day, which she attributes to taking Zoloft in the morning. Is extremely tired between 8 and 10 P.M. but responsibilities do not allow earlier retirement. Care of 4-year-old prevents rest and relaxation on the weekends.

Cognitive-perceptual pattern: Subjective hearing problem. Client states that voices are muffled in a noisy environment. Needs to be spoken to directly. No problem hearing if no environmental noise. No tinnitus. Auditory tests in past have been reportedly normal. Wears magnifying prescription eyeglasses during work hours for accommodation spasm; otherwise, vision is 20/20 bilaterally. No short-term memory loss. No difficulty learning. Attention span good. No reported episodes of confusion.

Self-perception–self-concept pattern: "I feel good about myself now." "I've done a pretty good job." Client believes she takes good care of herself and is aware of the importance of maintaining her medication regime, seeing her primary physician every three months, and seeing her social worker bimonthly. "If I don't maintain I will slip and I won't ever let myself get to that point again without seeking help." The depression has caused her to think of herself first and therefore take better care of herself. She considers herself worthy of living a happy, healthy, and productive life.

Role-relationship pattern: Lives with boyfriend and his 4-year-old son. Her relationship with her boyfriend is loving and supportive. Her relationship with her boyfriend's son is good. At 4 years of age, the boy requires a lot of the client's love and attention, which she gives willingly. She is very pleased with these relationships. Her family members and friends are supportive. She enjoys socializing with her friends. Her close friends, boyfriend, and family members are aware of her medical diagnoses, the treatment she receives and the potential drug side effects. She enjoys her work at the computer firm and relates well to her employer and co-workers. She is responsible for her boyfriend's son as well as shopping, cooking, and household maintenance.

Sexuality-reproductive pattern: Client is sexually active and has no problems. Menstrual cycle is 28 days and normal with some dysmenorrhea (unchanged). Due to her history of PID and endometriosis her fertility is uncertain. She does not take birth control pills.

Coping–stress tolerance pattern: Client's life has changed dramatically within the past year. An eight-year relationship ended and she is now living with a new boyfriend and his son. As a result of her depression she is more open with her feelings and expresses them more effectively to her friends, family members, boyfriend, and social worker. She believes she could not have made it through her depression without their support. Her attitude towards her diagnoses and treatment is, "It's part of my life; that's the way it is."

Value-belief pattern: Client strongly believes that you should treat others as you would want to be treated. She believes selfishness is healthy if there is no intent to harm another. She believes she is as deserving as the next person. She believes that she has control over her life and both physical and mental well-being. She believes in seeking whatever means necessary for greater well-being. When the odds were against her she pulled through. She feels a sense of personal triumph and newfound strength.

Screening Examination

Blood pressure = 118/68 (nonpostural); pulse = 84 and regular rhythm; respiration rate = 18 and regular rhythm with no abnormal breath sounds; temperature = 98.2; weight = 145 lbs; height = 5 ft, 6 in. Well-groomed and well-dressed. Alert and oriented to person, place, and time. Calm affect with no evidence of nervousness, restlessness, irritability, or tremor. Able to comprehend questions and information. Asks appropriate questions. Maintains eye contact with normal attention span. No evidence of confusion or short-term memory deficits. Speaks English. Normal hair distribution with no hair loss or thinning. Oral mucosa pink and somewhat dry; no lesions; no bleeding. Natural teeth with some recession of gum line.

Hearing is good in quiet environment; no tinnitus. Wears magnifying glasses for work only; no blurred vision. Skin is normal with some bruising on legs but otherwise no lesions or color changes; no excessive sweating. Gait is normal; able to perform ADL without limitations.

CASE 3

Case S. G.

(Adapted from a case by Anne T. Ferguson)

Age: 76 years. Marital status: widowed. Highest grade achieved: unknown. Vocational status: homemaker/retired. Race: white. Religion: Catholic.

Allergies: contrast dye, Demerol.

Medical diagnosis: status post vaginal suspension of the bladder neck; status post suprapubic tube placement.

History of present illness: History of frequent urinary tract infection and urinary incontinence for 15 to 20 years. Attempted to control incontinence with muscle exercises and external devices. Felt incontinence was affecting life activities and was progressively more frequent so presented for surgical intervention one week ago. Sent home from hospital postop with suprapubic tube intact and scheduled bladder training program with visiting nurse assistance. Current *E. coli* UTI being treated with Bactrim DS 1 tab PO bid × 10 days.

Past medical history: Presented to primary care physician three years ago with complaints of frequent indigestion; diagnosed with gastroesophageal reflux disorder and prescribed Zantac 150 mg PO bid. Recently diagnosed with hypertension and was started on Zestril (dose unknown) but secondary to side effect of persistent dry cough medication was changed recently to Calan SR 180 mg PO qd. Hypertension has been well controlled since this medication was started two months ago. Other health problems include history of bronchitis and pneumonia, bilateral cataracts—s/p left eye cataract removal 3 months ago, right breast biopsy × 5 (familial history of breast cancer), status post cholecystectomy, hysterectomy/oophorectomy (secondary to fibroid tumors) in 1967, and appendectomy in 1968.

Current medications: Bactrim DS 1 tab PO bid × 10 days; Zantac 150 mg PO bid; Calan SR 180 mg PO qd; ASA 2 tabs for occasional headache.

Assessment

Health perception–health management pattern: Has good understanding of and maintains current medication regimen. Is a very active citizen and considers herself fairly healthy despite the recent and past surgeries and illnesses. Generally seeks health care when she perceives that an illness is affecting her lifestyle. She is a nonsmoker and rarely drinks alcohol. States she usually takes 2 aspirin tablets for occasional headaches. Is able to understand importance of bladder training program and seems to have a good understanding of proper procedures involved.

Nutrition-metabolic pattern: Eats 3 meals a day. Tries to limit salt, fat, and sugar intake. Drinks a large amount of water and two cups of coffee per day. Weight and height stay unchanged. Appetite is good. No further complaints of indigestion since taking Zantac. No swallowing difficulty. No skin lesions or rashes. Skin is pink, warm, and dry. Suprapubic drain site is clean and without exudate. Bilateral lower abdominal surgical incisions are healing well.

Elimination pattern: Since beginning Calan SR patient has had extreme difficulty with constipation despite taking a stool softener once daily and increasing her fluid intake. Prior to taking Calan she did not have much difficulty with her bowels. Stool is brown and without blood. Bladder training program is going well and patient has begun voiding approx. 30 to 90 mL on her own with suprapubic tube residuals of 150 to 400 mL. Urine is clear yellow in color without sediment or blood. Patient reports no burning or incontinence since the surgery.

Activity-exercise pattern: States she tires easily since surgery but has sufficient energy to perform desired activities. She baby-sits for her grandchildren occasionally, is socially active in her elderly housing community, and states she is constantly on the go—driving, visiting, or shopping.

Sleep-rest pattern: Patient is generally rested and ready for activities after sleep. Patient has no difficulty falling asleep, sleeping, or awakening and uses no aids. Does not require a nap during the day.

Cognitive-perceptual pattern: Patient uses one hearing aid for everyday use and wears glasses for all activities. No memory problems and demonstrates an excellent learning capacity.

Self-perception–self-concept pattern: Patient states, "This doesn't affect me at all, I hardly know it's there—if this surgery works I'll feel a lot better—I can do more things." Patient seems to have had a self-perception impairment and therefore sought surgery and is hoping the surgery will improve her self-perception. The incontinence was affecting her life more than the suprapubic tube.

Role-relationship pattern: Patient has been widowed for three years and is adjusting well. Lives alone in elderly housing. Has two sons, who both live in town. Patient is particularly close with one son, his wife, and two grandchildren—recovered postop at their home before returning to her apartment. This family is very supportive of patient. Patient is independent in driving, shopping, all ADL, and all household maintenance. Patient has close friends in town and visits frequently.

Sexuality-reproductive pattern: Patient states she is not sexually involved. She is a gravida 8 para 2.

Coping–stress tolerance pattern: Patient states, "Not a lot of things bother me—I have a strong support in my son and his family if I need anything."

Value-belief pattern: Patient states that her religion is important to her.

Screening Examination

Pulse 70, regular rhythm and strong. BP 160/80. Respirations 18, deep regular rhythm. Lung sounds clear bilaterally. Temp 98 PO. Height 5 ft 5 in. Weight 148 lbs. Well-kept, clean in appearance. Oral mucous membrane pink and intact. No natural teeth, dentures intact (top and bottom). Alert and oriented × 3 spheres. Speech comprehendable and clear. Normal attention span. Hearing is adequate with use of hearing aid. Wears prescription glasses, no difficulty in reading. All extremities equal and strong muscle strength. No peripheral edema. Skin dry without rash or lesions. Gait is normal. Posture good. Independent in all ADL and household maintenance. Laboratory tests (significant); BUN 19; creatinine 0.8; cholesterol 234; T. Bili 0.2; Alk Phos 135; SGOT 114; WBC 15.4; Hgb/Hct 12.2/37; platelets 304.

CASE 4

Case M. H.

(Adapted from a case by Joyce Barkin)

Age: 48-year-old white female. Marital status: widow. Highest grade achieved: high school graduate. Vocational status: data entry worker for printing company.

Medical diagnoses: interstitial lung disease, essential hypertension, hypothyroidism, Crohn's disease.

History of present illness: One year ago patient first became aware of dyspnea on exertion. SOB occurred after walking up to office on second floor (previously not a problem). Noted lots of paper dust at work, with windows usually closed. Shortly thereafter was laid off. Six months later again aware of similar SOB while doing temporary work at a construction site. Dust and dirt from building materials present. Saw a cardiologist for "palpitations." Spirometry was done which revealed a vital capacity 60 percent of predicted. A diagnosis of asthma was made and Atrovent 2 puffs bid was prescribed. Used Atrovent for two months with no noticeable improvement; stopped on her own. After a complete cardiac and medical evaluation, patient was begun on metoprolol 50 mg with resolution of palpitations. No improvement in dyspnea, has gradually progressed to SOB while walking from bed to bathroom. Was referred to pulmonologist; CXR, lab studies—eosinophil count and pulmonary function tests—confirmed a restrictive defect with a reduced diffusing capacity; diagnosis of interstitial lung disease was made.

Past medical history: Five years ago a diagnosis of essential hypertension, which was well controlled with nonpharmacologic treatment of diet, exercise, weight reduction, limited alcohol. At the same time a diagnosis of hypothyroidism. Replacement therapy initiated with Synthroid 100 μg daily increased from initial dose of 50 μg. Fourteen years ago, diagnosis of Crohn's disease followed by gastroenterologist.

Family history: Mother is alive and healthy, takes medication for hypertension. Father died at age 62; he was a smoker who quit at age 35. His autopsy showed "early emphysema." Two siblings are alive and well, although both have a history of persistent cough. No history of cancer in immediate family.

Allergies: Penicillin "rash."

Current Medications: Synthroid 100 μg daily; metoprolol 50 mg daily; sulfasalazine 3 g daily.

Assessment

Health perception–health management pattern: Patient is discouraged and confused about persistent and increasing SOB; patient does not smoke, never did. She has one or two alcoholic drinks per month. Her exercise regimen of three 30-min walks per week has been discontinued for past 4 months due to increasing DOE. No c/o colds or flu. Denies use of home remedies. Practices self breast exam inconsistently.

Nutrition-metabolic pattern: Follows a low-cholesterol, low-fat diet. Usually eats poultry or fish as source of protein. Most meals are prepared at home. Limits salt intake. Has a high-fiber intake (fruits/vegetables). Admits fluid intake is low, less than 1 L of water per day; drinks two cups of caffeinated coffee in A.M. Total caloric intake is about eighteen hundred calories per day. Appetite is good. Lost 25 lb (intentionally) 6 years ago, works to keep weight WNL. Dentition is good, sees her dentist twice a year. Skin turgor is good. Cholesterol levels are normal. Has had a mammogram in the past year.

Elimination pattern: No urinary problems. Urine is clear; no burning, frequency, or incontinence. Patient is on maintenance bowel therapy. Patient has been in remission for 3 years. However, Crohn's disease is active; patient has diarrhea (5 to 10 episodes per day) and LLQ pain. Does not use laxatives. Has a daily bowel movement, no discomfort, brown soft stool; patient does home guaiac once a month for three consecutive stools.

Activity-exercise pattern: Patient feels she does not have enough energy for exercise beyond her ADL. SOB interferes with activities. Recreation is spent with friends and mother. Has not been working for 4 months. She is able to complete full self-care and appears neat and well-groomed. Patient wants to be able to exercise. Hobbies include sewing and gardening. Lifestyle is becoming more sedentary; watches television a lot.

Sleep-rest pattern: Patient has no difficulty falling asleep; does not use any aids. Often takes a nap during the day; orthopnea not present; does not wake SOB. Sleeps for 8 to 9 h uninterrupted most nights.

Cognitive-perceptual pattern: Patient is near-sighted; sees ophthalmologist every two years; denies problems with hearing, smell, taste, or touch. No memory loss. Language skills are intact. No difficulty with decision making.

Self-perception–self-concept pattern: Patient states, "I am tired of not being able to catch my breath." She is very discouraged over present illness. It has interfered with ability to work and recreate. Patient is usually pleasant, eager to have resolution of current medical problem.

Role-relationship pattern: She feels she has good friends in the area. Her mother and she are very compatible. They live close to each other. She feels she may depend on her mother too much because of her illness. She is close with her siblings and their children. She describes her family as a loving Irish family.

Sexuality-reproductive pattern: Patient is not sexually active. She wishes she had had children. Visits the gynecologist for annual Pap smear. Patient is postmenopausal.

Coping–stress tolerance pattern: Current illness is a source of stress; patient is not sure which way to proceed. Major source of support is her mother.

Value-belief pattern: Patient has a strong Catholic faith; many activities are centered around her church.

Screening Examination

Well-groomed, neat, and clean. Skin is intact without evidence of bruising or discoloration. Mucous membrane is pink and moist. Good dentition. Patient is 5 ft 5 in. and weighs 145 lb. Temperature is 98.0 PO. Wears glasses. No evidence of any optic disc changes. Hearing is good. Sense of smell is intact. Pulse is 80 regular; B/P is 130/84; respirations are 24. She is in mild respiratory distress at rest; there is a frequent nonproductive cough. Nodes WNL; thyroid not enlarged; no evidence of JVD. Chest is clear. No evidence of cyanosis or edema; 2+ clubbing. Gait and posture are normal. Fine motor movements intact. Muscle strength is +3 (out of 4). Maintains eye contact. Oriented to time, person, and place. Reflexes are intact.

CASE 5

Case A. B.

(Adapted from a case by Judith Shindul-Rothschild)

A 53-year-old man is escorted into the emergency room for an evaluation by the police. The patient is cooperative and says he wants help. He is disheveled, has filthy clothes and matted hair, and smells of urine. He is carrying a shopping bag that he says contains all his possessions. The police report that the patient was standing in the middle of a busy intersection screaming that he was the "messiah" and asking motorists to pray for peace.

Although the patient denies any psychiatric history, he speaks fondly of his many "friends" at the state hospital. He refuses to give his name or address, insisting that he is a messenger from God. He constantly taps his feet and has very poor eye contact. His hands are so tremulous he has difficulty holding a cup to take a drink of water. He licks his lips repeatedly throughout the interview. He cannot remember what he did today, but does remember he was born in East Boston. He does acknowledge hearing voices but denies any suicidal or homicidal ideation and refuses to go into any detail about what the voices are saying to him. He complains that his head hurts above his left ear.

When going through the patient's belongings, the clinical specialist finds an old prescription bottle for Haldol that expired two years ago. The patient says he stopped taking those pills because he "couldn't think straight." With further prodding he acknowledges that he used to get "shots" at the clinic from "Betsy the nurse" but couldn't be more specific. He does remember staying at the Pine Street Inn when taken there by the police if it's "really cold outside." He denies any recent alcohol or substance abuse; however he does have slurred speech, blood-shot eyes, and a jaundiced appearance.

Treatment Issues

1. What medical issues would you consider and what laboratory tests would you order?
2. How would you assess for tardive dyskinesia?

CASE 6

Case B. A.

(Adapted from a case by Judith Shindul-Rothschild)

B. A. is a 52-year-old divorced African-American male who owns an auto parts business. His chief complaint is, "I'm having a heart attack." He awoke in the middle of the night, gasping for breath, sweating, shaking, and experiencing pal-pitations. He states that he took his pulse, which was 120. It was his third attack of the week and the tenth that month that had awakened him from sleep. His pre-vious history reveals high blood pressure, diabetes controlled by diet, and migraine headaches. He states that these episodes began 2 years ago, but he's been afraid to come to the hospital because he doesn't want to be told he needs an operation.

Medicine in the ER rules out an MI but keeps B. A. overnight for observation. You see B. A. the next day for evaluation. As you gather more of a history, you learn that these attacks actually started when he was 12 years old, but he could control them with ingestion of beer. The immediate precipitant to these recurrent attacks varied, but they were associated with going to unfamiliar places and being in an enclosed space such as an elevator. B. A. states that only in the past 2 years have the attacks awakened him at night, and he finds that he has to drink more beer to calm himself down than in the past.

When you inquire if there have been any stressful events in his life in the past few years, B. A. adamantly denies any problems. He states that his divorce from his wife was amicable and that he sees his two daughters frequently. His business is booming; in fact he was recently awarded a large government contract to pro-vide auto parts for military bases throughout the United States. When you inquire if the additional travel has presented any problems for B. A., his mood suddenly shifts and his voice becomes tremulous and he begins to visibly perspire.

As you inquire more about B. A.'s drinking, you find that when he anticipates he will have an "episode" he can consume upwards of three six-packs of beer. He states that maybe he is an alcoholic, but if he didn't drink, he wouldn't be able to function at all. B. A.'s weekly consumption of beer varies widely depending upon how "jittery" he feels.

Treatment Issues

1. What are the co-morbid factors you would need to consider before making the diagnosis of panic disorder?
2. How would you combine psychopharmacy and cognitive-behavioral approaches?
3. What are the multicultural factors you should consider when planning B. A.'s care?

CASE 7

Case J. W.

(Adapted from a case by Debra Swerda)

Age: 24.

Allergies: no known allergies.

Reason for visit: Client here for "a Pap and to get a prescription for birth control pills."

Past illnesses/hospitalizations: Medical: had chickenpox and the mumps as a child. Surgical: wisdom teeth extraction in 1987; 3 stitches in right pinky finger from a cut in 1972.

Assessment

Health perception-health maintenance pattern: Client views her health as "very good." "I have never really been sick. I don't even really get colds or the flu very often." Client does not smoke and denies use of recreational drugs. Occasional glass of wine when out for dinner or out with friends. Client presently not on any prescribed medications. Takes Tylenol occasionally and takes ibuprofen for menstrual cramps. Does monthly SBE; uses seatbelts. No family history of cancer.

Nutrition-metabolic pattern: Client states her appetite is "very good." "I could eat all the time. My friends call me the garbage can because I can always finish what they can't eat." Sample diet related: client eats a well-balanced diet from all four food groups; does not take vitamins. Good fluid intake; good calcium intake. Client is responsible for her own meal preparation and states that she is very conscientious about her diet. Weight is stable. No family history of diabetes mellitus.

Elimination pattern: Regular bowel movement daily; no c/o constipation or diarrhea; does not use or require laxatives. Has no difficulties with voiding; no history of UTI.

Activity-exercise pattern: Client states she is "very conscientious about my diet and exercise." Client runs 1 to 2 miles, 3 to 4 times a week. Also does aerobic exercises and plays racquetball and tennis. Recreational activities include going to the movies, going out with friends, and reading. Client tolerates all activities well with no physical limitations or difficulties. Client is very well informed and educated about her diagnosis. Client states her family history is negative for heart disease or hypertension.

Sleep-rest pattern: Averages about 7 to 8 h of sleep per night. Sleeps in own room; denies difficulty with sleeping, falling asleep, or staying asleep. "I'm a sound sleeper. I'm out like a log and sleep all night." Presleep activities include a warm bath or shower and watching TV or reading. Perception of rest upon waking is "good." Does not require rest periods during the day.

Cognitive-perceptual pattern: Client is alert and oriented × 3 spheres. States has 20/20 vision; no changes in sight, hearing, taste, or smell. No changes in or difficulty with memory. No change in sensory integrity; does not get headaches or have difficulty with sense of balance. Able to articulate well; affect appropriate.

Self-perception–self-concept pattern: Client appears relaxed, comfortable, and very honest and open during examination. States, "I take good care of myself and my body and I feel good about myself. Things are going very well in my life. I have no complaints or concerns."

Role-relationship pattern: Presently involved in a steady relationship with a boyfriend she has been seeing for the past six months. Feels good about the relationship. Client has just recently started a new job, which she states is going very well and she is very happy with. States that most of her family lives in Florida, but that she is very close to both her parents and her two brothers. States she talks to them at least once a week and that she has a very close relationship with her mother. One of her brothers lives nearby and client sees him often.

Sexuality-reproductive pattern: Gravida 0 para 0. Onset of menses at age 12 to 13 years; regular periods every 28 to 32 days; flow 3 to 4 days; last menstrual period one month ago. States she usually has mild cramping day 1 and 2 of onset of period, which is relieved with ibuprofen. Has just become sexually active in the last 3 weeks with present steady boyfriend of six months. Has had sexual intercourse twice and they have used condoms. Would like to have a Pap and obtain birth control pills today. Last gynecologic exam and Pap smear were done two years ago and they were negative. States history of STD is negative.

Coping–stress tolerance pattern: Client states she does not really have any difficulty coping with stress or problems. States, "I don't usually feel very stressed or get upset. Things are going well in my life and I'm quite happy." Client exercises regularly and states that exercise makes her feel good and helps relieve any stress or tension that she may be feeling.

Value-belief pattern: Client is Catholic. "We always attended church regularly, but I don't always go to church every Sunday now." States she feels she has a strong faith and belief in God.

Review of Systems

General: J. W. views her health as "very good." Has not had any major illnesses.

Integument: Fair complexion; no eruptions or rashes of the skin; no disorders of the hair or nails.

Head: No c/o headaches; no history of trauma.

Eyes: Normal vision. 20/20; no diplopia or other visual disturbances; last eye examination one year ago.

Ears: Normal hearing; no tinnitus; no infections; occasional cerumen.

Nose: No epistaxis, discharge, or sinusitis.

Mouth, gums, and teeth: Teeth in good repair; visits dentist twice a year; last dental examination and teeth cleaning 3 months ago; no major problems.

Throat and neck: Very infrequent sore throat; no neck stiffness or pain; no hoarseness.

Breasts: No masses, discharge, or bleeding.

Resp: No SOB, dyspnea, cough, or wheeze; has infrequent colds, maybe one a year; no therapy other than Tylenol.

CV: No chest pain, palpitation, hypertension, or vascular disease. No family history of heart disease or hypertension.

GI: Appetite very good; one BM every day; no melena; no jaundice or ulcers; no nausea.

GU: No dysuria, hematuria, nocturia, UTI, or STD.

GYN: Gravida 0 para 0. Onset of menses age 12 to 13; regular periods every 28 to 32 days; flow 3 to 4 days; last menstrual period one month ago; has mild cramping day 1 and 2 of onset of period, relieved with ibuprofen. Became sexually active 3 weeks ago. Last Pap 2 years ago; negative. No history of UTI or STD.

Musc: No muscle weakness, joint pains, or cramps.

NP: No syncope, vertigo, or dizziness; intelligent and well-oriented in 3 spheres; sensorium intact; no paresthesias; pleasant, cheerful, and cooperative affect; appropriate mood; no apparent depression.

Lymph-hemat: No adenopathy; no bleeding disorders.

Endocrine: Tolerates heat and cold; no glycosuria, polydipsia, or excessive sweating.

Physical Examination

VS: T 98.7 P 68 R 16 BP 110/70 HT 5 ft 9 in. WT 152 lb.

General: J. W. is an alert, well-developed 23-year-old woman appearing about stated age; in no acute distress.

Skin: Fair complexion, good turgor; warm; no excoriations or lesions.

Hair: Normal distribution and consistency.

Nails: No deformities; nailbeds pink with good capillary refill; no clubbing.

Head: Symmetrical; normocephalic; normal hair distribution.

Face: No muscle weakness; appropriate facial expression.

Eyes: External eye structures symmetrical, without lesions; lashes and brows present; lacrimal apparatus nontender to palpitation, no excessive tearing; conjunctivae moist and clear; lens clear; sclera white; no defects of cornea or iris; PERRLA; can read newsprint 12 in. away; EOM normal; no nystagmus or strabismus. Fundi red reflex-clear, no fundal lesions; discs round, flat, cup normal; AV ratio normal, no AV nicking; retina has no hemorrhage or exudates; macula normal.

Ears: No masses or lesions of auricles or canals; tragus and auricle nontender to palpitation; no discharge; both TM pearly grey, shiny, no perforations; light reflex intact and landmarks discernible; able to identify whispered voice; Weber test normal with no lateralization; Rinne positive AC>BC.

Nose: Nostrils patent bilaterally; no masses or tenderness; no septal deviation or perforations; mucosa pink and intact; no rhinitis at present.

Mouth: Mucosa and gingivae pink; tongue moist and shiny, and midline without tremor during protrusion and movement; no lesions seen or palpated on oral mucosa, tongue, or palate; can clench teeth. Teeth in good repair.

Pharynx: Mucosa pink, no lesions; tonsils present; gag reflex intact; uvula and soft palate rise in midline with phonation "ah."

Neck: Full normal ROM and strength; no vein distention; carotid pulses equal and of good quality, no bruits; trachea in midline; thyroid not palpable, no bruits; no lymphadenopathy.

Thorax: Chest movements symmetrical, full expansion equal bilaterally; AP to lateral diameter 1:2; no tenderness; no visible masses; no adenopathy.

Lungs: Fremitus equal bilaterally; lung fields clear and resonant throughout; breath sounds clear; vocal sounds normal; no rales, rhonchi, or rubs.

Breasts: Symmetrical; no dimpling or edema; no changes in breast shape with movement; no nipple retraction or discharge; no tenderness, palpable masses, or nodules on examination.

Heart: No visible heaves or retractions on anterior chest; no heaves, thrills or rib retraction with palpation; PMI palpable at left 5th ICS; regular rhythm, rate 68 beats/minute; normal S1 and S2; no extra heart sounds, murmurs, gallops, or rubs.

Abdomen: Abdomen flat, with well-developed musculature; skin intact without lesions; no visible masses, pulsations, or hernias; normal bowel sounds in all four quadrants, no bruits; nontender to light and deep palpation; no masses; liver, spleen, and kidneys not palpable.

Back: Normal ROM; no spinal tenderness; no CVA tenderness.

Extremities: No skin, hair, or nail abnormalities; no venous dilation; radial, brachial, femoral, popliteal, posterior tibial, and dorsalis pedis pulses all palpable and equal; no masses or tenderness; no lymphadenopathy; fingers and toes dry and warm to touch; normal gait; full ROM; muscle strength intact; Romberg negative.

Genitalia: External: Normal pubic hair, no labial swellings or lesions, normal clitoris; introitus admits two fingers; no urethral redness, swelling, or discharge; Skene's and Bartholin's glands not inflamed; perineum clean and intact; no scars. Internal: Vagina: mucosa intact, moist, and pink; no bulging or masses. Uterus: anteverted, midline; average size, regular shape, mobile, normal consistency. Cervix: nonparous cervical os, pink and midline. Adenexa: tubes not palpated, ovaries not enlarged, slight tenderness. Cul-de-sac: no palpable cystocele or rectocele; no bulging, tenderness, or masses. Discharge: slight, clear discharge; no odor. Pap: Cervical scraping with cytobrush, endocervical swab, and vaginal pool swab performed and slides sent to the lab.

Rectal: Declined by client.

Neurologic: Cerebral function: alert and responsive, memory and orientation intact; appropriate behavior and speech. CN: i-xii grossly intact. Cerebellar function: finger-to-nose, heel-to-shin coordination intact; gait normal; Romberg negative. Motor system: no atrophy, weakness, or tremor. Sensory system: intact to light touch, pin prick; proprioception; and vibration sensation.

Reflexes: normal

1. What are the patient variables (present or absent) that are important in deciding if this patient should be prescribed oral contraceptives?
2. What further lab tests are indicated?

CASE 8

Case D. W.

(Adapted from a case by Kathleen B. O'Donnell)

Age: 42. Marital status: Married. Children: ages 10 and 12. Education: college degree.

Employment: salesman (recent promotion to district manager).

Present medical history: hypertension; hypercholesterolemia; sinusitis (amoxicillin-resistant).

Childhood illnesses: chickenpox; strep throat; asthma.

Allergies: NKDA.

Current medications: Mevacor 20 mg PO qd; Captopril 12.5 mg PO bid; Advil 200 to 400 mg PO prn.

History of present illness: Pleasant 42-year-old white male presents with 2-week history of sinus pressure, postnasal drip, slight sore throat especially at night, mild cough, fever, and green mucus from nose. Denies any ear pain. Had similar episode last year that did not respond to amoxicillin or Biaxin. Did have an excellent response to Ceftin.

Assessment

Health perception-health management pattern: Patient had not had a general physical exam in years and finally went after the persistent encouragement from his wife and since his brother had recently been diagnosed with hypertension (HTN). PE revealed that patient had HTN and elevated cholesterol. Was followed for three months with his BP without a change despite a modification in patient's lifestyle habits. Patient was started on HCTZ with a minimal response (for 6 weeks). Was then switched to Captopril 12.5 mg PO bid with a better response. D. W.'s cholesterol was followed for about one year without a response, despite a low-fat diet. Patient was also being followed by a dietician at this time. Was started on Lopid 600 mg PO bid without response after a 6-week check. Was then started on Mevacor 20 mg PO qd with a good response. Patient views his health as not as good as it used to be but feels that by going to the doctor and by changing his lifestyle habits will improve his health. States that he feels a lot of pressure to achieve, especially with his children approaching their teen years and eventually college years. Wears a seat belt. Immunizations are up to date; last tetanus two years ago. Has started walking on the weekends. Has recently been promoted at work and feels like he is under a lot of pressure. Finds it hard to "live healthy" when he's so busy at work. Quit smoking one year ago; smoked 1 to 2 packs a day for 20 years. Drinks 1 glass of wine or beer 4 or 5 times a week (has cut down; did drink every day). Patient denies the use of OTC cold medications. Does use Advil on a prn basis.

Nutrition-metabolic pattern: Patient is overweight. Tends to eat on the run or eat out a lot with his clients. Has increased his water intake to 6 glasses a day. Drinks 3 to 4 cups of coffee a day. Visits a dentist every year. Has been following a low-fat diet but tends to "sneak" donuts. Has reported a decreased appetite with his recent sinus infection.

Elimination pattern: Denies any problems with voiding. Denies an interrupted stream. Denies any constipation. Does not use laxatives. Notices a slight decrease in urinary output since he stopped taking the HCTZ.

Activity-exercise pattern: Patient denies any SOB, chest pain, or feelings of fatigue when not sick. Has tried to increase exercise by walking with his wife and by taking the stairs when at work. States it's hard to exercise due to the winter season and due to his busy work schedule. Recreational activities include watching his sons play sports and watching football.

Sleep-rest pattern: Patient reports that he normally gets a good night of sleep and that he generally feels well-rested. Has not been able to sleep over the past few days due to his sinus pain and due to his nagging cough. Usually sleeps 7 h a night. Does not use a sleeping medication.

Cognitive-perceptual pattern: Patient denies any deficits in hearing, vision, taste, or smell. Does not wear glasses. No changes in his memory and is able to make decisions easily. Learns best through reading. Denies any sensory changes. Patient monitors his blood pressure at home.

Self-perception–self-concept pattern: Patient is pleasant, somewhat tense, with a sense of humor. Generally feels good and is looking to improve his health. Feels in control of his life. Does not like to get sick and wishes he had gone to the doctor for his sinus infection sooner.

Role-relationship pattern: Has been married for 15 years. Would like to spend more time with his wife. Has a good relationship with his sons. Gets along with co-workers. Has recently been promoted. Has been with his company for 20 years. Does report concern about his BP and cholesterol because he wants to see his children grow up.

Sexuality-reproductive pattern: Has a monogamous relationship. Has had decreased sexual activity due to his sinus infection. Does not report any difficulty in maintaining an erection. Does not perform testicular exams. Uses condoms for birth control.

Coping-stress tolerance pattern: Patient can usually cope with stress. Does feel tense at times. Can talk things over with his wife. Listens to the radio and watches comedies when tense.

Value-belief pattern: Patient states that he gets what he wants out of life. Practicing Catholic. Values his family, religion, and health.

Screening Examination

General: A & O × 3. Appropriate behavior. Slightly overweight, good hygiene.

VS: T 99.6, NSR 80, BP 135/82 HT 5 ft 10 in. WT 195 lb (has lost 15 lb over past year).

Skin: No rashes or lesions; good turgor.

Hair: Well-groomed. Normal distribution.

Head: Symmetrical.

Sinus: Frontal and maxillary tenderness. Not able to transilluminate sinuses.

Eyes: Conjunctivae injected, no exudates.

Ears: TM nl; canals nl.

O/P: Erythematous, no exudate.

Nose: Erythematous, inflamed turbinates. Green mucus.

Nodes: nl.

Lungs: Inspiratory wheezes noted about base of lungs.

Breasts: Symmetrical.

Heart: Apical HR 72 NSR S2>S1 aortic and pulmonic S1>S2 apex area.

ABD: Soft, nontender, B.S. in 4 quads.

Back: nl curvature, full ROM.

Extremities: 2+ pulses bilateral and about radial, brachial, femoral, popliteal, posterior tibialis, dorsalis pedialis. Normal ROM.

Strength grade 5 bilat. No joint tenderness. Sensorium intact, proprioception intact. Vibration sensation intact. Normal gait. Romberg negative. Phalan's absent.

Testes: Deferred.

Rectal: Deferred.

Neuro: CN i-xii grossly intact.

Reflexes: nl. Babinski's absent.

CASE 9

Case B: Sr. Mary Mary

(Adapted from a case by Debra Swerda)

Age: 74; female

Allergies: aspirin and aspirin-containing products; they cause severe GI irritation.

Reason for visit: "I have been feeling miserable for about one month now. I had a cold and the flu about one month ago and I just haven't felt well since." Client had strep throat at that time and was treated with a course of Penicillin VK. "My throat has been very sore again for the past 5 days and now my nose is running and I had a temperature of 100 yesterday." Client also c/o chills and feeling warm for the past 3 days.

Past illnesses/hospitalizations: Medical: hypertension; high cholesterol; arthritis in right knee.

Surgical: tonsillectomy as a child; hysterectomy May 1990 for abnormal post-menopausal bleeding.

Assessment

Heath perception–health maintenance pattern: Client states that her health has always been "very good." "It's just this last month. I can't seem to get rid of this cold." Client has a history of hypertension and is on Lopressor 50 mg bid. Presently on no other prescription medications; takes Tylenol occasionally, but no other OTC medications. Client denies smoking, alcohol use. Client does do monthly SBE.

Nutrition-metabolic pattern: Client has high cholesterol; last cholesterol level 3 months ago was 220 mg/dL. Sample diet related: good intake of foods from all four food groups; client presently on a low-cholesterol, low-fat diet. States she is compliant with the diet and has also lost 10 lb over the past 3 months while on the prescribed diet. Client takes one multivitamin a day. Client is responsible for the preparation of her own food and does not add salt to preparation of food. Has hypertension which is well-controlled on medication and with diet. Good fluid and calcium intake; drinks at least 8 to 10 glasses of fluid per day. States appetite is "good." Other than intentional weight loss, no fluctuations in weight.

Elimination pattern: Daily bowel movement pattern with no c/o constipation; does not use laxatives. Client states she drinks plenty of fluids and watches her diet so as not to have any problems with constipation. States occasionally has nocturia, but associates this to the fact that she drinks a lot of fluids and has increased her fluid intake due to her cold. No c/o dysuria, hematuria, or frequency.

Activity-exercise pattern: Client walks about one mile a day for exercise; does not participate in any other regular forms of exercise. States, "I'm too old to be jumping around exercising." Has arthritis in right knee that has not limited or affected client's physical abilities. Client does not require or take medication for the arthritis. Recreational activities include being involved with many organizations and groups with the church; client also volunteers full time to teach people English as a second language. States she finds prayer, meditation, and reading relaxing; enjoys these activities daily.

Sleep-rest pattern: Client states she averages about 8 hours of sleep a night. Sleeps in own room. Awakens 1 or 2 times at night to void; no difficulty getting back to sleep or sleeping otherwise. Presleep activities include nightly reading and prayer. Perception of rest upon waking is "good." Client does not require rest or nap periods during the day.

Cognitive-perceptual pattern: Client is alert and oriented × 3 spheres. Client is nearsighted and wears corrective glasses; last eye examination 4 months ago; no other visual disturbances or problems. No changes in sight, hearing, taste, or smell. No perceived changes or difficulty with memory. No changes in sensory integrity; does not get headaches or have difficulty with sense of balance.

Self-perception–self-concept pattern: Client appears relaxed, comfortable, and very pleasant and talkative during examination. Sister states that she enjoys her life and is especially enjoying the volunteer work that she does now. States she has "a good life with wonderful family and friends."

Role-relationship pattern: Client is a Sister. States she "enjoys her life serving the people of the church and community." "I have always been happy with my decision to join the sisterhood and I have never had any regrets." Client is a retired schoolteacher who now does volunteer work full time. Client states she has a wonderful and supportive family and many friends.

Sexuality-reproductive pattern: Sister has never married and leads a celibate life. Had a hysterectomy one year ago for abnormal menopausal bleeding; has not had any further problems since the surgery.

Coping–stress-tolerance pattern: Client states, "I think I cope with life and problems very well. I have always had a lot of support from family, friends, and very importantly from God." Client states she finds consolation for her problems with meditation and prayer.

Value-belief pattern: Client has devoted her life to the Catholic church and considers herself "very religious." "I have a strong faith in God and the church." Client is involved with many religious activities and prays daily.

Review of Systems

General: Sr. M. M. considers her health has "always been very good, except for the last month or so. I just can't seem to get rid of this cold or flu." Has never had any serious illnesses; no major weight changes.

Integument: Fair complexion; no eruptions or rashes of the skin; no disorders of the hair or nails.

Head: No c/o headaches; no history of trauma.

Eyes: Has myopia; wears corrective glasses; no diplopia or other visual disturbances; last eye examination four months ago.

Ears: Normal hearing; no tinnitus; no infections; occasional cerumen.

Nose: No epistaxis, discharge, or sinusitis.

Mouth, gums, and teeth: Wears upper and lower dentures; new dentures one year ago; no major problems.

Throat and neck: Has been having sore throats for the past month; had strep throat one month ago, treated with penicillin VK; no neck stiffness or pain; no hoarseness.

Breasts: No masses, discharge, or bleeding.

Resp: No SOB, dyspnea, cough, or wheeze; has colds about 1 or 2 times a year; this year a viral infection has persisted, no other therapy other than Tylenol and fluids; takes one multivitamin a day.

CV: No chest pain, palpitation; has hypertension, on Lopressor 50 mg bid; has hypercholesterolemia; no other vascular problems.

GI: Appetite good; one BM every day; no melena; no jaundice or ulcers; no nausea.

GU: No dysuria, hematuria; occasional nocturia, 1 or 2 times a night.

GYN: Gravida 0 para 0; client had a complete hysterectomy May 1990 for abnormal post-menopausal bleeding; last gynecologic exam about 8 months ago.

Musc: No muscle weakness; has arthritis in right knee—no physical limitations, does not require medications.

NP: No syncope, vertigo, dizziness; intelligent and well-oriented in 3 spheres; sensorium intact; no paresthesias; pleasant, cheerful, and cooperative affect; appropriate mood; no apparent depression.

Lymph-hemat: No adenopathy; no bleeding disorders.

Endocrine: Prefers the temperature to be warm, but is tolerant of heat and cold; no glycosuria, polydipsia, or excessive sweating.

Physical Examination

VS: T 99.7 P 88 R 18 BP 140/68 HT 5 ft 3 in. WT 150 lb.

General: Sr. M. M. is an alert, 72-year-old woman appearing about stated age; in no acute distress.

Skin: Fair complexion, good turgor; warm; no excoriations or lesions; has a well-healed scar on abdomen from hysterectomy one year ago.

Hair: Normal distribution and consistency.

Nails: No deformities; nail beds pink with good capillary refill; no clubbing.

Head: Symmetrical; normocephalic; normal hair distribution.

Face: No muscle weakness; appropriate facial expression.

Eyes: External eye structures symmetrical, without lesions; lashes and brows present; lacrimal apparatus nontender to palpitation, no excessive tearing; conjunctivae moist and clear; lens clear; sclera white; no defects of cornea or iris; PERRLA; can read newsprint 12 in. away with corrective glasses; EOM normal; no nystagmus or strabismus. Fundi: Red reflex—clear, no fundal lesions; Discs round, flat, cup normal; AV ratio normal, no AV nicking; Retina—no hemorrhage or exudates; macula normal.

Ears: No masses or lesions of auricles or canals; tragus and auricle nontender to palpitation; no discharge; both TM pearly grey, shiny, no perforations; light reflex intact and landmarks discernible; able to identify whispered voice; Weber test normal with no lateralization; Rinne positive AC>BC.

Nose: Nostrils patent bilaterally; no masses or tenderness; no septal deviation or perforations; mucosa pink and intact; no rhinitis at present.

Mouth: Mucosa and gingivae pink; tongue moist and shiny and midline without tremor during protrusion and movement; no lesions seen or palpated on oral mucosa, tongue, or palate; can clench teeth. Dentures in good repair.

Pharynx: Mucosa slightly reddened, no exudate, no lesions; tonsils absent; gag reflex intact; uvula and soft palate rise in midline with phonation "ah."

Neck: Full normal ROM and strength; no vein distention; carotid pulses equal and of good quality, no bruits; trachea in midline; thyroid not palpable, no bruits; no lymphadenopathy.

Thorax: Chest movements symmetrical, full expansion equal bilaterally; AP to lateral diameter 1:2; no tenderness; no visible masses; no adenopathy.

Lungs: Fremitus equal bilaterally; lung fields clear and resonant throughout; breath sounds clear; vocal sounds normal; no rales, rhonchi, or rubs.

Breasts: Symmetrical; no dimpling or edema; no changes in breast shape with movement; no nipple retraction or discharge; no tenderness or palpable masses or nodules on examination.

Heart: No visible heaves or retractions on anterior chest; no heaves, thrills, or rib retraction with palpation; PMI palpable at left 5th ICS; regular rhythm, rate 88 beats per min; normal S1 and S2; no extra heart sounds, murmurs, gallops, or rubs.

Abdomen: Abdomen soft and slightly obese; no visible masses, pulsations, or hernias; skin intact without lesions, well-healed scar on abdomen from hysterectomy; normal bowel sounds in all 4 quadrants, no bruits; nontender to light and deep palpation; no masses; liver, spleen, and kidneys not palpable.

Back: Normal curvature; normal ROM; no spinal tenderness; no CVA tenderness.

Extremities: No skin, hair, or nail abnormalities; no venous dilation; radial, brachial, femoral, popliteal, posterior tibial, and dorsalis pedis pulses all palpable and equal; no masses or tenderness; no lymphadenopathy; fingers and toes dry and warm to touch; normal gait; full ROM; muscle strength intact; Romberg negative.

Genitalia: Declined by client—client will be seeing gynecologist in 2 months for exam.

Rectal: Declined by client.

Neurologic: Cerebral function: alert and responsive, memory and orientation intact; appropriate behavior and speech. CN: i-xii grossly intact. Cerebellar function: finger-to-nose, heel-to-shin coordination intact; gait normal; Romberg negative. Motor system: no atrophy, weakness, or tremor. Sensory system: intact to light touch, pin prick; proprioception and vibration sensation.

Reflexes: Normal.

CASE 10

Case Mrs. M.

(Adapted from a case by Cecilia M. Mullen)

Mrs. M. is a 60-year-old woman. She lives with her husband in their own suburban home. She has three grown children, two of whom live in nearby towns and one on the West Coast. She has four grandchildren. She is a retired seamstress; highest grade level is high school graduate. She uses a private physician for check-ups and drug-level monitoring but is also seen in an outpatient rehab clinic. Medical diagnosis: seizures, s/p right PCA CVA (six months ago).

Medical history: Longstanding history of COPD, on Theodur 400 mg PO qd and Atrovent 2 puffs qid. 1991—epiglottal Ca, s/p radiation therapy with no recurrence by CT scan. One year ago c/o SOB, left side numbness and admitted to hospital. Dx: CVA, or unknown etiology, no hx of HTN. Placed on Coumadin 5 mg PO qd. Cardiac work-up revealed mild LV dysfunction, no critical CAD, no A fib. Two weeks later, while still in the hospital, patient experienced a grand mal seizure and was placed on Dilantin 300 mg PO qd. Patient was discharged to home several weeks later with outpatient physical and occupational therapy for residual left side weakness. Six months later Coumadin therapy was lowered to alternate 5 mg with 2.5 mg every other day. Two weeks ago patient experienced headache and nausea while on vacation. Was seen by a local doctor, who obtained medical history from patient's physician. Dilantin was decreased to 200 mg qd based on "toxic side effects from Dilantin," according to patient, and was told to see primary physician in a few weeks. Currently patient c/o headache, right frontotemporal location, and neighbor noted left head turning with gaze preference. EMTs were called, and upon arrival, patient experienced a grand mal seizure. Dilantin level = 3.4 (normal 10 to 20). Theodur level = 10.8 (normal 10 to 20). PT = 15.5 (1-1/2 times control). Patient was loaded with Dilantin and Valium in the ER and Dilantin dose was increased to 300 mg qd. Head CT scan showed no new infarct or changes. After admission to ICU and then to neurology unit for neurologic and drug-level monitoring, patient was discharged to home with follow-up in the neurology clinic in three to four weeks.

Drug Therapy: Present medications: Theo-Dur 400 mg PO qd; Atrovent 2 puffs qid; Coumadin 5 mg alternating with 2.5 mg PO qd; Dilantin 300 mg PO qd.

Assessment

Health perception–health management pattern: Patient maintains medication regimen and seeks medical treatment to maintain health. An example of this is seeing a doctor while on vacation for symptoms she felt uncomfortable with. She keeps her appointments with primary physician and does not seek out multiple doctors for multiple opinions. She quit smoking when confronted with lung disease, which shows a willingness to manage own health. She understands the continued need for medication administration even when feeling well. She maintains her physical and occupational therapy appointments to increase her strength. She desires to regain some of the mobility lost when she experienced her CVA.

Nutritional-metabolic pattern: Gums appear intact, no abscesses apparent. Patient eats a well-balanced diet, but must sit upright while eating to prevent choking secondary to epiglottal relaxation due to radiation therapy and partial facial weakness. Husband is primary food preparer, but patient assists. Neighbors and relatives help with food shopping. Patient does not usually experience nausea or vomiting, diarrhea, or anorexia but does seek medical advice when these occur. Fluid intake includes juice and water with meals, 1 to 2 cups of tea a day. No skin lesions or discolorations. No alopecia noted. No cuts or bruises noted, although skin color is dark and light bruises may not be noticeable. Hct normal.

Elimination pattern: Daily bowel movements. Stool guaiac negative. No hemorrhoids. Urine clear, heme negative. No urinary incontinence. Bathroom is on same floor as living space so is easily accessible to patient despite her impaired mobility.

Activity-exercise pattern: Patient states she feels more fatigued since her CVA. She is left with weakness of the left arm preventing patient from sewing, which was a much enjoyed hobby of hers. She verbalizes her displeasure of the limitation and hopes to regain enough strength to allow her to complete some small sewing projects. She has slight weakness of lower left extremity, but patient walks without the assistance of a cane or device without difficulty. Her activity is limited more by her COPD. She becomes SOB with exertion and must take frequent rest periods. The use of Atrovent inhalant helps to alleviate SOB associated with activity. She is able to vacation with husband and friends and is a regular at church socials. She does not drive a car; her husband and friends are available for her needs.

Sleep-rest pattern: Patient states she needs naps during the day and sleeps intermittently at night. Total sleep time is about 8 h per day. Perhaps relaxation periods should be encouraged rather than naps to promote night sleep. No sleeping aids are used.

Cognitive-perceptual pattern: No hearing difficulties. Wears reading glasses. Denies blurred vision. Although patient is not highly educated, she has a basic understanding of her medical diagnosis, her medications, and the changes that have recently occurred in her life. She verbalizes her concerns well. Her husband, although not formally educated, has a basic understanding of the relationships of her medications. He knew that "when she takes all these different medicines, if you change one then that's going to change the others—no one told me, I just figured."

Self-perception–self-concept pattern: Patient views herself much differently since the stroke. She is depressed frequently and "feeling sorry for myself." She seeks out the comfort of friends and the church to help lift her spirits. She feels she contributes less to her marriage than she used to and that sometimes she is a burden to her husband and friends. She has seen a psychiatrist intermittently to talk with him and that has helped her to understand her feelings and that this is normal following a stroke. She appears to be in the process of coming to terms with her illness, and she needs support and positive feedback from health care providers.

Role-relationship pattern: Patient is very close to her husband and three children. Patient depends on husband for driving, shopping, household maintenance, and medication administration. Husband is in good health. Two children also help with those duties although they are grown with their own families. Patient has many friends whom she is close to and who help her out in many ways, both emotionally and physically. Mrs. M. continues to be actively involved in social activities with husband and friends at the church.

Sexuality-reproductive pattern: Patient appears to be uncomfortable with the subject of sexuality. When asked if she continues to be intimate with her husband, she simply states, "We are close."

Coping–stress tolerance pattern: Patient is notably distressed by the changes in her life over the past six months. She has experienced a debilitating illness, she had to quit her job and her hobby, she is dependent on others, and she suddenly finds herself taking medications throughout the day. Patient states that even cancer did not change or disrupt her life like this stroke has. She is coping well at the present time by following prescribed regimes and seeking the support of those close to her.

Value-belief pattern: Mrs. M. strongly values religion as essential to coping with her illness. She prays frequently to God for strength and finds comfort in the church and those associated with her church. Her social life revolves around the church and the people who belong to it. It has been part of her life since birth and is a source of strength to her.

Screening Examination

Alert and oriented, cooperative with assessment. Direct eye contact present. Appears neat and clean, slightly anxious throughout interview and examination. Very talkative. Oral mucosa and gums intact, no lesions. No dentures or missing teeth. Slight left facial weakness and drooping. Swallow response intact without aspiration noted. Left hemiparesis. Left arm with moderate gross motor strength and weak fine motor skills. Patient performs activities with right hand; needs increased concentration with use of left hand. Not able to pick up small objects with left hand. Left leg with moderate strength. DTR hyperreflexic on left. Gait is slow but steady; no ataxia.

Functional ability is independent for toileting and bathing. Needs assistance with dressing for zippers and tying. Needs assistance with home maintenance, shopping. Ambulates independently but likes to have someone nearby "in case I need them."

Breath sounds are diminished throughout; no crackles. RR 24, possibly baseline or due to anxiety or talking. No cough. O_2 sat 96% on room air. HR 92 without ectopy. BP 140/70. Abdomen soft. No c/o N/V, positive bowel sounds, stool guaiac negative. No bruising or rash noted; skin intact. Appetite fair. Afebrile. Weight 54 kg; Height 5 ft 3 in.

CASE 11

Case B. V.

(Adapted from case by L. Delaney)

Age: 78. Sex: male. Marital status: married. Religion: Jewish.

Education: High school equivalent. Work history: Retired clerical worker.

Current physicians: internist, urologist.

Allergies: None known.

Medical diagnoses: IDDM, HTN, gout, chronic renal insufficiency, congenital deafness, new CHF.

History of present illness: Was readmitted to VNA upon referral from internist after prescription of Lasix 40 mg PO qd for peripheral edema 3+ to 4+ with significant weight gain. This is fourth referral since beginning insulin therapy 9 years ago. Most admissions have been related to his diabetes management and compliance.

Current medications: Captopril 25 mg PO bid; allopurinol 300 mg PO qd; Mylanta 30 cc PO prn; Lasix 40 mg PO qd; Humulin 70/30 80 U SC every A.M.

Assessment

Health perception–health management pattern: B. V. reports feeling that his health is deteriorating. Seems to feel powerless in his ability to control his diabetes. Shrugs off most questions, comments, or suggestions. Overwhelmed by multiple health problems. Has always been dependent on family for contact with outsiders. Lets wife answer most questions. Wears Medic Alert bracelet.

Nutritional-metabolic pattern: Wife reports following 1800-calorie ADA meal plans at home; states, "I can't control what he eats outside." (Patient shrugs.) Weight 193 lb. Ten-pound weight loss reported since starting Lasix 2 weeks ago. Random BS 360 (patient shrugs). Patient generally has had at least one concentrated sweet food item per day; seems to view each item as "just this once." Takes Lasix with OJ. Adequate potassium intake; fair roughage intake; good fluid intake. FBS around 200.

Elimination pattern: Reports daily BM, formed, soft, dark brown. Denies constipation, diarrhea, hemorrhoids, or rectal bleeding. Notes increased urinary output after taking last Lasix. No urinary hesitancy or urgency. Nocturia once per night.

Activity-exercise pattern: Very sedentary life style. Apartment is dark and cluttered. Patient uses canes to steady ambulation; needs assistance to leave apartment due to decreased sensation in both legs, fine tremors, and poor activity tolerance. Attends deaf elderly community group once weekly by handicapped van. Does not perform any exercise. No gout attack in over three years.

Sleep-rest pattern: Reports 6 to 8 h each night. Usual bedtime is 9 to 10 P.M. No difficulty with sleep onset. Reports feeling tired most of the time. Uses one pillow. Reports satisfaction with quality and quantity of sleep. Sleep disturbed by nocturnal diuresis only; no difficulty falling back to sleep. Keeps urinal at bedside.

Cognitive-perceptual pattern: Deaf since birth. Can lip-read. Speech is difficult to understand, especially at first. Has TTY machine for telephone communication. Wife is also deaf and can lip-read; her speech is very clear. Sister frequently acts as go-between and is very involved in his care. Taste and smell intact. Vision impaired, wears glasses, has early diabetic retinopathy. Apartment kept very dark. Memory intact. Patient frequently communicates through note-writing or defers to wife to answer questions.

Self-perception–self-concept pattern: B. V. sees himself as needing care. Wife and sister are very concerned and both "fret" over him. Patient appears to shrug off their concerns, but does not discourage them.

Role-relationship pattern: Patient is married, has no children. Patient frequently defers to wife when asked a question. Reports relationship as caring "although she nags." Also very close to younger sister who lives nearby with her family. Sister is not hearing impaired and apparently has served as his contact both before and since his marriage.

Sexuality-reproductive pattern: Patient underwent TURP four years ago for BPH. TURP successful, no recurrence, sees urologist yearly. No children, married later in life.

Coping–stress tolerance pattern: Patient and wife are very close to his sister and her family. Patient seems to have always been to a birthday or wedding or holiday party, either with family or at the deaf community center. This is generally where he eats his sweets. Patient anxious, overwhelmed, passive.

Value-belief pattern: Patient and his wife are both Jewish. They belong to a nearby temple and generally attend on high holidays only. Patient does state his faith is important to him, keeps up to date on Jewish and Israeli affairs by reading weekly Jewish newspaper.

Physical Examination/Review of Systems

VS: 120/70; 80 regular; 20; T 98.4; Height 5 ft 5 in.; Weight 193 lb; NKDA.
Skin: Warm, dry, no lesions; LE skin appears drier, cooler, paler.
Head: No trauma, headaches. Hair thinning, gray, male pattern baldness.
Eyes: Diabetic neuropathy; wears glasses; no cataracts; PERRLA; no s/s infection; irritation; conjunctivae moist. Last ophthalmic exam 3 months ago.

Ears: Deaf since birth; no infections, inflammation, discharge.

Nose: Patent bilaterally; no bleeding or discharge. Reports seasonal allergies decreasing with age. No polyps or obstruction.

Mouth: Upper and lower partial dentures. Last dental appointment 1 year ago. Gums pink; slight odor to breath; tongue midline; mucosa moist; no lesions; taste diminished.

Throat: No soreness; no c/o pain or stiffness. No lymphadenopathy.

Chest: Symmetrical, good expansion. Lungs clear. Reports DOE. Occasional dry cough. Slight kyphosis. No pain or hemoptysis. Rate 20.

Heart: S1>S2. No murmurs or gallops Rate 80, regular, NSR, BP 120/70. Recent onset left-sided CHF. Denies chest pain or palpitations. Hx HTN. Electrolytes WNL.

GI/Abdomen: Remarkable for obesity. No hepatomegaly or splenomegaly. No pain or indigestion reported. No scars or deviations. Appetite good. BM qd, + bowel sounds. No hemorrhoids or rectal bleeding. No adenopathy.

GU: Increased urinary output with Lasix. No testicular masses; does not perform TSE. Hx BPH, TURP. No hematuria, hesitancy, or urgency. Nocturnal diuresis × 1/noc. Mild renal failure; BUN 22 mg/dL; creatinine 1.8 mg/dL; uric acid 5.0 mg/dL.

Neuro: Memory intact, affect appropriate, A&O × 3. Denies syncope, vertigo. Muscle weakness bilaterally. Fine tremors both upper extremities. Decreased sensation to both LE. Denies pain, paresthesia. Ambulates with cane. Needs assistance for lengthy trips or vehicle transfers. Congenital deafness. Balance fair.

Vascular: 1+ bilateral peripheral edema. Started on Lasix qd, 10-lb weight loss. Extremities slightly pale and cooler, pulses intact. Peripheral vascular and retinal changes noted. No clubbing.

Cholesterol 190.

CASE 12

Case A. G.

(Adapted from a case by Kathleen Salerno)

A. G. is a 60-year-old white, Catholic female of Irish descent who is married with 3 grown children. She has a business school diploma, does office work part time, and babysits 3 grandchildren 2 days each week.

Her past medical history includes asthma at age 12, ruptured appendix and appendectomy at age 15, a single episode of ulcerative colitis at the age of 27, when pregnant, 3 normal vaginal births, shingles, osteoarthritis and rheumatism, and asthmatic bronchitis.

She is highly allergic to penicillin and sulfa drugs with anaphylaxis-type reaction.

Family history is negative for lung, renal, hepatic, and autoimmune diseases and diabetes. Her mother had coronary artery disease and MI after the age of 60 and osteoarthritis. Her father had rheumatic heart disease. Both are deceased. There are three siblings, all living. A brother has a history of Crohn's disease and a sister has a history of basal cell cancer.

A. G. comes in today for a physical examination and evaluation of her home medication management of chronic asthmatic bronchitis and osteoarthritis.

History of Present Illness

Asthma was first diagnosed at age 12 and treated with prn adrenalin injections and "Kellogg's Asthma Relief," which she describes as an incense used for inhalation and effective in the management of the disease. Asthma attacks subsided at the age of 21 but recurred 10 years ago with a bronchitis attack requiring treatment with IV steroids, antibiotics, and aminophylline. Discharged on tapering prednisone, Theo-Dur prn, inhalers prn, and cough suppressants prn. During a similar hospitalization 4 years ago, she was placed on ceftriaxone IV in the hospital and discharged home on usual medications plus PO ciprofloxacin. Rehospitalized soon after discharge with a fever of unknown origin. Drug fever was questioned, but A. G. has since received both ceftriaxone and ciprofloxacin without noted problems. At this time theophylline products were discontinued because of sudden chest discomfort (cardiac origin was ruled out). Home nebulizer treatments were prescribed, along with the inhalers, tapering prednisone, and a cough suppressant.

For past 4 years has had arthritis and rheumatism. Naprosyn and Lodine tried separately over this time period, without effect. Began on Voltaren a year ago with good symptom relief. Three months ago was hospitalized with pneumococcal pneumonia and a high fever. A. G. feels the pneumonia was related to the albuterol nebulizer treatments she was taking at home. Soon after her hospitalization, vials of albuterol were recalled by the manufacturer after they were found to contain bacteria (although not pneumococcus). The vials that she had at home were from the lot that was recalled. Hypotension and dehydration complicated her recovery. She was rigorously rehydrated but developed transient elevated liver enzymes and amber urine. A consulting gastroenterologist implicated volume depletion and Voltaren as the cause. Voltaren was held for a few weeks and resumed when the LFTs improved. The pneumonia was treated with ceftriaxone and then ciprofloxacin successfully. A. G. has been well since.

Current Medications

Voltaren 75 mg PO bid (with food)
Vanceril 4 inh qid (with spacer)

Atrovent 2 inh qid
Intal 2 cc bid via nebulizer and prn to qid total
Albuterol 0.5 cc bid via nebulizer and prn to qid total
Quinamm 1 tab PO at hs
lorazepam 0.5 mg PO bid prn anxiety (seldom used)
Tylenol 1000 mg PO prn (usually taken qhs)

Assessment

Health perception–health management pattern: Knowledgeable about medications and uses. Sees primary care provider every 4 months. Drinks one cup of coffee per day and no other caffeinated foods. Quit smoking 10 years ago but smoked 2 packs per day for 35 years prior to that. One alcoholic beverage per week. Has health insurance with deductible and prescription coverage with a copayment. No herbal or home remedies used.

Nutrition-metabolic pattern: Good appetite. 3 meals daily. Eats beef 2 times per week and 5 eggs per week. Cholesterol is 192 and has never been a problem. Drinks 8 glasses of water each day. No swallowing difficulties, food intolerances, food allergies, or gastrointestinal upset. Wounds heal quickly. She is overweight and attempts to diet on a nutritionally balanced program, usually Weight Watchers, from time to time.

Elimination pattern: Urine clear, yellow. Daily bowel movements are formed, brown, without blood. Diarrhea precedes bouts of bronchitis.

Activity-exercise pattern: Joint swelling and tenderness helped with Voltaren. Must pace activities because of asthma. Knows activity limitations. Tries to walk for 1 h at least every other day. Likes to read, visit friends, or watch TV in her spare time.

Sleep-rest pattern: Rises early. Sleeps well; tired by the end of the day. Adequate energy for activity when well. Takes Quinamm and Tylenol for painful leg cramps at night, with good effect.

Cognitive-perceptual pattern: Hears well. Glasses for reading. No difficulty with learning and remembering.

Self-perception–self-concept pattern: Discouraged with self when sick. Would like to lose weight but has always had difficulty. States she would feel better if she had a full-time job, outside of home. Laid off 4 years ago.

Role-relationship pattern: Lives with 59-year-old husband, who is retired. He is in fair health and able to care for himself. A. G. is depended upon for the household management and also to babysit her grandchildren 2 days per week. Close relationship with three grown children who live close by. Many supportive friends. Good relationship with siblings, but they live far away. Husband sometimes angry when A. G. is sick and must curb activities.

Sexuality-reproductive pattern: Menopause at age 51. No supplemental hormones or calcium supplements. Monogamous relationship. Routine mammograms and Pap smears. Complains of vaginal dryness.

Coping–stress tolerance pattern: Difficulty coping with bronchospasm when acutely ill. Very anxious during exacerbations of asthma and is helped by lorazepam. Copes well with daily living and does not use tranquilizers routinely.

Value-belief pattern: Devout Roman Catholic with much faith in prayer. Values family, friends, quiet time, and feeling well. Religious beliefs do not interfere with health-seeking behavior.

Screening Assessment

Well-groomed, clean appearance. Alert, oriented, with clear speech and appropriate attention span. Pupils equal and reactive. Tongue midline, buccal membranes moist. Teeth intact—partial plate. Lungs clear; diminished breath sounds bilateral bases. Respiratory rate 20 per minute. Apical pulse 78, regular. No edema, clubbing, or cyanosis of extremities. Extensive varicosities of both legs noted. No bruising or petechaie noted. Generalized weakness of extremities and tenderness of left elbow. No joint swelling observed. Adequate range of motion. Abdomen soft, non-tender; positive bowel sounds. Height 5 ft 5 in. Weight 214 lb.

CASE 13

Case A. C.

(Adapted from a case by Lisa Kennedy Sheldon)

Age: 45-year-old white male. Marital status: single. Occupation: unemployed. Allergies: phenothiazine intolerance due to anticholinergic activity.

Reason for visit: follow-up depression and back pain. "I need more amitriptyline and Tylenol #3 for my back pain."

Past illnesses/hospitalizations: medical: nodular goiter (for 15 years); post traumatic stress disorder (incest survivor); depression due to PTSD; substance abuse; left testicular seminoma (one year ago); degenerative joint disease (L3 to L5) Surgical: s/p appendectomy (18 years ago); s/p left orchiectomy and radiation therapy for testicular seminoma (one year ago); s/p rhinoplasty (1 year ago).

Current medications: amitriptyline 150 mg PO qh; Tylenol #3 one tablet PO q 4 h; Synthroid 0.15 mg PO qd; Motrin 800 mg PO tid.

Assessment

Health perception–health management pattern: A. C. says he is "doing okay" today. No suicidal thoughts at this time and has been seeing his counselor every 2 weeks. He states that he feels like he's having trouble with his near vision. He also continues to have problems with an obsessive-compulsive disorder that manifests itself now with hair cutting. He spends several hours a day cutting his hair. He will be seeing a psychopharmacologist at the counselor's next week and has been advised to stay on his amitriptyline until then. Has smoked 2 packs per day for 20 years. Has smoked marijuana 3 to 4 puffs every day for many years. Drinks a few beers occasionally but gets "stomach upset." Cocaine use in the past but none since 1989. He is not currently driving and he stopped using his Moped in June 1994 because he could not "handle it anymore."

Nutrition-metabolic pattern: Appetite poor. Weight down 10 lb over the last 20 years. Appears thin and hunched over. Prepares simple foods like soup and sandwiches. Sometimes he eats better when his friends come over. Fluid intake good. Drinks 1 or 2 cups of coffee daily. He does not like to cook.

Elimination pattern: Bowel movement once or twice a day. No problems with constipation and no laxative use. Some dribbling when finishing urination. Up at night to urinate frequently but in small amounts.

Sleep-rest pattern: A. C. has difficulty falling asleep and usually stays up until 3 or 4 A.M. and arises at 11 A.M. Watches TV or writes songs prior to going to sleep. He feels "tired" most of the time.

Activity-exercise pattern: Does not engage in any exercise program. Friends drive him or he walks or takes bicycle to appointments. Has had chest pains in past when pushing a wheelchair and when riding his bicycle. Chest X-ray showed left ventricular hypertrophy. EKG showed axis deviation and abnormal sinus rhythm. He enjoys writing songs and playing Scrabble with friends.

Cognitive-perceptual pattern: Finds his vision blurry lately. Scheduled to go to eye clinic in two weeks for evaluation. No change in hearing, taste, or smell. Complains of headaches of increasing severity over the last 2 years and he believes this is because of his vision. He sometimes has numbness in his hands and legs. Has had back pain since a bike accident in 1973. Duration and intensity vary. Spinal x-ray shows mild degenerative changes at L3 and L4. Has had two episodes of loss of consciousness upon arising from a sitting position and both times he states his head was the first thing to hit the floor. Articulates well and frequently. He is very talkative and relates stories in great detail. He is somewhat fidgety and appears distressed. Eye contact is intermittent. He uses amitriptyline at bedtime for his "depression and PTSD." Oriented × 3. Completed 2 years of college until "social issues" forced him to leave.

Self-perception–self-concept pattern: Sees self as "male incest survivor," suffering from PTSD due to relationship with father. This abuse occurred from ages 3 to 14 years. Has had suicidal and patricidal thoughts in the past. Currently, he does not want to hurt himself. He can do only "menial work" because of his "developmental problems." His "music compositions and inventions and business plans" keep him going.

Role-relationship pattern: Lives alone in rented house. Estranged from father and mother since he revealed the sexual abuse at age 17. Contact with brother in area is periodic. Has friends who come over to visit and play Scrabble. Broke up with "alcoholic girlfriend of five years," 1-1/2 years ago. Currently unemployed and seeking disability and Medicaid because he does not want to be "homeless." Previously employed as a companion for Child Health Services and as a taxi driver.

Sexuality-reproductive pattern: No current sexual relationship. No children because he is "afraid of what I might do to them." Complains of left groin pain at site of orchiectomy.

Coping–stress tolerance pattern: Sees himself as an "incest survivor" with PTSD who cannot do "meaningful work." Angry with father for disowning him and for the sexual abuse. Feels suicidal often although not currently. He likes his current counselor and has some friends and an incest survivors group that he finds supportive. He also finds himself with many physical ailments and symptoms, which he focuses on daily. Finds composing songs relaxing. He states he needs "psychiatric and medical help to do anything."

Value-belief pattern: Does not attend any religious service. Continues to be angry with family because of incest. Believes that his music, inventions, and business ideas will solve his problems once he makes "some connections."

Review of Symptoms

General: Many complaints today. "Back pain" continues and he wants more Tylenol #3 and doesn't want to "go to streets" for it. Also complaining of groin pain at site of orchiectomy. Not suicidal currently. "I think my thyroid is smaller."

Integument: No rashes. Multiple variegated moles on upper chest and back which A. C. worries are cancerous.

Head: C/o headaches for 2 years.

Eyes: Complains of difficulty seeing close work or reading.

Ears: Normal hearing. No tinnitus.

Nose: No drainage. Feels lightheaded (s/p rhinoplasty) and feels this is because of his "newly aerated sinuses."

Mouth, gums, teeth: Complaining of dryness in mouth; chews gum to alleviate this. Teeth intact. Prior gingivitis. Last saw dentist 7 years ago.

Throat and neck: Large thyroid for 25 years. No complaints of sore throat, hoarseness. No pain in the neck.

Breasts: No enlargement or masses. Small mole over left breast worries A. C., and he feels it could be cancer.

Respirations: Some SOB with exertion. No wheezing. Occasional cough which is productive of dark colored sputum. No pain on inspiration.

CV: C/o chest pains in past. None currently.

GI: No appetite. Regular BMs—2 per day. Soft, no melena.

GU: Voids frequently at night in small amounts. No burning or hematuria.

Muscular-skeletal: Complains of back pain. Has had previous right shoulder pain.

NP: Has had recent "lightheadedness" since rhinoplasty. Prior syncopal episodes but not in last month. Intelligent, very verbal man who is oriented × 3. Affect appears somewhat depressed with many somatic complaints. Has described numbness in hands and feet.

Lymph–hematological: No adenopathy. No abnormal bleeding.

Endocrine: Goiter for 25 years with Synthroid replacement. "Hates" the cold weather.

Physical Examination

VS: T 97.6 PO P 96 R 17 BP 118/70 HT 71-1/2 in. WT 171 lb.

General: Somewhat disheveled-appearing man who appears younger than age with slouched-over posture and fidgeting with hands. Clothes appear dirty and he has strong body odor.

Skin: Many moles on chest and back. No pain or change in moles noticed recently, but A. C. has been very concerned about skin cancer.

Hair: Coarse, thick hair cut very short.

Nails: Bitten nails, crusty and swollen cuticles. Pink nail beds.

Head: Symmetrical, normocephalic; c/o increasing headaches and two incidents of falling on head in the past.

Face: Downcast eyes. No muscle weakness.

Eyes: Pupils equal and reactive to light and accommodation. No retinal field problems. Sclera white.

Ears: Canals with moderate amount of cerumen. Both TM gray and mobile.

Nose: No drainage; s/p right septal repair 2 months ago. No deviation of septum on exam. Membranes with 1+ erythema.

Mouth: Teeth intact, no apparent caries. Gums pink and smooth but somewhat dry. Tongue protrudes at midline, no tremor.

Neck: 4+ enlarged thyroid, symmetric.

Lungs: Clear to auscultation. No cough or difficulty breathing at this time.

Breasts: No enlargement or masses noted.

Heart: Irregular rate of 96, PMI at 5th intercostal space, midclavicular line.

Abdomen: No hepatosplenomegaly.

Back: Complaining of back pain in lumbar region over vertebrae L3 to L5 when pressure put over area.

Extremities: No decreased sensation in hands or feet. Pulses present. Reflexes normal.

Genitalia: Left orchiectomy scar present; clean and well-healed. Penis without lesions. Other testicle smooth and mobile, no lumps or nodules.

Rectal: Deferred on patient request.

CASE 14

Case W. T.

(Adapted from a case by Cara Jean Yamamoto)

W. T. is a 57-year-old white male who returns to clinic after 2 months c/o "respiratory infection" and coughing up approximately 1 to 2 weeks. Unresolved with Bactrim 80/400 bid. Increased SOB and wheezing. Able to sleep only 3 to 4 h in naps. Denies chest pain, dizziness, palpitations. No headaches. Regular BM. No problems voiding. Occasional "upset stomach" related to theophylline (according to patient); resolves on its own. Edema in lower extremities without change.

Medicines (as reported by patient): Azmacort 2 puffs qid; taking tid; Lasix 40 mg 2 tabs bid (80 mg total qd); Atrovent 2 puffs q4; Isosorbid 20 mg 2 tabs qid; metaproterenol 20 mg qid; metaproterenol 2 puffs q 4–6 (not using often); MVI 1 tab bid; NTG SL 0.4 mg (hasn't needed); SLO-K 8 meq 2 tabs bid (32 meq total); prednisone 5 mg 4 tabs q A.M. (taking 2 tabs A.M., 2 tabs P.M.); theophylline (Uniphyl) 400 mg q hs [taking 1 A.M. and 300 mg Slo-Bid (leftover) in P.M. total 700 mg qd]; Bactrim 80/400 bid 12/21/89 (Taking tid for 1½ weeks).

Weight 333.75 lb (decreased from 339.5 three months ago). BP R (large cuff) sitting 162/94, R standing 154/90. AP 106 regular. R 28 to 32. Inspiratory and expiratory wheezes throughout. No decrease in adventitious BS following cough. S1>S2 (pulm) no murmur noted. Skin warm and dry. LE dry, 2–3+ edema, dermatitis. No open lesions noted.

CASE 15

Case Mrs. Jones

(Case by Susan Chase)

Mrs. Jones, a 50-year-old woman who works as an office manager is a new patient to you, complaining of chest pain on exertion. She is a 40-pack-per-year smoker, is normal weight for height, and has no other medical problems. She is not diabetic and her lung sounds are clear. Her blood pressure is 148/88. Pulse rate 84. She never engaged in regular physical exercise and is afraid to now because of chest pain which she experiences as a burning ache in her left chest and shoulder. Her EKG at rest is normal.

What pharmacological choices are you considering?

Sublingual nitroglycerin 0.3 mg, for chest pain. Instruct her to place the tablet under the tongue and rest. Patient may experience headache. If pain is not eliminated, she may repeat dose two times. If she still has pain, she should seek emergency care.

Metoprolol succinate, 50 mg, bid. Take with meals.

Consider aspirin, 80 mg per day, as a platelet aggregation inhibitor to prevent thrombosis.

What nonpharmacologic measure do you suggest?

Of primary importance is a smoke cessation program. After pain is controlled, based on results of stress test, she should begin a walking program. If she is more comfortable, she can do this in a supervised setting such as a cardiac rehabilitation type program.

If Mrs. Jones were diabetic, would you change anything?

Choose calcium channel blocker instead of beta blocker.

Mrs. Jones is getting relief from her pain using sublingual nitroglycerin, but she is taking tablets several times a day. What could you offer her?

Suggest a nitroglycerin patch, such as Minitran 0.1 mg/hr. Remove patch at bedtime. Place new patch in morning.

CASE 16

Case Mr. Whitney

(Case by Susan Chase)

Mr. Whitney is a 70-year-old man who is retired. His daughter brings him to the clinic with increased shortness of breath, difficulty sleeping after 2 or 3 h because of breathing problems, recent weight gain, and puffy ankles. His heart rate is 92 and blood pressure 160/94. He had an MI two years before. He has crackles that do not clear with coughing and 2+ pitting ankle edema. He has an S3 sound heard over the mitral area. Currently, he is taking digoxin 0.25 a day and Lasix 40 mg a day, ordered by family doctor who is now retired.

What pharmacological approach do you select?

Provided renal function is intact, HCTZ 25 mg twice a day can be safely given to elderly patients. Monitor potassium and digoxin level. If renal function is impaired, loop diuretics such as Lasix may be required.

Quinapril, 5 mg bid. ACE inhibitors can reduce afterload and therefore reduce workload on the heart. Monitor renal function.

CASE 17

Case Mrs. Brown

(Case by Susan Chase)

Mrs. Brown, a 40-year-old African-American female comes to your office after having her blood pressure screened at church and the nurse telling her that her pressure was elevated. Her BP today is 160/94. Mrs. Brown is the mother of 4 and grandmother of 2, who live nearby. She works as a secretary, and she is overweight.

How do you manage her initially?

Nonpharmacologic measures are suggested, such as salt restriction and increased exercise.

Begin a weight loss program. Have her return in one month for evaluation.

She returns in one month with an 8-pound weight loss and a pressure of 160/90. What is your approach?

Begin her on HCTZ 50 mg daily.

If, after one month her pressure is still not below 140/90, consider adding a calcium channel blocker, which works better with African-Americans than beta blockers. As another alternative, you could also increase her HCTZ dosage. This option would be less expensive.

CASE 18

Case Mr. Davis

(Case by Susan Chase)

Mr. Davis is a 75-year-old man with longstanding congestive heart failure. He has an irregular pulse with a rate of 116, and a blood pressure of 96/66. His EKG reveals atrial fibrillation. He has just moved here to live with his daughter and does not have any of his prior medications. How would you approach his management?

Determine digoxin level. Most likely he would have been on digoxin in the past. Based on this result, order digoxin, which will decrease his ventricular response to the atrial fibrillation. Consult with a cardiologist and try to obtain old medical records.

Determine his prothrombin time. Patients with chronic atrial fibrillation have reduced rates of cerebrovascular accidents when anticoagulated.

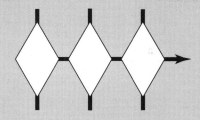

Appendixes

MEDWATCH FORM

THERAPEUTIC DRUG MONITORING

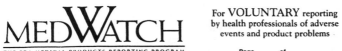

For VOLUNTARY reporting
by health professionals of adverse
events and product problems

Form Approved: OMB No. 0910-0291 Expires: 12/31/94
See OMB statement on reverse

FDA Use Only (MB)

Triage unit
sequence #

THE FDA MEDICAL PRODUCTS REPORTING PROGRAM

Page _____ of _____

A. Patient information

1. Patient identifier	2. Age at time of event:	3. Sex	4. Weight
	or _____	☐ female	_____ lbs
	Date of birth:		or
In confidence		☐ male	_____ kgs

B. Adverse event or product problem

1. ☐ **Adverse event** and/or ☐ **Product problem** (e.g., defects/malfunctions)

2. Outcomes attributed to adverse event (check all that apply)

☐ death _____ (mo/day/yr)
☐ life-threatening
☐ hospitalization – initial or prolonged

☐ disability
☐ congenital anomaly
☐ required intervention to prevent permanent impairment/damage
☐ other:

3. Date of event (mo/day/yr)	4. Date of this report (mo/day/yr)

5. Describe event or problem

6. Relevant tests/laboratory data, including dates

7. Other relevant history, including preexisting medical conditions (e.g., allergies, race, pregnancy, smoking and alcohol use, hepatic/renal dysfunction, etc.)

PLEASE TYPE OR USE BLACK INK

C. Suspect medication(s)

1. **Name** (give labeled strength & mfr/labeler, (if known)

#1

#2

2. Dose, frequency & route used	3. Therapy dates (if unknown, give duration) from/to (or best estimate)
#1	#1
#2	#2

4. **Diagnosis for use** (indication)

#1

#2

6. Lot # (if known)	7. Exp. date (if known)
#1	#1
#2	#2

9. **NDC #** (for product problems only)

—   —

5. **Event abated after use stopped or dose reduced**

#1 ☐ yes ☐ no ☐ doesn't apply
#2 ☐ yes ☐ no ☐ doesn't apply

8. **Event reappeared after reintroduction**

#1 ☐ yes ☐ no ☐ doesn't apply
#2 ☐ yes ☐ no ☐ doesn't apply

10. **Concomitant medical products** and therapy dates (exclude treatment of event)

D. Suspect medical device

1. **Brand name**

2. **Type of device**

3. **Manufacturer name & address**

4. **Operator of device**
☐ health professional
☐ lay user/patient
☐ other:

5. **Expiration date** (mo/day/yr)

6.
model # _____
catalog # _____
serial # _____
lot # _____
other # _____

7. **If implanted, give date** (mo/day/yr)

8. **If explanted, give date** (mo/day/yr)

9. **Device available for evaluation?** (Do not send to FDA)
☐ yes   ☐ no   ☐ returned to manufacturer on _____ (mo/day/yr)

10. **Concomitant medical products** and therapy dates (exclude treatment of event)

E. Reporter (see confidentiality section on back)

1. **Name, address & phone #**

2. **Health professional?**
☐ yes ☐ no

3. **Occupation**

4. **Also reported to**
☐ manufacturer
☐ user facility
☐ distributor

5. If you do NOT want your identity disclosed to the manufacturer, place an " X " in this box. ☐

Mail to: MEDWATCH
5600 Fishers Lane
Rockville, MD 20852-9787

or FAX to:
1-800-FDA-0178

FDA Form 3500 (6/93)

Submission of a report does not constitute an admission that medical personnel or the product caused or contributed to the event.

451

ADVICE ABOUT VOLUNTARY REPORTING

Report experiences with:
- medications (drugs or biologics)
- medical devices (including in-vitro diagnostics)
- special nutritional products (dietary supplements, medical foods, infant formulas)
- other products regulated by FDA

Report SERIOUS adverse events. An event is serious when the patient outcome is:
- death
- life-threatening (real risk of dying)
- hospitalization (initial or prolonged)
- disability (significant, persistent or permanent)
- congenital anomaly
- required intervention to prevent permanent impairment or damage

Report even if:
- you're not certain the product caused the event
- you don't have all the details

Report product problems – quality, performance or safety concerns such as:
- suspected contamination
- questionable stability
- defective components
- poor packaging or labeling

How to report:
- just fill in the sections that apply to your report
- use section C for all products except medical devices
- attach additional blank pages if needed
- use a separate form for each patient
- report either to FDA or the manufacturer (or both)

Important numbers:
- 1-800-FDA-0178   to FAX report
- 1-800-FDA-7737   to report by modem
- 1-800-FDA-1088   for more information or to report quality problems
- 1-800-822-7967   for a VAERS form for vaccines

If your report involves a serious adverse event with a device and it occurred in a facility outside a doctor's office, that facility may be legally required to report to FDA and/or the manufacturer. Please notify the person in that facility who would handle such reporting.

Confidentiality: The patient's identity is held in strict confidence by FDA and protected to the fullest extent of the law. The reporter's identity may be shared with the manufacturer unless requested otherwise. However, FDA will not disclose the reporter's identity in response to a request from the public, pursuant to the Freedom of Information Act.

The public reporting burden for this collection of information has been estimated to average 30 minutes per response, including the time for reviewing instructions, searching existing data sources, gathering and maintaining the data needed, and completing and reviewing the collection of information. Send your comments regarding this burden estimate or any other aspect of this collection of information, including suggestions for reducing this burden to:

Reports Clearance Officer, PHS
Hubert H. Humphrey Building,
Room 721-B
200 Independence Avenue, S.W.
Washington, DC 20201
ATTN: PRA

and to:
Office of Management and
Budget
Paperwork Reduction Project
(0910-0230)
Washington, DC 20503

Please do NOT
return this form
to either of these
addresses.

FDA Form 3500-back   **Please Use Address Provided Below – Just Fold In Thirds, Tape and Mail**

**Department of
Health and Human Services**
Public Health Service
Food and Drug Administration
Rockville, MD 20857

Official Business
Penalty for Private Use $300

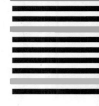

NO POSTAGE
NECESSARY
IF MAILED
IN THE
UNITED STATES
OR APO/FPO

BUSINESS REPLY MAIL
FIRST CLASS MAIL   PERMIT NO. 946   ROCKVILLE, MD

POSTAGE WILL BE PAID BY FOOD AND DRUG ADMINISTRATION

MEDWATCH
**The FDA Medical Products Reporting Program
Food and Drug Administration
5600 Fishers Lane
Rockville, MD 20852-9787**

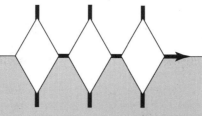

THERAPEUTIC DRUG MONITORING (TDM)*

Selective drugs are monitored by serum and urine for the purposes of achieving and maintaining therapeutic drug effect and for preventing drug toxicity. Drugs with a wide therapeutic range (window), the difference between effective dose and toxic dose, are not usually monitored. Drug monitoring is important in maintaining a drug concentration–response relationship, especially when the serum drug range (window) is narrow, such as with digoxin and lithium. Therapeutic drug monitoring (TDM) is the process of following drug levels and adjusting them to maintain a therapeutic level. Not all drugs can be dosed and/or monitored by their blood levels alone.

Drug levels are obtained at peak time and trough time after a steady state of the drug has occurred in the client. Steady state is reached after four to five half-lives of a drug and can be reached sooner if the drug has a short half-life. Once steady state is achieved, serum drug level is checked at the peak level (maximum drug concentration) and/or at trough/residual level (minimum drug concentration). If the trough or residual level is at the high therapeutic point, toxicity might occur. Careful assessment is needed by both physical and laboratory means.

TDM is required for drugs with a narrow therapeutic index or range (window); when other methods for monitoring drugs are noneffective, such as blood pressure (BP) monitoring; for determining when adequate blood concentrations are reached; for evaluating client's compliance to drug therapy; for determining whether other drugs have altered serum drug levels (increased or decreased) that could result in drug toxicity or lack of therapeutic effect; and for establishing new serum-drug level when dosage is changed.

Drug groups for TDM include analgesics, antibiotics, anticonvulsants, antineoplastics, bronchodilators, cardiac drugs, hypoglycemics, sedatives, and tranquilizers. To conduct TDM effectively, the laboratory must be provided with the following information: the drug name and daily dosage, time and amount of last dose, time blood was drawn, route of administration, and client's age. Without complete information, serum drug reporting might be incorrect.

*Revised by Ronald J. Lefever, R.Ph., Pharmacy Services, Medical College of Virginia, Richmond, VA.

SOURCE: Kee JL: *Laboratory and Diagnostic Tests with Nursing Implications*, 4th ed. Stamford, CT: Appleton & Lange, 1995. Used with permission.

Drug	Therapeutic Range	Peak Time	Toxic Level
Acetaminophen (Tylenol)	10–20 µg/mL	1–2½ hours	>50 µg/mL Hepatotoxicity: >200 µg/mL
Acetohexamide (Dymelor)	20–70 µg/mL (should be dosed according to blood glucose levels)	2–4 hours	>75 µg/mL
Alcohol	Negative		Mild toxic: 150 mg/dL Marked toxic: >250 mgL
Alprazolam (Xanax)	10–50 ng/mL	1–2 hours	>75 ng/mL
Amikacin (Amikin)	Peak: 20–30 µg/mL Trough: ≤10 µg/mL	Intravenously: ½ hour Intramuscular: ½–1½ hours	Peak: >35 µg/mL Trough: >10 µg/mL
Aminocaproic Acid (Amicar)	100–400 µg/mL	1 hour	>400 µg/mL
Aminophylline (see Theophylline)			
Amiodarone (Cordarone)	0.5–2.5 µg/mL	2–10 hours	>2.5 µg/mL
Amitriptyline (Elavil)	125–200 ng/mL	2–12 hours	>500 ng/mL
Amobarbital (Amytal)	1–5 µg/mL	2 hours	>15 µg/mL Severe toxicity: >30 µg/mL
Amoxapine (Asendin)	200–400 ng/mL	1½ hours	>500 ng/mL
Amphetamine: Serum	20–30 ng/mL		0.2 µg/mL
Urine		Detectable in urine after 3 hours; positive for 24–48 hours	>30 µg/ml urine
Aspirin (see Salicylates)			
Atenolol (Tenormin)	200–500 ng/mL	2–4 hours	>500 ng/mL

Drug	Therapeutic Range	Peak Time	Toxic Level
Bromide	20–80 mg/dL		>100 mg/dL
Butabarbital (Butisol)	1–2 µg/mL	3–4 hours	>10 µg/mL
Caffeine	Adult: 3–15 µg/mL Infant: 8–20 µg/mL	½–1 hour	>50 µg/mL
Carbamazepine (Tegretol)	4–12 µg/mL	6 hours (Range 2–24 hours)	>9–15 µg/mL
Chloral Hydrate (Noctec)	2–12 µg/mL	1–2 hours	>20 µg/mL
Chloramphenicol (Chloromycetin)	10–20 mg/L		>25 mg/L
Chlordiazepoxide (Librium)	1–5 µg/mL	2–3 hours	>5 µg/mL
Chlorpromazine (Thorazine)	50–300 ng/mL	2–4 hours	>750 ng/mL
Chlorpropamide (Diabinese)	75–250 µg/mL	3–6 hours	>250–750 µg/mL
Clonidine (Catapres)	0.2–2.0 ng/mL (Hypotensive effect)	2–5 hours	>2.0 ng/mL
Clorazepate (Tranxene)	0.12–1.0 µg/mL	1–2 hours	>1.0 µg/mL
Cimetidine (Tagamet)	Trough: 0.5–1.2 µg/mL	1–1½ hours	Trough: >1.5 µg/mL
Clonazepam (Klonopin)	10–60 ng/mL	2 hours	>80 ng/mL
Codeine	10–100 ng/mL	1–2 hours	>200 ng/mL
Dantrolene (Dantrium)	1–3 µg/mL	5 hours	>5 µg/mL
Desipramine (Norpramin)	125–300 ng/mL	4–6 hours	>400 ng/mL
Diazepam (Valium)	0.5–2 mg/L 400–600 ng/mL	1–2 hours	>3 mg/L >3000 ng/mL
Digitoxin (Rarely administered)	10–25 ng/mL	Noticeable: 2–4 hours Peak: 12–24 hours	>30 ng/mL
Digoxin	0.5–2 ng/mL	PO: 6–8 hours IV: 1½–2 hours	2–3 ng/mL

(continued)

Drug	Therapeutic Range	Peak Time	Toxic Level
Dilantin (see Phenytoin)			
Diltiazem (Cardizem)	50–200 ng/mL	2–3 hours	>200 ng/mL
Disopyramide (Norpace)	2–4 µg/mL	2 hours	>4 µg/mL
Doxepin (Sinequan)	150–300 ng/mL	2–4 hours	>500 ng/mL
Ethchlorvynol (Placidyl)	2–8 µg/mL	1–2 hours	>20 µg/mL
Ethosuximide (Zarontin)	40–100 µg/mL	2–4 hours	>150 µg/mL
Flecainide (Tambocor)	0.2–1.0 µg/mL	3 hours	>1.0 µg/mL
Flurazepam (Dalmane)	20–110 ng/mL		>1500 ng/mL
Gentamicin (Garamycin)	Peak: 6–12 µg/mL Trough: <2 µg/mL	IV: 15–30 minutes	Peak: >12 µg/mL Trough: >2 µg/mL
Glutethimide (Doriden)	2–6 µg/mL	1–2 hours	>20 µg/mL
Haloperidol (Haldol)	5–15 ng/mL	2–6 hours	>50 ng/mL
Hydromorphone (Dilaudid)	1–30 ng/mL	½–1½ hours	>100 ng/mL
Ibuprofen (Motrin, etc.)	10–50 µg/mL	1–2 hours	>100 µg/mL
Imipramine (Tofranil)	150–300 ng/mL	PO: 1–2 hours IM: 30 minutes	>500 ng/mL
Isoniazid (INH, Nydrazid)	1–7 µg/mL (Dose usually adjusted based on liver function tests)	1–2 hours	>20 µg/mL
Kanamycin (Kantrex)	Peak: 15–30 mg/mL Trough: 1–4 mg/mL	PO: 1–2 hours IM: 30 minutes– 1 hour	Peak: >35 mg/mL Trough: >10 mg/mL
Lead	<20 µg/mL Urine: <80 µg/ 24 hours		>80 µg/mL Urine: >125 µg/ 24 hours

Drug	Therapeutic Range	Peak Time	Toxic Level
Lidocaine (Xylocaine)	1.5–5 μg/mL	IV: 10 minutes	>6 μg/mL
Lithium	0.8–1.2 mEq/L	½–4 hours	>1.5 mEq/L
Lorazepam (Ativan)	50–240 ng/mL	1–3 hours	>300 ng/mL
Maprotiline (Ludiomil)	200–300 ng/mL	12 hours	>500 ng/mL
Meperidine (Demerol)	0.4–0.7 μg/mL	2–4 hours	>1.0 μg/mL
Mephenytoin (Mesantoin)	15–40 μg/mL	2–4 hours	>50 μg/mL
Meprobamate (Equanil, Miltown)	15–25 μg/mL	2 hours	>50 μg/mL
Methadone (Dolophine)	100–400 ng/mL	½ to 1 hour	>2000 ng/mL or >0.2 μg/mL
Methyldopa (Aldomet)	1–5 μg/mL	3–6 hours	>7 μg/mL
Methyprylon (Noludar)	8–10 μg/mL	1–2 hours	>50 μg/mL
Metoprolol (Lopressor)	75–200 ng/mL	2–4 hours	>225 ng/mL
Mexiletine (Mexitil)	0.5–2 μg/mL	2–3 hours	>2 μg/mL
Morphine	10–80 ng/mL	IV: immediately IM: ½–1 hour SC: 1–1½ hours	>200 ng/mL
Netilmicin (Netromycin)	Peak: 0.5–10 μg/mL Trough: <4 μg/mL	IV: 30 minutes	Peak: >16 μg/mL Trough: >4 μg/mL
Nifedipine (Procardia)	50–100 ng/mL	½ to 2 hours	>100 ng/mL
Nortriptyline (Aventyl)	50–150 ng/mL	8 hours	>200 ng/mL
Oxazepam (Serax)	0.2–1.4 μg/mL	1–2 hours	
Oxycodone (Percodan)	10–100 ng/mL	½–1 hour	>200 ng/mL
Pentazocine (Talwin)	0.05–0.2 μg/mL	1–2 hours	>1.0 μg/mL Urine: >3.0 μg/mL

(continued)

Drug	Therapeutic Range	Peak Time	Toxic Level
Pentobarbital (Nembutal)	1–5 µg/mL	½–1 hour	>10 µg/mL Severe toxicity: >30 µg/mL
Phenmetrazine (Preludin)	5–30 µg/mL (Urine)	2 hours	>50 µg/mL (Urine)
Phenobarbital (Luminal)	15–40 µg/mL	6–18 hours	>40 µg/mL Severe toxicity: >80 µg/mL
Phenytoin (Dilantin)	10–20 µg/mL	4–8 hours	>20–30 µg/mL Severe toxicity: >40 µg/mL
Pindolol (Visken)	0.5–6.0 ng/mL	2–4 hours	>10 ng/mL
Primidone (Mysoline)	5–12 µg/mL	2–4 hours	>12–15 µg/mL
Procainamide (Pronestyl)	4–10 µg/mL	1 hour	>10 µg/mL
Procaine (Novocain)	<11 µg/mL	10–30 minutes	>20 µg/mL
Prochlorperazine (Compazine)	50–300 ng/mL	2–4 hours	>1000 ng/mL
Propoxyphene (Darvon)	0.1–0.4 µg/mL	2–3 hours	>0.5 µg/mL
Propranolol (Inderal)	>100 ng/mL	1–2 hours	>150 ng/mL
Protriptyline (Vivactil)	50–150 ng/mL	8–12 hours	>200 ng/mL
Quinidine	2–5 µg/mL	1–3 hours	>6 µg/mL
Ranitidine (Zantac)	100 ng/mL	2–3 hours	>100 ng/mL
Reserpine (Serpasil)	20 ng/mL	2–4 hours	>20 ng/mL
Salicylates (Aspirin)	10–30 mg/dL	1–2 hours	Tinnitis: 20–40 mg/mL Hyperventilation: >35 mg/dL Severe toxicity: >50 mg/dL
Secobarbital (Seconal)	2–5 µg/mL	1 hour	>15 µg/mL Severe toxicity: >30 µg/mL

Drug	Therapeutic Range	Peak Time	Toxic Level
Theophylline (Theodur, Aminodur)	10–20 µg/mL	PO: 2–3 hours IV: 15 minutes (Depends on smoking or nonsmoking)	>20 µg/mL
Thioridazine	100–600 ng/mL	2–4 hours	>2000 ng/mL
Timolol (Blocadren)	3–55 ng/mL	1–2 hours	>60 ng/mL
Tobramycin (Nebcin)	Peak: 5–10 µg/mL Trough: 1–1.5 µg/mL	IV: 15–30 minutes IM: ½–1½ hours	Peak: >12 µg/mL Trough: >2 µg/mL
Tocainide (Tonocard)	4–10 µg/mL	½–3 hours	>12 µg/mL
Tolbutamide (Orinase)	80–240 µg/mL	3–5 hours	>640 µg/mL
Trazodone (Desyrel)	500–2500 ng/mL	1–2 weeks	>4000 ng/mL
Trifluoperazine (Stelazine)	50–300 ng/mL	2–4 hours	>1000 ng/mL
Valproic Acid (Depakene)	50–100 µg/mL	½–1½ hours	>100 µg/mL Severe toxicity: >150 µg/mL
Vancomycin (Vanocin)	Peak: 20–40 µg/mL Trough: 5–10 µg/mL	IV: Peak: 5 minutes IV: Trough: 12 hours	Peak: >80 µg/mL
Verapamil (Calan)	100–300 ng/mL	PO: 1–2 hours IV: 5 minutes	>500 ng/mL
Wafarin (Coumadin)	1–10 µg/mL (Dose usually adjusted by 1 to 2.5 × control)	1½–3 days	>10 µg/mL

INDEX

Page numbers followed by *f* indicate figures; page numbers followed by *t* indicate tables.

ISBN 0-07-105485-5

90000

9 780071 054850